D0984839

Neurosurgical Ethics in Practice: Value-based Medicine

Ahmed Ammar • Mark Bernstein
Editors

Neurosurgical Ethics in Practice: Value-based Medicine

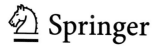 Springer

Editors
Ahmed Ammar, MBChB, DMSc,
FICS, FACS, FAANS
Department of Neurosurgery
King Fahd University Hospital
Dammam University
Al Khobar
Saudi Arabia

Mark Bernstein, MD, MHSc, FRCSC
Division of Neurosurgery
Toronto Western Hospital
University of Toronto
Toronto, ON
Canada

ISBN 978-3-642-54979-3   ISBN 978-3-642-54980-9   (eBook)
DOI 10.1007/978-3-642-54980-9
Springer Heidelberg New York Dordrecht London

Library of Congress Control Number: 2014943517

Printed on acid-free paper

Springer is part of Springer Science+Business Media (www.springer.com)

The editors dedicate this book to their wives and daughters, and to patients everywhere.

Preface

Modern medical practice is dominated by technology and evidence based medicine emphasizing the importance of scientific data to guide our daily practice. But through the years, as medicine has crossed different cultures and borders, it has been and will be always be the ultimate value-based activity, much of which is not necessarily based in evidence. Through history the practice of medicine in Ancient Egypt, Ancient China, India and other old civilizations was deeply connected with the religious and social values of these societies at that time. It is important to note and remember that physicians and surgeons are not allowed to practice medicine before taking the Hippocratic Oath which has become an essential part of Graduation Ceremonies of Faculties/Schools of Medicine all over the world.

Over the years, medical ethics has attracted the attention of philosophers, theologians, researchers, and scholars. It has become an independent and well-studied branch of ethics, called bioethics. Most hospitals all over the world have established their own ethics committees. All professional medical and surgical (including neurosurgical) societies have their own ethics committees as well. However new challenges constantly arise with the expansion of technology and changes in patients' level of knowledge and expectations which require vigilant attention to the ethical dimensions of what we do.

Good neurosurgical practice is not only based on evidence, skills, and modern equipment but also on good values and ethical approaches to problems (i.e. value-based medicine). Young neurosurgeons learn about ethical issues in neurosurgery largely through observation of the behavior of their staff who can act as role models, but there do exist more formal processes for approaching ethical dilemmas which we try to demonstrate in the book.

This book is the first to discuss different ethical issues in the daily practice of the neurosurgical practitioner. It is written by neurosurgeons about everyday ethical challenges we face. It is intended for neurosurgeons and neurosurgery trainees all over the world. Neurosurgical practice shares many common issues with other medical and surgical practices, but there are important issues that are quite specific to neurosurgical practice due to the nature of the patients, and the fact that neurosurgeons deal with the organ which contains the psyche and the soul of patients. Having said that, this book would certainly be useful to surgeons of all stripes, especially those in training, and medical students as well.

Special features of this volume include:

1. All chapters are relatively brief, written in simple language, and easily digestible.
2. All chapters have a maximum of two co-authors and are written by practicing neurosurgeons with an interest in ethics as sole or senior author or both authors.
3. All chapters follow the same format and structure and have been heavily edited to be as internally congruous as possible to enhance the readability and knowledge transfer.
4. Different ethical topics are discussed following introduction of the topic by one or more illustrative cases encountered during everyday neurosurgical practice.
5. "Pearl Boxes" highlight short important lessons.
6. An attempt is made to show the process by which ethical dilemmas can be approached, as the "single right answer" often does not exist in ethics (or in surgery!).
7. The book avoids as much as possible the use of deep philosophical principles and language and heavy bibliographies, and tries to adhere to the daily language of neurosurgeons in clinical practice.

The book is divided into five thematic parts.

Part I is introductory and has chapters on generic ethical issues like the classical ethics principles and theories and cross-cultural nuances in ethics.

Part II deals with patients' rights and includes chapters on specific patients' rights, informed consent, privacy and confidentiality, families' rights, and children's rights.

Part III deals with issues around the end of life, and brain death, important issues in all of medicine and perhaps particularly in neurosurgery. This is such an important area that there are two closely related overlapping chapters (Chaps. 8 and 9).

Part IV deals with the duties of neurosurgeons and has chapters on specific neurosurgeons' duties, workplace ethics, surgical innovation, research ethics – both in elective and emergency settings, neuroethics, errors, and surgical education.

Part V deals with the intersection of neurosurgery and society and includes chapters on priority setting, conflict of interest, medicolegal issues, and neurosurgeons interacting with the media.

The editors thank all the chapter contributors; Ms. Elizabeth Orthmann and Ms. Inga von Behrens at Springer; Hanan Ammar, Lujain Ammar, Dr. Ahmed Abdelfatteh, and Janice Liwanag (Al Khobar); and Lynn Nowen and Lee Bernstein (Toronto). We sincerely hope this volume can provide guidance and information to practitioners of our noble profession, in countries around the word and at every level of experience.

Al Khobar, Saudi Arabia   Ahmed Ammar, MBChB, DMSc, FICS, FACS, FAANS
Toronto, ON, Canada   Mark Bernstein, MD, MHSc, FRCSC

Contents

Part IV   Neurosurgeons' Duties

Part V   Neurosurgeons and Society

Contributors

Ahmed Ammar, MBChB, DMSc, FICS, FACS, FAANS Department of Neurosurgery, King Fahd University Hospital, Dammam University, Al Khobar, Saudi Arabia

Mark Bernstein, MD, MHSc, FRCSC Division of Neurosurgery, Toronto Western Hospital, University of Toronto, Toronto, ON, Canada

T.H.R. de Jong, MD Department of Neurosurgery, Erasmus MC University Medical Center, Rotterdam, CA, The Netherlands

Tania DePellegrin, MHSc Joint Center of Bioethics, University of Toronto, Toronto, ON, Canada

Karen M. Devon, MD, MSc, FRCSC Division of General Surgery, Women's College Hospital, University Health Network, University of Toronto, Toronto, ON, Canada

James Downar, MD, MHSc, FRCPC Division of Respirology/Critical Care, Toronto General Hospital, Toronto, ON, Canada

Divisions of Critical Care and Palliative Care, University of Toronto, Toronto, ON, Canada

George M. Ibrahim, MD Division of Neurosurgery, Department of Surgery, Institute of Medical Science, University of Toronto, Toronto, ON, Canada

Vijendra K. Jain, MCh Department of Neurosurgery, Max Super Specialty Hospital, New Delhi, India

Yoko Kato, MD, PhD Department of Neurosurgery, Fujita Health University, Toyoake, Aichi, Japan

Erwin J.O. Kompanje, PhD Intensive Care Medicine, Erasmus MC University Medical Center, Rotterdam, The Netherlands

Nir Lipsman, MD Division of Neurosurgery, University of Toronto, Toronto, ON, Canada

Department of Surgery, University of Toronto, Toronto, ON, Canada

Adefolarin O. Malomo, MB, BS, MHSc, FWACS Departments of Surgery
and Human Anatomy, University of Ibadan, Ibadan, Nigeria

Department of Neurological Surgery, University College Hospital, Ibadan, Nigeria

Patrick McDonald, MD, MHSc, FRCSC Section of Neurosurgery,
Winnipeg Children's Hospital, Winnipeg, MB, Canada

Department of Surgery, University of Manitoba, Manitoba Institute of
Child Health, Winnipeg, MB, Canada

Daniel Mendelsohn, MD, MSc Division of Neurosurgery,
University of British Columbia, Vancouver, BC, Canada

Michael Reid Addenbrooke's Hospital, University of Cambridge School
of Clinical Medicine, Cambridge, UK

Geert Seynaeve, MD, MPH, MMPhR Department of Occupational Health
and Safety, Free University Brussels, Brussels, Belgium

Jeffrey M. Singh, MD, FRCPC Division of Respirology,
Interdepartmental Division of Critical Care Medicine,
Toronto Western Hospital, University of Toronto, Toronto, ON, Canada

Ta-Chih Tan, MD Division of Pediatric Neurosurgery,
Department of Pediatrics, HSK-Wiesbaden, Wiesbaden, Germany

Ross Upshur, MD, MSc Division of Clinical Public Health,
Clinical Research, Bridgepoint Health, Dalla Lana School of Public Health,
Toronto, ON, Canada

Department of Family and Community Medicine, University of Toronto,
Toronto, ON, Canada

Part I

Introduction to Ethics

Brief History of Bioethics

Ahmed Ammar

1.1 Introduction

Bioethics is a composite term derived from the Greek words for life and ethics. It can be defined as the systematic study of the moral dimensions, including moral vision, decisions, conduct, and policies of the life sciences and health care, employing several methodologies in an interdisciplinary setting (Reich 1995). It is about doing right or doing what ought to be done. Bioethics can be discussed in philosophical terms, in theological terms, and through actual case studies (Jonsen et al. 1998; Pence 1995). Various types of ethical reasoning systems, such as principles, relativism, situational ethics, and theories such as utilitarianism and deontology, offer approaches to bioethical dilemmas.

Practicing ethics in both medicine and surgery means that when a doctor is faced with a choice, he/she should choose to do that which will be best for the patient and/or is the "right" thing to do. However, being well intentioned alone is not enough for the clinician, as there are an unusually large number of gray areas, and the morally preferable course of action to be followed is not always clear or self-evident. There are very many situations in which the doctor is called upon to make difficult ethical choices, including end-of-life issues, informed consent, and research ethics. Each of these situations tests not just the physician's medical expertise but also his/her virtue, honesty, maturity, and thoughtful awareness of the implications of his/her decision.

> **Pearl**
> Bioethics can be defined as the systematic study of moral challenges in medicine, including moral vision, decisions, conduct, and policies related to medicine.

A. Ammar, MBChB, DMSc, FICS, FACS, FAANS
Department of Neurosurgery, King Fahd University Hospital, Dammam University, 40121, Al Khobar 31952, Saudi Arabia
e-mail: ahmed@ahmedammar.com

A. Ammar, M. Bernstein (eds.), *Neurosurgical Ethics in Practice: Value-based Medicine*, DOI 10.1007/978-3-642-54980-9_1, © Springer-Verlag Berlin Heidelberg 2014

1.2   History of Medical Ethics

Although the very first practice of medicine is undocumented, it is generally accepted that the first widespread tradition of medicine, with specialties developing, was in Ancient Egypt. Medicine in Ancient Egypt was practiced in temples, and controlled by religion; thus, the question of ethics did not arise. It is believed that Imhotep, who was a high religious priest, architect (he built the first pyramid), astrologer, poet, and later on in life a chief minister (2630 B.C.), built and ran the first school of medicine in the backyard of a temple as an indication of the close relationship between religion and medicine.

The Law Code of Hammurabi, King of Babylon in1800 B.C., is considered as the first law code which included punishment for medical malpractice (Walsh 2010).

The first documented use of medicine in Ancient Greece appears around 800 B.C., although Hippocrates was not born until around 460 B.C.

The date at which the Hippocratic Oath was penned is debatable, and very few historians believe that Hippocrates was its soul author (Edelstein 1943). The oath was broadly split into two areas. The first dealt with respecting teachers and passing medical knowledge to new generations – this part is probably the part inspired by Hippocrates. The second part covered the principle that a doctor must always do his best for his/her patients, never harm them, recognizing his/her own limitations, and never cause them injustice. It also included a portion on dignity and preserving patients' secrets. At the time it was introduced, all physicians were bound by it. Over time the Hippocratic Oath was abandoned, and many schools of medicine did not require doctors to recite or follow it.

In ancient India, the ethical approach to the patient was based on compassion due to the influence of the Hindu religion. The doctors enhanced the concept of treating all patients with dignity and respect and practiced different methods for healing the body and mind. The Sanatana Dharma or verdict religion traditions and teachings were used to heal the mind and body. The earliest known protagonists of Indian medicine based their work on these ancient texts about spiritual philosophy and ethics (Singh and Saradananda 2008).

The word "taoist" in ancient Chinese science and medicine has been explained as a frame of mind and source of perplexity with special reference to the relationship between science and religion. Medicine was not an exception; thus, the roots of medical practice in ancient China can be traced to Chinese religion (Bowman and Hui 2000).

In Early Jewish medical history, medical ethics were clearly observed. These ethics mainly followed traditional rabbinic law (halakha). Jewish medical ethics were mainly applied ethics. Scholars and rabbis believed in God's power to heal all diseases and illness and practiced medicine according to that belief (Halperin 2004; Goldsand et al. 2001).

Early Christianity inherited Greek and Roman culture and teachings including medical knowledge. The morals and values of Hippocrates and Galen dominated medical practice in the early Christian period. The Vatican used Canon law to control medical practice by monks and nuns. John Paul II wrote in 1998: "Catholic bioethics engages the intellect through reason at one end and through faith on the other. Faith complements reason." The influence of the great religions continues to have a powerful effect in modern bioethics (Coward and Sidhu 2000; Daar and alKhitamy 2001; Ellerby et al. 2000; Markwell and Brown 2001; Pauls and Hutchinson 2002).

A strong resurgence of interest in medical ethics arose in the modern era as a result of several highly visible egregious breaches of ethics, which, unlike many other ethical dilemmas encountered on a daily basis, left no ambiguity as to the immorality of the acts. Thus, developed the field of bioethics, the formalization of the four overriding principles (Beauchamp and Childress 2001), and the application of philosophy to the addressing of ethical challenges in medicine (Arras et al. 1999; Kant 1993; Mill 1991; Rawls 1971). A brief examination of arguably the two most visible violations of medical ethics deserves mention.

> **Pearl**
> The virtue and good intentions of doctors and other health care providers cannot be solely relied upon to produce ethically desirable results. Ethical dilemmas, especially nowadays, are so nuanced and complex that systems for approaching these dilemmas are needed.

1.3 Nazi Medical War Crimes

Following WWII, revelations of the extent of Nazi "medical experimentation" on prisoners shocked the world. These experiments were performed on thousands of concentration camp prisoners and included practices such as injecting people with gasoline and live viruses, immersing people in ice water, and forcing people to ingest poisons. These experiments were performed, if not devised, by doctors. The doctors were subsequently tried in Nuremburg, and as a result, a code of practice for medical research was established (Nuremberg Military Tribunal 1996; Trials of War Criminals 1949).

1.4 Tuskegee Syphilis Study

From 1930 to 1972, a study was carried out in Tuskegee, Alabama, only on black males, examining the natural history of untreated syphilis. Early in the study, it became clear that the rate of complications in infected men was much higher than in the control group. By the mid-1940s, it was apparent that the death rate among the infected individuals was twice as high as among controls. At this time it was already known that penicillin was effective in the treatment of syphilis, but the study continued and the patients were unaware of the possibility of treatment with the antibiotic (Levine et al. 2012).

Following reports of the Tuskegee study, it became clear that the Nuremburg code of practice was insufficient to protect patients. The Congress established the National Commission for the Protection of Human Subjects of Biomedical and Behavioral Research, and they issued the Belmont Report in 1979 (National Commission for the Protection of Human Subjects 1978). This report identified basic medical principles such as autonomy, beneficence, and justice. Although the report was to establish a code of practice for medical research, those three ethical elements were also applied to the code of practice for treating patients. The World Declaration of Helsinki followed in 2000 (World Medical Association Declaration of Helsinki 2000).

> **Pearl**
> Modern codes of bioethics largely arose from egregious ethical breaches such as the Tuskegee experiment and the Nazi doctors' war crimes during the Second World War.

1.5   The Hippocratic Oath

The Hippocratic Oath articulates a commitment by the physician to do his/her best for the patient, cause no harm, and not cause injustice to the patient. It may represent the first well-known code of ethics in the history of medicine. For centuries, the graduates of medical schools have sworn the Oath as the first step in starting their career as medical doctors. Most university authorities all over the world keep up the respected tradition. Often new graduates are reminded about the history of the oath to emphasize that the practice of medicine, since early history, is based on ethics and good values. History is not just a series of stories to entertain us but stories that teach us how to continue in our daily life. Therefore, throughout years of clinical practice, all medical practitioners should recall the Hippocratic Oath and keep it in mind in all they do. It should not be considered as simply part of the joyful celebration of graduation. Swearing the Hippocratic Oath or its modification is to swear to adhere to the medical ethical code and should be considered as the last important lesson in medical school and message to consider for life.

> **Pearl**
> Every medical physician or surgeon should still take the Hippocratic Oath very seriously and consider it a basic guide to follow good medical ethics in medical practice. It is simple and embodies at least three of the four modern bioethics principles – beneficence, nonmaleficence, and justice.

1.6   Value-Based Medicine

While the concept of patient-centered care has been around for over 60 years (Leino 1952), the concept of evidence-based medicine essentially revolutionized over 20 years ago the way clinicians weigh their treatment options and administer treatment to any given patient, or groups of patients (Oxman et al. 1993). But underlying all of clinical practice, however, must be value-based medicine, by which we mean the same attention is given to ethical dimensions of our treatment of patients as is given to the evidence bearing on the case (i.e., value in this sense refers to ethical or moral value). This area of consideration under the name bioethics has gained traction over the last 15–20 years. The key elements of value-based medicine which, like evidence-based medicine, inform our clinical decisions are shown in Fig. 1.1 and are:

1. Autonomy, in which the patient has the right to choose or refuse methods for the management of their medical problem. Neurosurgeons and medical doctors must recognize the correct practice of autonomy is to work with the patient as a partner in order to make decisions about the best method of treatment.

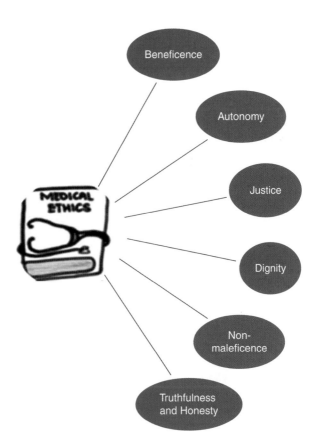

Fig. 1.1 Elements of value-based medicine

Fig. 1.2 Venn diagram showing the relationships of technical, strategic, and ethical medical care

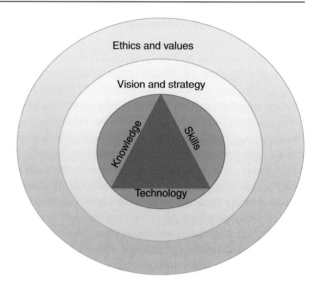

2. Beneficence, in which the physician or surgeon must consider the patient's benefit as the sole goal for the relationship with patient. The neurosurgeon should ask himself/herself honestly if the suggested method brings the most benefit for the patient.
3. Nonmaleficence, in which the neurosurgeon and the team have to do their best not to harm the patient. This risk of the proposed treatment should be minimized and explained to the patient very well, and every precaution should be taken to prevent it.
4. Justice, in which fairness and equality of medical care is applied for every patient, which includes distribution of the doctor's time and attention. Every patient has the right to receive the best possible and affordable medical care.
5. Dignity, which flows in both directions. In every treatment plan and every interaction, the patient and the treating team should be treated with respect and dignity.
6. Truthfulness and honesty, in which the relationship between a patient and the treating surgeon should be based on unconditional truth telling and honesty. The neurosurgeon should answer every patient's question honestly and should admit openly any mistakes made.

Figure 1.2 shows the relationship between ethics and values and other components of medical care.

The surgeon is first and foremost obliged to establish a relationship and rapport with the patient to understand their wishes and goals of treatment and to make them feel as comfortable as possible at a very frightening time. When discussing risks and benefits during informed consent, the neurosurgeon can gain valuable insight into the patient's culture and beliefs. Culture and belief play a vital role in the discussion of benefits and harm – while a particular course of treatment may present the best physical outcome, it may cause irreparable psychological damage if it goes against the patient's culture or moral standards. The neurosurgeon should assist the patient in weighing the benefits and harm, without asserting pressure or influence. Meaningful informed consent can only be reached when autonomy and beneficence work in tandem.

Conclusion

There is no doubt that history has great influence and impact on our daily lives. Human life is highly valued and respected in all ancient and modern civilizations. All religions without exception placed high value on human life, and medical practice in different periods of history was heavily influenced by religion. But ethical standards and norms cannot be written in stone and applied uniformly everywhere. They are now confronting more and more complex challenges, and ethical practices vary from culture to culture, religion to religion, country to country, city to city, and even hospital to hospital (e.g., depending on whether the hospital is a government/public hospital or private hospital).

If one is honestly treating a patient in the same way as he/she would like to be treated, he/she is likely following a code of ethical standards (notwithstanding cultural differences alluded to above). However, in many situations, the ethical dilemma is too nuanced and complex for this simplistic virtue-based approach. In the chapters following, ethical challenges confronted on a daily basis by all doctors, and specifically neurosurgeons, are examined using systems for addressing them.

References

Arras JD, Steinbock B, London AJ (1999) Moral reasoning in the medical context. In: Arras JD, Steinbock B (eds) Ethical issues in modern medicine, 5th edn. Mayfield Pub. Co, Houston

Beauchamp TL, Childress JF (2001) Principles of biomedical ethics, 5th edn. Oxford University Press Inc, New York

Bowman KW, Hui EC (2000) Bioethics for clinicians: 20. Chinese bioethics. Can Med Assoc J 163(11):1481–1485

Coward H, Sidhu T (2000) Bioethics for clinicians: 19. Hinduism and Sikhism. Can Med Assoc J 163(9):1167–1170

Daar AS, al Khitamy AB (2001) Bioethics for clinicians: 21. Islamic bioethics. Can Med Assoc J 164(1):60–63

Edelstein L (1943) The Hippocratic oath, text, translation and interpretation. The Johns Hopkins Press, Baltimore

Ellerby JH, McKenzie J, McKay S et al (2000) Bioethics for clinicians: 18. Aboriginal cultures. Can Med Assoc J 163(7):845–850

Goldsand G, Rosenberg ZR, Gordon M (2001) Bioethics for clinicians: 22. Jewish bioethics. Can Med Assoc J 164(2):219–222

Halperin M (2004) Milestones in Jewish medical ethics: medical-halachic literature in Israel, 1948–1998. Assia Jew Med Ethics 4(2):4–19

Jonsen AR, Siegler M, Winslade WJ (1998) Clinical ethics, 4th edn. McGraw-Hill, New York

Kant I (1993) Critique of pure reason. Orion Publishing Group, London

Leino A (1952) Planning patient-centered care. Am J Nurs 52(3):324–325

Levine RS, Williams JC, Kilbourne BA et al (2012) Tuskegee redux: evolution of legal mandates for human experimentation. J Health Care Poor Underserved 23(4 Suppl):104–125

Markwell HJ, Brown BF (2001) Bioethics for clinicians: 27. Catholic bioethics. Can Med Assoc J 165(2):189–192

Mill JS (1991) On liberty and other essays. In: Gray J (ed) John Stuart Mill on liberty and other essays. Oxford University Press, New York

National Commission for the Protection of Human Subjects of Biomedical and Behavioral Research (1978) The Belmont report: ethical principles and guidelines for the protection of human subjects of research. US Government Printing Office, Washington, DC

Nuremberg Military Tribunal (1996) The Nuremberg code. JAMA 276:1691

Oxman AD, Sackett DL, Guyatt GH (1993) Users' guides to the medical literature. I. How to get started. The evidence-based medicine working group. JAMA 270(17):2093–2095

Pauls M, Hutchinson RC (2002) Bioethics for clinicians: 28. Protestant bioethics. Can Med Assoc J 166(3):339–343

Pence GE (1995) Classic cases in medical ethics, 2nd edn. McGraw-Hill, New York

Rawls J (1971) A theory of justice. Bellknap Press, Boston

Reich WT (1995) Encyclopedia of bioethics. Simon & Shuster Macmillan, New York

Singh B, Saradananda S (2008) Ethics and surgical training in ancient India – a clue for current practice. S Afr Med J 98:218–221

Trials of War Criminals before the Nuremberg Military Tribunals under control council law (1949). No. 10, vol. 2. U.S. Government Printing Office, Washington, DC, pp. 181–182

Walsh J (2010) The popes and science: the history of the papal relations to science during the middle ages and down to our own time. Fordham University Press, New York

World Medical Association Declaration of Helsinki: ethical principles for medical research human subjects (2000) Edinburgh: World Medical Association. Available at: http:Involv//www.wma.net/en/30publications/10policies/b3/ing

Ethics Principles and Theories

2

Adefolarin O. Malomo and Mark Bernstein

2.1 Introduction

Ethics, the systematic study of morality, utilizes the contents of formal philosophy to explore its subject matter (MacIntyre 1971). Bioethics is ethics as applied to medicine, or value-based medicine. Bioethics provides an attempt to find the "right answer" when moral ambiguity exists in a medical situation. When one encounters a moral dilemma, there is often no one right answer, but bioethics can provide frameworks for analyzing the problem utilizing the ethical principles and theories. The ethical principles and theories have evolved from theological teachings and philosophical discourse. Some ethics problems may be resolved relatively easily by applying one or more principles or theories, but many are so complex and/or culturally nuanced, and in many situations, the "right" answer cannot be achieved. Some typical ethical dilemmas experienced by neurosurgeons around the planet include (1) how much to disclose to a patient about a complication and/or error, (2) how to obtain informed consent as ethically as possible, (3) how to ethically introduce innovation in care, (4) how to ethically teach trainees without compromising patient care, (5) how to prioritize competing interests in a system with finite resources, and (6) how to ethically perform clinical research involving patients. Many of these situations are discussed in this book, and all are approachable using the ethical theories and principles.

A.O. Malomo, MB, BS, MHSc, FWACS
Departments of Surgery and Human Anatomy, University of Ibadan, Ibadan, Nigeria

Department of Neurological Surgery, University of Ibadan, Ibadan, Nigeria
e-mail: ademalomo@yahoo.com

M. Bernstein, MD, MHSc, FRCSC (✉)
Division of Neurosurgery, Toronto Western Hospital, University of Toronto,
399 Bathurst Street, Toronto, ON M5T 2S8, Canada
e-mail: mark.bernstein@uhn.ca

A. Ammar, M. Bernstein (eds.), *Neurosurgical Ethics in Practice: Value-based Medicine*,
DOI 10.1007/978-3-642-54980-9_2, © Springer-Verlag Berlin Heidelberg 2014

2.2   Illustrative Case (Assisted Suicide)

Ms. Brava is a courageous woman 48 year old with a brain stem glioma. She has received radiation and chemotherapy but is progressing with loss of mobility and brain stem functions. She knows the disease will relentlessly rob her of her mobility, her ability to eat, and finally her ability to breathe without mechanical assistance, while her mind remains alert. She finds no dignity in such a life and wishes to circumvent an agonizing death through assisted suicide. She requests her physician to help her with an assisted suicide, but he reports he cannot as it is illegal. When she asks him how he personally feels about it, he responds "I'm personally conflicted, but you are my patient and really I want to help you, but taking a life is wrong." How does one approach assisted suicide from a personal, ethical, and societal perspective?

2.3   Approach to the Case

Arguments for and against assisted suicide using both ethics principles and theories can be simply applied as follows. Utilitarians may consider suicide as morally acceptable in the circumstances described as such would yield the best outcome to the largest number of people; it is noteworthy that utilitarians make no differences between such an act done actively or passively. Deontologists would forbid killing. Kant considered suicide inconsistent logically; individualists can consider it right only by considering that the patient has waved both the right to life and the negative right not to be interfered with. Communitarians would generally see it as a loss to society and shrink from it unless it was a community that traditionally allowed such. In principlism, autonomy would recommend respecting the patient's wishes. The principles of nonmaleficence and beneficence in this situation would have a different meaning for such patients than the traditional one and may be in favor of assisted suicide. The principle of justice would be to enable the incapacitated to obtain what is available to all else, in societies that allow suicide. Followers of ethics of care would be supportive of alleviating suffering. Religious ethics and traditional medical virtue ethics would forbid it (Beauchamp and Childress 2001; Arras et al. 1999).

> **Pearl**
> In medicine and in neurosurgery, there is often no one right answer to an ethical problem, but there is a systematic process for analyzing the problem to expose all the possible viewpoints and approaches and to make sure all stakeholders' voices are heard.

2.4   Discussion

Below is a brief introduction to the main ethical principles, theories, and other systems commonly used to ethically analyze moral dilemmas is presented. Most of them would be easily accessible to and usable by neurosurgeons in everyday practice. The theories are coherent, clear, comprehensive, complete, explanatory, prescriptive, and pragmatic statements about goodness in general and the rightness of an action. They are based in philosophy and are grounds from which ethical principles as mid-level frameworks can be drawn to furnish rules of action. Principles are also usually the main building blocks of various schools of ethics such as those of theological origin – Buddhist, Jewish, Christian, and Islamic (Deigh 2001; Beauchamp and Childress 2001). Theories are affected by the place, time, and culture. They have strengths and weaknesses, and areas of optimal application all of which will help their appreciation and application (Arras et al. 1999).

> **Pearl**
> Ethical analysis is highly dependent on religion and culture, for example, discussions of issues like assisted suicide and abortion are not possible in some settings. Cultural sensitivity is central to ethical discourse or even to the initial recognition of an issue as being ethically ambiguous.

2.4.1   Principlism

Principlism is a simplistic but useful system of ethical analysis derived from four principles of common morality. In principlism, we may need to look elsewhere to determine meanings and interpretations, in spite of these specifying rules. For instance, "good" and "harm" are not always clear in human and clinical situations, and in such cases, we need other resources to determine them.

The four principles consist of autonomy (free will or agency), beneficence (to do good), nonmaleficence (not to harm), and justice (fair distribution of benefits and burdens). Each is a prima facie principle, is equal to all the others, and may override others in different situations, but all remain important in considering execution of decision (Beauchamp and Childress 2001; Deigh 2001). The initial ethical analysis of most challenges faced by neurosurgeons can be carried out by examining how each of the four principles bears on the problem, especially the first three for most situations involving one patient as opposed to groups of patients. When the principles fall short, the ethical theories described below may help (especially utilitarianism and deontology).

Pearl

The four principles at the core of bioethics are autonomy, beneficence, mon-maleficence, and justice. Principlism is a simplistic but effective way of examining bioethical dilemmas.

2.4.2 Utilitarianism

This theory is usually associated with the philosophers Jeremy Bentham and John Stuart Mill. It determines the rightness of any action merely by its utility in producing happiness or a good outcome. Utilitarians calculate happiness and the best action is that which produces the greatest amount of happiness for the individual, community, or entities concerned, or the best outcome for the largest number of people. The calculus is, in principle, person, place, and time neutral. It is also mode neutral in the sense that some consequences can be produced by positive intervention or negative withholding of possible intervention. Utilitarians are concerned not about intentions or means, but the consequences of adopting the choice made (Beauchamp and Childress 2001; Arras et al. 1999; Mill 1991).

This theory is clear, definite, empirical, liberal, fair, and pragmatic and blends well with democratic concepts being originally aimed at improving public policy rather than personal "character." Utilitarianism admits to other values but argues that such values are real only to the extent that they are instrumental to producing happiness: they are all reducible to happiness. However, measuring or accurately projecting the probability of the purity, magnitude, and intensity of happiness even if we could agree on its exact nature is problematic. Also, most people, unlike utilitarians, would not agree that moral responsibility from positive acts and negative withholding of intervention are rationally, morally equivalent. It is also questionable whether morality can be strengthened in a society that pays little regard to intention and whether ends that maximize overall happiness at the expense of individual rights and even justice can be valid.

Rule utilitarianism can guide subordinate rules or policies which also guide acts broadly without reference to the calculus of individual acts. Act utilitarianism can be used to guide every individual act separately. A danger of act utilitarianism is that with differing individual capabilities and robustness, we can easily end up with inconsistencies and even the slippery slope. Strict rule utilitarianism, on the other hand, ignores the fact that every moral rule has exceptions. It is hard to frame rules that can account for all unusual situations. Rule utilitarianism need not collapse into act utilitarianism; it in principle does to exceptions what act utilitarianism does to minorities. Both rule and act utilitarianism ignore rights and justice and assume, probably unjustifiably, that all virtues are reducible to the instrumentality of producing happiness, or good outcome.

2.4.3   Kantian Deontology

Deontology is a moral theory that holds that true morals exist in the context of duty, being categorical imperatives, purely and absolutely binding from the mere sense of duty and not any other reasons of feelings, emotions, or ends, not even happiness. Deontologists have a morality that does its duty even if it makes the world end. The duty is to do the right thing irrespective of outcome, in direct contradistinction to utilitarianism. The challenge with deontology in modern medicine is the ambiguity of what constitutes the right thing, which is relative especially given the religious and cultural diversity of health care systems. Some basic tenets of Kant's philosophy are presented in Table 2.1.

Immanuel Kant was a rational purist – to him morality was binding in the sense of being an absolute, "categorical" imperative which a pure rational free will finds to be a duty. The will is authentic when absolutely free from self-interest and all other internal or external influences except pure practical reason; pure practical reason makes the free will good by making it transcend self-interest and all other

Table 2.1   Selected quotes from Kant essential to deontological ethical theory

1. "A good will is not good because of what it effects or accomplishes…Thus the moral worth of an action does not lie in the effect expected…"
2. The representation of an objective principle …is called a command, and the formula of the command is called an imperative. All imperatives are expressed by an ought…"
3. "… if the action would be good merely as a means to something else the imperative is hypothetical; if the action is represented as in itself good, …then it is categorical."
4. "There is therefore only a single categorical imperative and it is this: act only in accordance with that maxim through which you can at the same time will that it become a universal law."
5. "All rational beings stand under the law that each of them is to treat himself and all others never merely as a means but always at the same time as ends in themselves."
6. "Duty is that action to which someone is bound…To assure one's own happiness is a duty."
7. "Be an honourable human being…Do not wrong anyone."
8. "Freedom (independence from being constrained by another's choice), insofar as it can exist with the freedom of every other in accordance with universal law, is the only original right belonging to every man by virtue of his humanity."
9. "The greatest violation of a human being's duty to himself …is the contrary of truthfulness, lying …a lie…does not require what jurists insist upon adding for their definition that it must harm another…for it always harms another… inasmuch as it makes the source of right unusable."
10. "…beneficience is the maxim of making others' happiness one's end… To be beneficient, that is to promote according to one's means the happiness of others in need, without hoping for something in return, is everyone's duty."
11. "Every human being has a legitimate claim to respect from his fellow human beings and is in turn bound to respect every other."

Data from Kant (1996)

influences into universal commitment in a logically consistent way, for the mere duty of pursuing "good will." This for Kant was the nature, sum, and process of morality. Morality to him was purely a rational deduction of its own type: acting under a consistent maxim that one could will to be universal, derived through a process of pure practical reason by a perfectly free will, as an autonomous agent. A maxim that is purely rational, consistent, and universal is, of course, categorical in that it derives from a perfectly free "good will" and aims for nothing other than the "universalizable." Kant recognized other values, but separates them from the moral one. Understandably, his model of reason is like that in mathematics – maxim-based, ultrapure, and rigorous. For him, moral value can occur only in the context of morality as described above. Since morality is an abstract concept, it can be derived only by pure practical reason, not emotion, feeling, tradition, or consequences of following moral imperatives. Maxims derived from any of the mentioned factors or any other factor than pure practical reason would be hypothetical (Kant 1978, 1993, 1996).

To Kant, humans are moral agents because they are capable of pure practical reasoning to discern what moral maxims ought to be and have the freedom of will to choose them. So, humans ought to act as autonomous moral agents. On this rests their moral dignity and why they should never be used as mere means to an end but as ends in themselves, which is another maxim of his. Morality is a pure duty owed by humans as autonomous rational agents with wills free from all other influences.

Kant's abstract system based on idealized purist suppositions about reason and experiential freedom of the will has more of the purity of reason than reality or practice. This is obvious in health care settings. However, it overcomes the weaknesses of utilitarianism in respecting individuality and justice and extolling the values of rationality, freedom, equality, and independence. It focuses on "autonomy" "respect for persons," and integrity, primary responsibility, or duty. Later workers based on Kant's contributions, called Kantians, have extracted, adapted, and redeployed these concepts, sometimes in ways that are far from but reminiscent of Kant's usage (Secker 1999). For instance, in principlism, autonomy or respect for persons is now specified in the act of informed consent and also relates to maintenance of privacy and confidentiality. Kantian analysis of common medical problems can shed useful light on the morally ambiguous issues at hand (Bernstein and Fundner 2003; Bernstein and Brown 2004).

Pearl

The two dominant ethical theories are utilitarianism and deontology. Their difference can be simplistically demonstrated using the "life boat scenario." A ship sinks and 12 people find themselves in a lifeboat, but it is only safe to hold 10 for the time needed to get to shore. Utilitarians would invite two persons to leave so that two die but ten are saved. Deontologists would insist that none should leave so all 12 would die. Even though the outcome is worse, the duty to do the right thing, and not take a life, is honored.

2.4.4 Kantian Contractarianism

There are two main social contract theories: Hobbesian and Kantian. Contractarianism is an effort at formalizing society especially with respect to the content of social obligations and the motivation for fulfilling them. It is based on the mythical contract we have made with each other which we are morally obliged to keep. Only Kantian contractarianism will be discussed here. Kantians have extracted and reapplied in more practical ways, some of the terms and concepts used by Kant. One such Kantian in contractarian moral theory was developed by John Rawls whose consistent concern was more societal than individual. His starting assumption was that since as Kant said, we are all ends in ourselves, we are then all of equal moral status and should be treated as being equal, with fairness in society. His myth or model therefore starts from a presumed state of ignorance, where each and all are ignorant of their present or would be social advantages and those of others. In such a state, ordinary self-interest would dictate that one decides to give the best possible to everyone being considered, since any lot might end up as one's own (Rawls 1971). Rawls then went on to advocate equality of liberty, opportunity, and distribution of resources in that order of priority. In distribution of resources, he proposed that inequality in distribution of resources should only be such as is required by circumstances and as would make everyone happy. Rawls considered that behind the veil of ignorance, every rational being would be fair. This means that every situation in ethics (and in everything!) should be analyzed and judged without preknowledge about the stakeholders or preconceived notions by the evaluator – this way absolute fairness prevails. Rawls aimed at the goal of "justice as fairness" in his works where "justice" (and "right") precedes "goodness." Significantly, freedom, justice, and fairness are moral values which are usually considered important and relevant in health care services especially in respect of access to care and resource allocation (Beauchamp and Childress 2001; Arras et al. 1999; Kant 1978).

2.4.5 Rights-Based Theory

This is "liberal Individualism." It has old traces but has been worked into the fabric of present-day lives with implications for the health care sector.

Historically, John Locke advocated the concept that under the natural law, all humans have perfect freedom and protection from interference with their "properties" – lives, liberty, and possessions. Kant valued autonomous will. John Stuart Mill, in addition to his work on utilitarianism, advocated for freedom of conscience, taste, and association as well as freedom from public and religious interference beyond advice, instruction, persuasion, or avoidance at the most, except where the interests of others are injured, everyone being equally responsible and accountable in society. More recently added are civil rights causes, global declarations, national constitutions, laws, and policies. Today's liberalism came later.

Rights are usually based on more immediate rules that make them distinct and clear, rather than equally valid principles and theories. They can be social, moral, legal, or other types of rights. Although rights always entail obligations, moral obligations sometimes do not entail rights. For instance, the moral obligation for the wealthy to be generous or charitable to the needy does not imply the needy's right to be given, either at individual or national levels. It is often considered that rights are prior to obligation, but on this, the jury is still out. Also, rights can be positive when they require action, or negative when they prohibit interference with the owner of the right. Usually, the negative legal right to what a society considers immoral will not be backed by a positive legal right to receive public sponsorship in doing it.

Rights are not inherently complete and are more suited to legal than moral situations. Strikingly, the law usually trumps morality where rights dominate. Indeed, morality may require waiving of legal rights in order to foster a greater good than law. Rights and freedoms are vital fibers of human society when morality already exists as their context (Arras et al. 1999; Beauchamp and Childress 2001; Rutherford 2002).

2.4.6 Religious Ethics

Religions are socialized responses to spirituality and so are aspects of sociocultural development. Religion always has ethical implications and is probably itself an effort at ethical response; it influences moral considerations even in secular societies. Indeed, religion, moral philosophy, and law continue to influence the development of bioethics discussions. The clarity, distinction, and rigor of religious depositions tend to affect their inputs into general ethical discourses today. Religion tends to run deep in human experience, emotion, and expression, especially in severely challenging or overwhelming circumstances like neurosurgeons see on a regular basis.

The Christian idea of the Natural Law Theory was that God has detectably inscribed the law of creatures' nature. Natural law is therefore a part of the expression of Divine law. Through their rationality, for instance, humans are able to actively participate in Divine plans. Through the same, their "good" cannot be merely analogous to that of beasts, and so, through various principles, maxims, commandments, and others, the Roman Catholic Church teaching on marriage, sexuality, contraception, abortion, sanctity of human life, and others emerged. One of the Church's fundamental natural concepts is to do "good" and avoid "evil."

Religious ethics have their own narratives and myths which they adopt in their own genre of justification in developing their peculiar principles and theories. Practitioners need to pay appropriate attention to these in reasoning out the balance of good with patients of different religions and ideologies (Beauchamp and Childress 2001; Arras et al. 1999; Gadama 1999).

2.4.7 Communitarianism

This is community-based moral theory in which values are determined by the community and what is best for the community trumps what is best for an individual. This is particularly common in parts of South Asia and Africa. Generally, grand theories start by examining commonly held norms. Also, humans are fundamentally social and community creatures, and insight into community-based theories may help balance the extremes of others, individualism, for instance. This approach can be a survival device because actual threat level affects optimal freedom and individualistic behaviors allowable. Challenges attributable to liberal individualism, especially in the West are partly responsible for the current popularity of communitarianism.

Communitarians' lives are geared towards full self-realization in the community. Their ethos is towards "both and," not "either or"; not "I and you" but "we and us." Native communitarians lack written grand theories because their literature is typically oral and their theories embedded in narratives, social norms, and sanctions. Communitarians see their universe as an extension of their own reality – they are a mere speck in its vastness, but its vastness is a real extension of themselves which they may learn properly to engage. The focal entity is neither the individual nor the majority but the community; the tool is not pure reason or rigorous analysis but ongoing culture and tradition. The sense of oneness of all runs through. The valid contents of mutual belonging and cooperative living to achieve clearly defined common ends through common values are approaches which can help inform the model of "medical community." This latter understanding drives many current philosophical communitarians. Some philosophical communitarians completely reject the entire contents of liberalism, while others tolerate some strands of individualism in context.

Rights are meaningless without the context of real obligation to others. However, as we seek to emphasize communal sense of being, we should watch out for the shy underdogs and greedy domineering aggressors and seek also the virtues of assertiveness in participation, codetermination, and joint ownership in communities (Beauchamp and Childress 2001; Arras et al. 1999; Etzioni 2001).

2.4.8 Feminist Ethics

Feminist ethics developed in response to sociopolitical and economic concerns about female disadvantaged perception, position, status, roles and the undervaluation of femaleness in traditional patriarchal world views and values. In spite of the various eighteenth- and nineteenth-century efforts, various oppressions of women and the unjust lower rating of femaleness and female dispositions persisted. In the more successful twentieth-century efforts, it is still clear that females can suffer from class, race, and disability disadvantages and even injustices, especially in certain specific parts of the world. Such issues have informed the concerns of feminist movements and ethics. There are several schools of feminist ethics (Beauchamp and Childress 2001; Arras et al. 1999; Mackinnon 2009; Tessmann 2009).

2.4.9 Ethics of Care

This approach emphasizes interconnectedness, caring motives, emotional commitments, compassion, fidelity, love, and acceptance of responsibility to act on behalf of dependents. It opposes overly impersonal, deserting, indifferent, and individualistic systems. It is most relevant in the setting of close family situations or at most in communitarian systems (Beauchamp and Childress 2001; Arras et al. 1999; Bradshaw 1996).

2.4.10   Virtue Ethics

This includes multiple old subsystems in which groups, ideologies, and religions have a list of excellences called virtue, that is, virtuous personality traits. Aristotle discussed some virtues – temperance, courage, justice, wisdom, and practical reason. He recommended teaching a life of doing what is noble through upbringing and good habits. A virtuous person acts based on reason, habit, and developed character, because the virtues tend to be their own justification. Aristotle's virtuous man is the constant canon, and we know what to do in virtue ethics by knowing what virtuous persons in those circumstances would do (Arras et al. 1999; Hursthouse 2006; McCammon and Brody 2012). There is still ambiguity in relying on any neurosurgeons's virtues because (1) virtues are relative dependent on culture, religion, personality, experience, etc., and (2) even if we are virtuous, we cannot always know the correct thing to do in some situations due to their complexity – we cannot rely on virtue alone.

> **Pearl**
> A neurosurgeon's virtue alone cannot be relied upon – many ethical dilemmas are too complex and/or culturally nuanced.

2.4.11   Casuistry

This is more of a procedure than theory or principle of ethics. It is a bottom-up approach like in legal reasoning. It involves defining a case and choosing a paradigmatic case like it, determining their moral similarity and differences, determining the rules and principles involved in the paradigmatic case and relating it to the case at hand, and clarifying decisions if necessary under the light of overarching theories (Beauchamp and Childress 2001; Fiester 2006).

> **Conclusion**
> The practice of neurosurgery is challenging intellectually, manually, emotionally, and psychologically. Ethically ambiguous and/or challenging situations arise on an almost daily basis. One cannot be expected to always know the right answer. Sometimes legal precedent helps us; for example, most neurosurgeons do not have to consider a patient request about assisted suicide as it is illegal in

the vast majority of jurisdictions in the world. However, some ethical dilemmas are timeless and universal, and there will arise new ones in the future with innovative treatments, such as developments with deep brain surgery, gene therapy, and changes in legal and social norms, like legalization of assisted suicide in more parts of the world. One cannot be prepared for every new situation, but a working knowledge of the basic bioethical approaches to assessing a problem can be invaluable to the practitioner.

Acknowledgment We thank Sylvia O. Malomo and A.D. Faraye for their help.

References

Arras JD, Steinbock B, London AJ (1999) Moral reasoning in the medical context. In: Arras JD, Steinbock B (eds) Ethical issues in modern medicine, 5th edn. Mayfield Pub Co, Houston

Beauchamp TL, Childress JF (2001) Principles of biomedical ethics, 5th edn. Oxford University Press Inc, New York

Bernstein M, Brown B (2004) Doctors' duty to disclose error: a deontological or Kantian ethical analysis. Can J Neurol Sci 31:169–174

Bernstein M, Fundner R (2003) House of healing, house of disrespect: a Kantian perspective on disrespectful behaviour among hospital workers. Hosp Q 6:62–66

Bradshaw A (1996) Yes! There is an ethics of care: an answer for Peter Allmark. J Med Ethics 22:8–12

Deigh J (2001) Ethics. In: Audi R (ed) The Cambridge dictionary of philosophy, secondth edn. Cambridge University Press, Cambridge

Etzioni A (2001) On communitarian approach to bioethics. Theor Med Bioeth 32:363–374

Fiester A (2006) Casuistry and the moral continuum. Evaluating animal biotechnology. Politics Life Sci 25(1–2):15–22

Gadama H (1999) Hermeneutics Religion and Ethics (trans Weinsheimer J). Yale, Yale University

Hursthouse R (2006) Applying virtue ethics to our treatment of other animals. In: Welchman J (ed) The practice of virtue. Hackett Publishing Company, Cambridge, MA

Kant I (1978) Critique of practical reason. Bobbs-Merrill Educational Publishing, Indianapolis

Kant I (1993) Critique of pure reason. Orion Publishing Group, London

Kant I (1996) Practical philosophy. Cambridge University Press, Cambridge

MacIntyre A (1971) A short history of ethics. Routledge and Kegan Paul, London

Mackinnon CJ (2009) Applying feminist, multicultural, and social justice theory to diverse women who function as caregivers in end-of-life and palliative home care. Palliat Support Care 7(4):501–512

McCammon SD, Brody H (2012) How virtue ethics informs medical professionalism. HEC Forum 24(4):257–272

Mill JS (1991) On liberty and other essays. In: Gray J (ed) John Stuart Mill on liberty and other essays. Oxford University Press, New York

Rawls J (1971) A theory of justice. Bellknap Press, Boston

Rutherford MB (2002) A bibliographic essay on individualism. The Hedgehog Rev Spr 02: 116–127

Secker B (1999) The appearance of Kant's deontology in contemporary Kantianism: concepts of patient autonomy in bioethics. J Med Philos 24(1):43–66

Tessmann L (2009) Introduction. In: Tessmann L (ed) Feminist ethics and social and political philosophy: theorizing the non ideal. Springer, New York

Cross-Cultural Ethics

3

Ahmed Ammar and Mark Bernstein

3.1 Introduction

Medical ethics, although generally universal, are interpreted differently in different places. Values are also relative so that value-based medicine is subject to the relativity of religious beliefs, cultural milieu, politics, laws, geography, and others. How should ethical differences be managed? In order to answer that question, it is important to understand what causes the differences.

Most anthropologists agree that an important part of the definition of culture is the thoughts, behaviors, and customs of the group. All of these have an impact on the interpretation and implementation of medical ethics. One commentator stated that primary cultural values are transmitted to a culture's members by socialization and parenting, education, and religion. There are also secondary factors that affect ethical behavior – they include differences in the systems of laws across nations, accepted human resource management systems, organizational culture, and professional cultures and codes of conduct (Pitta et al. 1999). Another commentator articulated that ethical relativism theorizes that morality is relative to the norms of one's culture. The perception of whether an action is wrong or right is dictated by acceptable norms in the society in which it occurs (Wong 1986).

Many classic cultural differences in societies resulting in unusual and challenging patient relationships with the medical profession have been eloquently documented in single case studies such as those involving native or aboriginal people in northern

A. Ammar, MBChB, DMSc, FICS, FACS, FAANS (✉)
Department of Neurosurgery, King Fahd University Hosptial, Dammam University,
40121, Al Khobar 31952, Saudi Arabia
e-mail: ahmed@ahmedammar.com

M. Bernstein, MD, MHSc, FRCSC
Division of Neurosurgery, Toronto Western Hospital, University of Toronto,
399 Bathurst Street, Toronto, ON M5T 2S8, Canada
e-mail: mark.bernstein@uhn.ca

A. Ammar, M. Bernstein (eds.), *Neurosurgical Ethics in Practice: Value-based Medicine*,
DOI 10.1007/978-3-642-54980-9_3, © Springer-Verlag Berlin Heidelberg 2014

Canada (McDonald 2006) and the Hmong people who emigrated to the USA (Fadiman 1997). Qualitative research methodology has been successfully used to explore cultural and religious influences, like end-of-life care in ethnic minority groups (Donovan et al. 2011). More egregious examples of cultural differences in medical practice across the planet include practices which are considered heinous and even illegal in some parts of the world and are commonplace in others, like female genital mutilation (Kopelman 2013). There is considerable sociocultural controversy over male circumcision as well, although obviously not at the same level.

Currently, in almost every hospital, in some countries more than others, medical, paramedical staff, and patients from different nationalities, holding different faiths and beliefs, and from very different backgrounds work together in harmony. What allows these differences to be tolerated is a sound organizational ethic in the institution and the central and overriding aim by all parties to work for the best interest of the patient. Below are several examples of ethical challenges for which cultural, religious, ethnic, and geographic differences may have major influence on how patients and families react to these common problems.

3.2   Illustrative Case 1 (Privacy of Person)

An elderly lady from an Arab Gulf State with a cauda equina syndrome from a spinal tumor required urgent admission to a North American hospital where she was visiting her son. She requested a room in an all female ward. Initially the nurses were insulted by her request. No all female ward beds were available in the hospital so the patient accepted admission to the mixed ward.

3.3   Illustrative Case 2 (Privacy of Information)

A middle-aged Italian woman was admitted to a hospital in Saudi Arabia, complaining of weakness in both lower limbs. A gentleman identifying himself as family inquired about her condition and was told all of the medical facts pertaining to her case, without the doctors obtaining consent from the patient.

3.4   Approach to These Cases

The patient has the right to privacy and his/her dignity should be respected. However, the perception and implementation of those rights vary according to culture. In the case of the Arabic lady, her culture made her extremely sensitive to being on the same ward as an unrelated male. However, she would have considered it perfectly normal to have her husband informed of the details of her case, without prior permission. Conversely, the Western lady felt that her right to privacy was infringed, because in Saudi Arabia, it is considered unusual to not reveal details to a male relative of a female patient. However, this patient would not have felt uncomfortable in a mixed ward.

The patient has the right to choose the place he or she believes will provide the best medical care for that particular medical problem, within reasonable limits. In the case of the Arab woman, she had to make a choice between the place where she could receive what she considered to be the best medical care and her cultural sensitivities.

> **Pearl**
> It is important to understand the culture and values of patients in order to maintain their dignity and privacy. The patient must also consider the ethics of the treating organization. In order for the best medical care to be provided, both the patient and health care providers must be willing to compromise within certain limits.

3.5   Illustrative Case (Touching)

A neurosurgery resident is attending the clinic with a neurosurgeon in a large teaching hospital in a North American city. He enters the room of a new female patient, who has been referred with the diagnosis of Chiari malformation. He instinctively extends his hand for a handshake as he usually does and then notices she is wearing a head scarf. The patient recoils from this gesture. She is sorry she has embarrassed him but feels she must adhere to the laws of Islam.

3.6   Approach to the Case

In observant Muslim and Jewish religion and law, it is forbidden for a person to physically touch a person of the opposite sex past the age of puberty who is not a close relative, like a spouse or child (Bernstein 2007). This is in direct contradistinction to most other cultures and religions where physical touching is acceptable and even often seen as beneficial, especially in the relationship between a patient and a health care provider. These are diametrically opposed customs for greetings which are at the same time both ethically sound, depending on one's religious beliefs. Even during the medically necessary parts of the examination, consent for touching a patient is implicit, but the physician should explicitly ask the patient's permission with: "May I touch you." Strictly, this practice should extend to all patients of both sexes and all religions and at all times.

> **Pearl**
> Physicians should not offer a handshake to a religious Muslim or Jewish patient of the opposite sex. They should always be respectful of modesty and privacy of patient's bodies and not take this for granted because of the doctor-patient relationship.

3.7   Illustrative Case 3 (End-of-Life Issues)

A 21-year-old victim of a car accident with a severe closed head injury was admitted to the ICU. The patient rapidly deteriorated and was declared brain dead within 24 h. The patient's family asked for any treatment anywhere with money being no object. They refused to accept that their loved one was dead making it impossible to discuss organ donation or termination of ventilation.

3.8   Approach to the Case

Death is as much a part of life as birth. Birth is universally accepted as being joyous, whereas the attitude to terminality and death varies from culture to culture and even within cultures. Quality during life and dignity in death are among the fundamental rights of every human.

Comparison of the reaction of Thai and American families to patients dying in ICU yielded the observation that in Thailand, families of dying patients often advocate for aggressive ICU care in order to pay their debt of life. Their reasoning is apparently based on process, not outcome. Many Americans may similarly see the process of providing care as in some ways more important than cure (Stonington 2013). Doctors in many cultures also do not accept the determination of death by neurological endpoints (Hamdy 2013). In Western culture, some have chosen suicide rather than wait for death from a terminal disease (Ammar 1997) and at minimum many, including those with terminal brain tumors, are open to the conversation about assisted suicide (Lipsman et al. 2007).

Many people still find the idea of brain death difficult to understand. The person delivering such bad news has to appreciate and understand the deep values, faiths, and beliefs of the patient and family and approach them gently. Since they associate the word "death" with the cessation of all life functions, a patient who is being ventilated, has a heartbeat, and is possibly exhibiting reflex posturing definitely does not fit the "normal" definition of dead. So, in cases of brain death, it is even more important to take into account knowledge of the family's culture and beliefs, in order to make it easier for them to accept the news. Religious factors obviously impact families' views toward brain death and subsequently organ donation (Oliver et al. 2012).

> **Pearl**
> Facing death is the ultimate situation where deep values and faith of most humans prevail. Neurosurgeons must be tolerant to patients' belief systems, within reason. Acceptance of the concept of brain death should be promoted in order to alleviate a patient's indignity, avoid wasting precious health care resources, and improve the availability of organs for transplantation.

3.9   Illustrative Case 4 (Litigation)

A 55-year-old religious patient was operated for L4-5 microdiscectomy. The neurosurgeon misinterpreted the localizing X-ray and removed the L5-S1 healthy disc. Shortly after, the mistake was discovered, and the L4-5 disc was also removed. The patient recovered well with no complaints. Following the surgery, the neurosurgeon informed the patient of the mistake and expected the patient to sue him; he was surprised that the patient did not. Months later, the patient was asked why he did not sue the neurosurgeon. The answer was "the neurosurgeon had no intention to make that mistake, it is God's will."

3.10   Approach to the Case

Medical litigation statistics vary widely from country to country. In the USA medical litigation is frequent, whereas in countries such as India and China, it is less common. Many cultural factors, such as societal ethics, the value of work, faith, the law, societal hierarchy, and the position of the medical doctor in that structure, all influence the decision to litigate. In societies where the medical doctor has achieved very high status in society, litigation is less likely. Similarly, deep religious conviction that complications of surgery, including death, are God's will leads to acceptance of the mistake rather than litigation. Conversely, in societies where surgical specialists are seen merely as very well-paid technicians, there is less tolerance for errors and an expectation that the doctor can perform miracles if paid enough. In these societies medical litigation is more common.

Honesty, one of the basics of medical ethics was observed and practiced in this case. The neurosurgeon did not hide or deny his mistake. The patient may have forgiven the error, because he became pain free and returned to work, and although appreciating the honesty of the neurosurgeon the outcome of no legal action may have been different if the patient had not enjoyed good pain relief from the procedure. However, it is likely that faith and a deep belief in destiny may direct patients to forgive doctors for errors.

It is likely that every neurosurgeon is likely to be sued if he/she continues to practice until the age of 65; however, this is clearly not the case in every country (Jena et al. 2011). Patients have the right to complain if they do not receive the expected medical care. Irrespective of the possibility of litigation, neurosurgeons should strive to always do the right thing and to provide the best possible care.

> **Pearl**
> Honesty and patient respect should always be strictly observed. The patient has the right to complain, but these complaints should not stop progress in medical practice. Honesty and responding to complaints is more challenging in some cultures and religions than others.

3.11   Illustrative Case (Problems Arising from Inadequate Resources)

In a hospital in a large city in sub-Saharan Africa, a hot waiting room is over-crowded with people, most of whom are standing. Slowly they are seen over a period of about 5 h. In each examining room are two small desks and four chairs. A senior resident sits behind one desk and a junior resident sits behind the other, both seeing patients at the same time. A third patient wanders in and one of the residents addresses her problems. A staff neurosurgeon comes in at the same time to comment on one of the cases.

3.12   Approach to the Case

This egregious lack of privacy, mainly driven by shortage of physical resources of enough examining rooms, would not be tolerated in resource-rich countries. Utilitarian ethics simply trumps Kantian deontology in the sense that in order for patients to be seen and to receive whatever care is available, the "right" thing by Western standards cannot be done (i.e., their being seen alone in privacy). In some cultures and settings, ethical shortcuts must be considered acceptable. Respect for persons is violated but this is necessary within this culture with insufficient infrastructure. Patients seem to accept this and tolerate it.

3.13   Illustrative Case (Gifts from Patients)

An elderly gentleman originally from eastern Europe now living in Canada is making his second visit to the neurosurgeon in the clinic. He has severe spinal stenosis and has come back after his MRI. The neurosurgeon tells him that he requires a lumbar decompression and offers to do it in a month. The patient shakes the neurosurgeon's hand vigorously, smiles widely, and says: "Thank you so much doctor, this is wonderful. If you can do it sooner that would be even better." As he leaves he forces an envelope into the neurosurgeon's hand. At the end of the day, he takes the envelope out of his lab coat pocket and opens it to find ten crisp $100.00 bills.

3.14   Approach to the Case

In Western culture, gifts above and beyond bottles of wine and the like are frowned upon and make surgeons, particularly those who are reimbursed by government or insurance companies, very uncomfortable. It is seen as representing a conflicting force which could alter the care given to the patient, which would be inherently unfair or unjust to other patients. Most doctors would wish to decline a too-generous gift but if they do so, they certainly insult the patient, in whose home culture this would be perfectly acceptable and possibly even expected. In the final analysis, it may be preferable for all doctors to just accept gifts with gratitude but make sure they do not act as a conflict of interest and give the patient special status (Bernstein and Upshur 2008).

3.15 Illustrative Case (Consent for Research)

A North American group of researchers is performing a study on the views and perceptions of patients being seen in a neurosurgery clinic in sub-Saharan Africa and being recommended an operation. The interview is conducted in the native dialect spoken in the city and translated into English by local neurosurgery residents for thematic analysis. Patients are adult males and females. Many of the patients come from rural areas and they need to ask the elders in their village for permission to answer the researchers' questions and to consent for the surgery.

3.16 Approach to the Case

Informed consent is the foundation of what physicians do, especially surgeons. How can we possibly cut into peoples' bodies, especially their brains without them understanding what we hope to achieve, how their symptoms will be helped, what complications might forever alter their quality of life, and other essential information. Consent for research is even more complex, and there have been many examples of less than perfect consent being obtained for research studies (Newman et al. 2011). It may be a generalization but informed consent in resource-rich settings is likely to be more rigorous and accountable than that in resource-poor settings (Kiguba et al. 2012; Knifed et al. 2008). Cultural differences and differing levels of sophistication in some societies may render these populations more vulnerable and contribute to suboptimal informed consent, and these differences must not be exploited (Newman et al. 2011; Simonds and Christopher 2013). Informed consent for research is an area in which cultural difference should arguably not be embraced and accepted but should be fought and rectified.

3.17 Illustrative Case (Access to Care)

A patient in the US undergoes surgery for a 4 cm convexity meningioma. Similar patients are treated the same week in Canada, Germany, Saudi Arabia, Ghana, Norway, and Brazil. All the operations go well and the patients are discharged 3, 1, 5, 7, 13, 6, and 6 days postoperatively, respectively. The patient's personal hospital bills are $32,000.00, $0.00, $23,000.00, $0.00, $278.00, $0.00, and $21,000.00, respectively.

3.18   Approach to the Case

Citizens in only a few countries like Scandinavians countries, Canada, Saudi Arabia, the UK, and a few other countries have essentially free access to every kind of health care, except elective nonessential surgery like cosmetic surgery. The evolution of these societies to embrace "socialized" medicine depends on politics, affluence, and other historical factors. In some of these countries, the burden of free health care means longer waiting periods for elective surgery than in nonsocialized systems. In other countries, the health insurance system is a selective system, the standard of care provided being linked to the ability to pay, i.e., a two-tiered system. This two-tiered system is cultural, being reinforced by a common belief that people deserve what they can pay for. These people would argue that if you fail to work, or are in a poorly paid job, then you should receive a lower standard of medical care. In most developing world countries, the free governmental health care system and public health insurance is inefficient. In order to receive standard and efficient health care, patients generally have to attend a private hospital or clinic. Several factors influence this global discrepancy in health care systems such as economy, social standards, level of education, availability of modern, well-equipped facilities staffed by well-trained medical and paramedical staff, and other factors. Neurosurgery is an expensive specialty of medicine making it less accessible in countries with poor economies. These cultural inequities will not be resolved quickly – it will take a lot of time and changes in leadership and governmental priorities and increasing engagement by nongovernmental organizations and individual groups (Howe et al. 2013).

There thus exists an ethical dilemma between the patient's right to receive the best possible medical care and the availability of such care and the expensive cost of the health care services. Not every country can provide the necessary budget for free, modern, and efficient health care systems. However, every patient, anywhere in the world should be entitled to the best available care. These inequities in care represent another example of cultural/societal differences which should not be embraced but should be fought.

> **Pearl**
> The patient's right to receive good and timely health care is a fundamental human right or should be considered as such. Justice suggests that all the health care resources should be equally distributed. Developing and maintaining a professional and modern health care system is expensive and outside the reach of some governments. Governments, the private sector, nongovernmental organizations, and individuals should cooperate to help find solutions to this problem.

3.19   Illustrative Case (Blood Transfusion in a Jehovah's Witnesses)

A 38-year-old woman presents with a subacute history over months of a weak right leg, and MRI shows a huge bilateral parasagittal meningioma. Surgery is required. She declares that she is a Jehovah's Witness and refuses blood transfusion. She requests surgery and accepts the prospect of death if uncontrollable blood loss occurs.

3.20   Approach to the Case

Most neurosurgeons have encountered such a case and they are taxing. Of course the right and autonomy of a consenting adult to refuse a treatment that people of most other cultures or religions would gladly accept is inviolable. Most surgeons may not understand or agree with such a decision, but they must respect it and, above all, honor the patient's wish. If they do not, it is a form of assault, they will be sued, and they will lose the suit. Interestingly, studies of such patients undergoing neurosurgical operations have generally revealed positive results (Suess et al. 2001). Certain proactive measures can be taken to reduce blood loss such as even more meticulous than usual attention to hemostasis and infiltration of the incision site with local anesthetic with epinephrine. The surgeon may also have to be mentally prepared to leave more tumor behind and/or convert the tumor removal into a two-stage operation.

3.21   Illustrative Case (Help with Dying)

A 69-year-old man with a biopsy-proven malignant glioma of the brain stem is progressively losing function, especially lower cranial nerves, in spite of treatment with radiation, temozolomide, and ventriculoperitoneal shunt (Fig. 3.1). He asks his health care providers to help him end his life with dignity before he can no longer control his main bodily functions.

3.22   Approach to the Case

The fifteenth century Latin text *Ars Moriendi* provided guidance to achieve a good death. The response to our patient's request is subject to geographically where he is located. A minority of countries/states allow assisted suicide particularly in Europe and the USA (Lavery et al. 1997; Steck et al. 2013), and many others are attempting to do likewise (Quebec to proceed with "dying with dignity" legislation 2013). In these jurisdictions patients, and specifically those with malignant brain tumors, appear to be open to discussing the legalization of assisted suicide (Lipsman et al. 2007). In other cultures such as the devoutly Muslim countries, assisted suicide is not possible, nor is even the conversation about it. It is clear that culture and geography play a large role in the legality and/or moral acceptability of assisted suicide.

Fig. 3.1 Axial T1 gadolinium-enhanced MRI of 69-year-old man (a physician) with progressive upper brain stem glioblastoma who requested help with assisted suicide. His request was denied as he lived in a jurisdiction where it is illegal

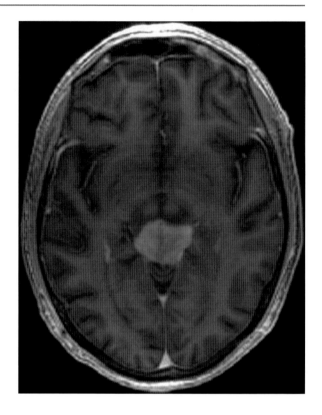

Conclusion

There is clearly ethical relativism in that what is considered morally acceptable or desirable in one culture/country/religion may be ethical unacceptable or undesirable in another. The above examples are by no means exhaustive but give a glimpse of how neurosurgeons all over the world may confront situations which are foreign to their way of thinking and to which they must strive to be as flexible and sensitive as possible. Examining multiple patients in one physical space would be unthinkable in the developed world but is morally acceptable in the parts of the developing world. While it would be morally unacceptable for a surgeon not to transfuse an average patient with excessive blood loss, it would be wrong and even illegal for him/her to transfuse a patient who is Jehovah's Witness against their expressed wishes. No matter how difficult to comprehend some situations may be, we must remember that at the center is an ill human being and a suffering family.

Ethical relativism can be defined as the theory which claims that because different societies have different ethical beliefs, there is no rational way of determining whether an action is morally right or wrong other than by asking whether the people of that society believe it is right or wrong (Bowman and Hui 2000; Coward and Sidhu 2000; Daar and al Khatamy 2001; Ellerby et al. 2000; Goldsand et al. 2001; Markwell and Brown 2001; Pauls and Hutchinson 2002).

Ethical relativism posits that there are no ethical standards that are absolutely true and that apply to people of all societies. Instead, relativism holds, something is right for the people in one particular society if it accords with their moral standards and wrong for them if it violates their moral standards.

Given that we live in and are surrounded by many different cultures and the distances between countries and places have diminished by the revolution in immigration, communication, and information, every effort should be made to understand and accept others. Diversity is reality and an inevitability and is to be celebrated, and hospitals present a good example of such a multicultural community, in which everyone comes together to all work for one goal – the best interest of the patient.

References

Ammar A (1997) Influence of different culture on neurosurgical practice. Childs Nerv Syst 13:91–94

Bernstein M (2007) Magic touch. Handling patients in a touchy age. Parkhurst Exch 15:22–23

Bernstein M, Upshur R (2008) Beware patients bearing gifts. Parkhurst Exch 16:72–73

Bowman KW, Hui EC (2000) Bioethics for clinicians: 20. Chinese bioethics. CMAJ 163(11):1481–1485

Coward H, Sidhu T (2000) Bioethics for clinicians: 19. Hinduism and Sikhism. CMAJ 163(9):1167–1170

Daar AS, al Khitamy AB (2001) Bioethics for clinicians: 21. Islamic bioethics. CMAJ 164(1):60–63

Donovan R, Williams A, Stajduhar K et al (2011) The influence of culture on home-based family caregiving at end-of-life: a case study of Dutch reformed family care givers in Ontario. Can Soc Sci Med 72(3):338–346

Ellerby JH, McKenzie J, McKay S et al (2000) Bioethics for clinicians: 18. Aboriginal cultures. CMAJ 163(7):845–850

Fadiman A (1997) The spirit catches you and you fall down. Farrar, Straus and Giroux, New York

Goldsand G, Rosenberg ZR, Gordon M (2001) Bioethics for clinicians: 22. Jewish bioethics. CMAJ 164(2):219–222

Hamdy S (2013) Not quite dead: why Egyptian doctors refuse the diagnosis of death by neurological criteria. Theor Med Bioeth 34:147–160

Howe KL, Zhou G, July J et al (2013) Teaching awake craniotomy in resource-poor settings and implementing it sustainably. World Neurosurg 80:171–174

Jena AB, Seabury S, Lakdawalla D et al (2011) Malpractice risk according to physician specialty. N Engl J Med 365:629–636

Kiguba R, Kutyabami P, Kiwuwa S et al (2012) Assessing the quality of informed consent in a resource-limited setting: a cross-sectional study. BMC Med Ethics 13:21

Knifed E, Lipsman N, Mason W et al (2008) Patients' perception of the informed consent process for neuro-oncology trials. Neuro-Oncology 10:348–354

Kopelman LM (2013) Make her a virgin again: when medical disputes about minors are cultural clashes. J Med Philos 39(1):8–25

Lavery JV, Dickens BM, Boyle JM et al (1997) Bioethics for clinicians: 11. Euthanasia and assisted suicide. CMAJ 156:1405–1408

Lipsman N, Skanda A, Kimmelman J et al (2007) The attitudes of brain cancer patients and their caregivers towards death and dying: a qualitative study. BMC Palliat Care 6:7

Markwell HJ, Brown BF (2001) Bioethics for clinicians: 27. Catholic bioethics. CMAJ 165(2):189–192

McDonald P (2006) There's a bug in your head. Hastings center report. p 7

Newman PA, Logie C, James L et al (2011) "Speaking the dialect": understanding public discourse in the aftermath of an HIV vaccine trial shutdown. Am J Public Health 101(9):1749–1758

Oliver M, Ahmed A, Woywodt A (2012) Donating in good faith or getting into trouble. Religion and organ donation revisited. World J Transplant 2(5):69–73

Pauls M, Hutchinson RC (2002) Bioethics for clinicians: 28. Protestant bioethics. CMAJ 166(3):339–343

Pitta DA, Fung H, Isberg S (1999) Ethical issues across cultures: managing the differing perspectives of China and the USA. J Consum Mark 16:240–256

Quebec to proceed with "dying with dignity" legislation (2013). http://www.cbc.ca/news/canada/montreal/quebec-to-proceed-with-dying-with-dignity-legislation-1.1307518

Simonds VW, Christopher S (2013) Adapting Western research methods to indigenous ways of knowing. Am J Public Health 103:185–192

Steck N, Egger M, Maessen M et al (2013) Euthanasia and assisted suicide in selected European countries and US states: systematic literature review. Med Care 51(10):938–944

Stonington SD (2013) The debt of life – Thai lessons on a process-oriented ethical logic. N Engl J Med 369:1583–1585

Suess S, Suess O, Brock M (2001) Neurosurgical procedures in Jehovah's Witnesses: an increased risk? Neurosurgery 49(2):266–272

Wong DB (1986) Moral relativity. University of California Press, Berkeley, p 248

Part II

Patients' Rights

Patients' Rights

4

Ahmed Ammar and Geert Seynaeve

4.1   Introduction

In the last few decades, evidence-based medicine has become the main basis of modern medical practice. But medical practice is also based on values and ethics, and value-based medicine should be as prominent as evidence-based medicine. There is no doubt that the observation of patient's rights is the cornerstone of modern medical practice and that most clinicians agree on what those rights are. However, in daily practice, there may be cases which pose a dilemma in medical ethics. Several international and national organizations, such as AANS (AANS Board of Directors. AANS Code of Ethics 2007), AMA (AMA Code of Ethics 2006), and WFNS and EANS (World Federation of Neurosurgical Societies 2007; European Association of Neurological Societies 2000), have issued special documents to recognize patients' rights. The patient has the right to receive the best possible and available treatment; know the details and natural history of the disease; know the different methods and options for treatment and the anticipated outcome of each; confidentiality, the right to be respected, and the right of preservation of dignity; know who is going to operate on him/her; choose, or at least to agree upon, the treating team and the surgeon; choose the method of treatment; refuse treatment; and others (Fig. 4.1).

A dilemma arises if the strict observation of one of the patient's rights, such as the right to choose the method of treatment or to refuse a procedure, is not honored, as this may hinder or prevent the provision of the best care for the patient. Providing

A. Ammar, MBChB, DMSc, FICS, FACS, FAANS (✉)
Department of Neurosurgery, King Fahd University Hospital, Dammam University,
40121, Al Khobar, 31952, Saudi Arabia
e-mail: ahmed@ahmedammar.com

G. Seynaeve, MD, MPH, MMPhR
Department of Occupational Health and Safety, Free University Brussels, Brussels, Belgium
e-mail: geert.seynaeve@attentia-cbmt.be

A. Ammar, M. Bernstein (eds.), *Neurosurgical Ethics in Practice: Value-based Medicine*,
DOI 10.1007/978-3-642-54980-9_4, © Springer-Verlag Berlin Heidelberg 2014

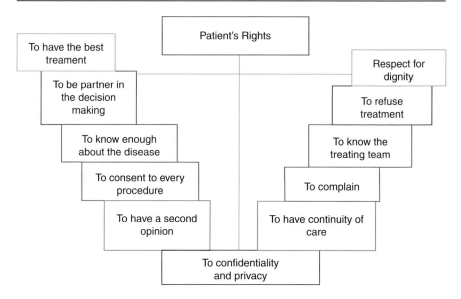

Fig. 4.1 The most important patients' rights

the best possible medical care for patients is not only the main task of every medical care provider but is also the essence and meaning of medical practice. Therefore, most practitioners believe that the most important right the patient may have is to receive the best possible medical treatment.

4.2   Illustrative Case (Patient's Right to Receive Bad News)

A 25 year-old male law student was admitted for biopsy of a tumor in the dominant thalamus. The biopsy showed glioblastoma multiforme. The treating consultant and resident informed the patient clearly about the nature of his disease and the prognosis of a likely unfavorable outcome. He was informed in detail about the planned course of treatment which included transfer to the oncology center for further management. A few hours later, the patient attempted to commit suicide.

4.3   Approach to the Case

It is ethically correct that the treating neurosurgeon informed the patient about the nature of the disease, the expected outcome, and the management plan. The treating teams are obliged as well to answer any question the patient and his/her family may have. However, the serious outcome of that case may raise a question about the skills of delivering the bad news to the patient. Patients have the right to have information delivered honestly but also with compassion and as much optimism as is honestly doable. Delivering bad news should be well planned according to clear understanding of the patient's psychology and expected reaction to such news. Sometimes it is advisable to ask close relatives to participate and be there during the delivery of bad news, although special precautions should be taken not to breach the patient's confidentiality and privacy. The neurosurgeon should also choose the best time for the patient and the place to deliver any serious knows. Enough time should be given for the patient and the family to ask and receive honest and clear answers. The culture and faith of the patient may play an important role in altering the response of the patient (Ammar 1997; Bahus et al. 2012; Guven and Sert 2010; Jotkowitz and Glick 2009).

4.4   Discussion

4.4.1   Patients' General Rights

There is not, and should not be, any conflict between patient's rights and the treating neurosurgeons' interests (Johnson and Johnson 2007). Patient's rights may be taken for granted. Most professional medical societies like WFNS and EANS have documents on patient's rights. In daily practice, many doctors, neurosurgeons, nurses, and patients may think that they know enough about patients' rights; however, a deeper knowledge of bioethics and ethical implications and concepts is not very clear to many neurosurgeons and patients. Therefore, from time to time, ethical questions and dilemmas may arise. The ethical code of the American Medical Association (AMA Code of Ethics 2006) summarizes the patient's rights as the following: "The right to receive information from physicians and to discuss the benefits, risks, and costs of appropriate treatment alternatives; the right to make decisions regarding the health care that is recommended by the physician; the right to courtesy, respect, dignity, responsiveness, and timely attention to health needs; the right to confidentiality; the right to continuity of health care and the basic right to have adequate health care."

The AMA code (AMA Code of Ethics 2006) as other ethical codes puts in practice the main ethical principles of patients' rights as the following: (a) autonomy, the patient has the right to refuse or choose his/her treatment (voluntas aegroti suprema lex); (b) beneficence, a practitioner should act in the best interest of the patient (salus aegroti suprema lex); (c) non-maleficence, "first, do no harm" (primum non nocere); (d) justice, concerns the distribution of scarce health resources and the decision of who gets what treatment (fairness and equality); (e) dignity, the patient and the person treating the patient have the right to be treated with dignity; and (f) truthfulness and honesty.

4.4.1.1 Right to the Best Treatment Available

Patients have the right to receive the best possible medical treatment. There are several levels of medical treatment which include:

(a) Access to proper and efficient medical facilities such as outpatient clinics and hospitals
(b) Opportunity to be admitted and adequately treated in the emergency ward in case of an emergency (in the unfortunate situation of a system in which the patient has to pay for health care privately, at minimum emergency, care must be a sacred right and guaranteed)
(c) Access to the best possible standard of care including surgery
(d) Access to adequate follow-up after discharge from the hospital

An uncommon but not rare difficult situation arises when a patient asks for inappropriate treatment (e.g., Gamma Knife radiosurgery for 74 metastases, spinal cord transplant, and surgery for a dominant thalamic hemorrhage in a 91 year-old with GCS 4). The surgeon must calmly and simply explain to the best of his/her ability why this request cannot be met, based on evidence, risk-benefit analysis, and/or availability of special resources (Weijer et al. 1998).

4.4.1.2 Right to Be Told the Truth

Every patient has the absolute right to receive honest and clear facts about his/her problem (Hebert et al. 1997). It is easy for neurosurgeons to be a bit "unclear" on some negative details, when they talk to patients; this is usually done to preserve the patient's feelings and sense of hope and sometimes to spare the neurosurgeon extra grief. But qualitative research studies have clearly documented that patients want the truth (Yu and Bernstein 2011). The pain of being told untruths would trump the pain of the truth for most patients although cultural differences may be at play in some cases.

4.4.1.3 Right to Know Enough About the Medical Problem

The treating physician or neurosurgeon should tell the patient all the available facts about the patient's medical problem that a reasonable person would want to know such as diagnosis, causes, different methods of treatment, the natural history with no treatment, complications, and expected outcome of each treatment options. Not every detail can or need be told, but certainly whatever the individual patient requests to know. This information should be given to the patient in simple understandable language avoiding complicated medical terms so the patient can understand, as best as possible and can digest the information. Mistakes and errors, which sometimes occur during the course of treatment, should be discussed in detail with the patient in honest and understandable language.

> **Pearl**
> Patient's rights must be preserved and respected, without exception. The patient has to be ethically and clearly educated about the medical problem in understandable language.

4.4.1.4 Right to Participate in Making the Decision About Treatment

To ensure the success of any treatment plan, the patient should be included as an important partner in making the decision. The patient has the right to choose, agree upon, and decide about every step of treatment along the course of the disease. In order to prepare the patient for making such decisions and be a true partner in fighting the patient's disease:

(a) The patient should receive all information about his/her medical problem.
(b) The patient should know the different options and alternatives for the suggested treatment.
(c) The patient should know the outcome of every method of treatment.
(d) The patient should have time to think about and discuss with his/her close relatives or friends about the medical conditions and management plan.
(e) The patient should know the quality of service in the hospital and the qualifications and experience of the treating team (if he/she asks).

> **Pearl**
> The patient should be considered as a partner in the treatment plan and be heavily involved in the decision-making process. If he/she waives that right, it should be respected and well documented.

4.4.1.5 Right to Consent to Every Procedure

The patient or the patient's decision-makers should consent to every procedure during the course of the treatment. With procedures with any risk, the patient should sign an informed consent form (e.g., surgery, radiation treatment). Verbal consent is generally adequate for less-invasive procedures such as venipuncture for blood tests or intravenous administration of fluids and insertion of urinary catheter.

4.4.1.6 Right to Confidentiality and Privacy

Confidentiality and privacy of all patients should be strictly respected. Every patient has the right to this unless he/she waives this right. The opportunities for potential abuse of these rights are rampant in the everyday life of a hospital in today's complex health-care systems. So, constant vigilance by the health-care team is needed, as well as the patient's self-advocacy to remind everyone to safeguard his/her privacy.

4.4.1.7 Right to Complain

Patients may feel during the course of treatment that the received treatment was not properly indicated, or properly executed, or there have been mistakes or errors in one way or another. The patient and the family should have the right to complain, at one or more of several levels:

(a) The patient may complain to the treating neurosurgeon. The treating consultant should listen and take the complaint very seriously and try to make certain the patient knows he/she has been heard and positively respond to the patient's concerns. If some corrective action is appropriate, the surgeon should try to take action to rectify the cause of complaint and keep the patient up to date on those actions. Many complaints go no further than this.

(b) Patients and their families have the right to complain to the hospital authorities (e.g., the public relations department or to an administrator). The hospital authorities should contact the treating team and discuss the complaints and work to solve any problems. It is advisable to arrange meetings between the treating team and the patient and his/her family to solve any conflict. Such a meeting should be held in a constructive environment of honesty, care, and understanding.

(c) Patients and their families have the right to complain to the surgeon's governing body such as the local College of Surgeons.

(d) The patient may sue any member of the treating team in the courts.

4.4.1.8 Right to Know Who the Treating Team Is

Building up a good professional relationship with patients and their families is very important for successful medical care. Such a relationship should be based on trust and honesty. So patients must know who is treating them and their qualifications and their experiences if asked. In case trainees are involved in part of the treatment under the supervision of senior consultants, patients must know that, although surgeons are generally poor at being explicit about this information (Knifed et al. 2008a, b). The patient should have the right to a second opinion, and the treating surgeon should be prepared to arrange this for the patient if asked to do so.

From time to time in every university surgeon's practice, a patient states a wish to have the consultant surgeon do the operation and not have the residents involved. This request is not compatible with the workings of a teaching hospital, and the patient should be gently explained how things work and that the consultant takes full responsibility to provide an excellent operation. This explanation is honest and is generally sufficient for most patients to proceed.

4.4.1.9 Right to Have One's Dignity Preserved

The patient's dignity is central to ethical medical practice. Preserving the patient's dignity is not only a basic human right but also important to ensure that the patient will follow medical instructions enabling the best outcome of his/her course of management. Besides the obvious large elements contributing to a patient's dignity, there are many small issues which can be very important in making patients feel valued and worthwhile such as not waiting too long in the neurosurgeon's waiting room and receiving an apology if they do wait too long or for other discourtesies.

Patients who feel respected and treated as a valuable human, equal to anybody else, will be able to make good decisions and positively cooperate with the treating team. A common cause for patient dissatisfaction is lack of communication and loss of dignity. While the dictionary definition of dignity is clear, dignity in daily medical practice is rather vague. The perspective of dignity may vary among the patient, neurosurgeon, and nursing staff, and the perspective may also vary according to culture, personality, self-evaluation, and expectation. Therefore, patients' culture, beliefs, and personality should all be taken into consideration. They should be treated with respect regardless of the state of mind or the severity of the neurosurgical condition. In order to secure ethical respect of patient's dignity, certain tools are available (Cheshire Dignity Assessment Tools 2009). At an organizational level, collaboration between clinical ethicists and risk management can lead to respectful patient care (Sine and Sharpe 2011).

Dignity should be spelled out clearly to avoid any ambiguous, vague application or misunderstanding among the hospital staff. Dignity is essentially concerned with how people feel, think, and behave in relation to the worth or value of themselves and others. To treat someone with dignity is to treat them as being of worth and value, in a way that is respectful of them as valued individuals.

4.4.1.10 Right to Have Education About Their Condition

Neurosurgeons around the world treat patients from different cultures and backgrounds and with different perspectives on medical problems and medical care. Culture, religion, health, and literacy levels each have a direct impact on the course of treatment. Patient education is an opportunity to distribute health information equally among diverse cultures and communities as a good example of justice, one of the fundamental ethics principles of medical practice.

Patient education should be a central philosophy of all treating teams. It is not uncommon to see patients who have incorrect information about their medical problems and about how health care functions in their area. Patient education is important and should be contributed by all members of the health-care team (Marks 2009; Redman 2011; Zanchetta and Bernstein 2004) – it is the duty of the treating neurosurgeon, nurses, and hospital administration to provide patients information. Special precautions must be taken to ensure that patient education is ethical. Feeding the patient incomplete facts or providing information on one form of treatment only, particularly when it influences the patient to agree to the procedure of choice of the treating surgeon, is not ethical. Online information is becoming more commonplace for patients (Bramall and Bernstein 2014).

> **Pearl**
> Providing patients with good-quality educational materials and websites is beneficial to them and to the health-care team, as an educated patient is a more satisfied patient who is likely to help navigate his/her medical treatment better than an uneducated one.

4.4.1.11 Right to Not Be Abandoned

Abandonment occurs when a neurosurgeon, without proper notice, unilaterally severs his professional relationship with a patient who is in need of continuing health care. This is rare. Also uncommon is the situation in which the neurosurgeon feels he/she cannot constructively care for the patient, usually because a loss of trust or a personality conflict, in which there is a formal process the neurosurgeon must follow. In this case, it is also the neurosurgeon's responsibility to find another surgeon for the patient (Bernstein and Upshur 2008; White and Wicclair 2012). If patients suffer injury or complications due to abandonment, the treating neurosurgeon should be held responsible.

4.4.1.12 Patients' Responsibility to Ensure Their Rights

Patients can be instrumental to ensuring that their rights are respected and should be active participants in their care, not passive recipients. Patients should ask about their rights and should have an understanding of the diagnosis commensurate with their ability to understand. The patient should understand the nature of his/her disease and know the details of his/her management and speak up whenever they perceive a gap in their understanding or communication with the treating team. Patient awareness and freedom to ask questions are important tools the patient should use to ensure his/her rights and to self-advocate.

4.4.2 Patient's Right to Refuse Treatment

4.4.2.1 Introduction

Refusal of treatment is a right of every patient, but it poses the greatest threat to the right to receive the best possible care. There are several causes for adult patients to refuse treatment or surgery, including the following:

1. The patient does not understand the seriousness of the medical problem or the consequences of refusal of treatment, either due to failure of the surgeon or simplicity of the patient.
2. The patient has had a previous negative experience with a previous surgical procedure.
3. The patient's religious faith trumps medical recommendation, as there are certain groups who refuse blood transfusion, surgical intervention, or even drug therapy.
4. The patient has a psychiatric problem such as severe depression or frontal lobe syndrome or some other psychological problems.
5. The patient has complete lack of trust in the treating team and/or the medical system.
6. The patient has decided to be treated elsewhere.

Refusal of the patient to receive treatment may be of several forms for different reasons (Glod 2010; Pope 2010). The refusal may take the form of absolute refusal to receive any treatment including surgery, or the patient may refuse surgical treatment but accept other forms of treatment, or the patient may simply be resistant to treatment, without absolute refusal.

The neurosurgeon or the treating physician facing such a challenge finds himself/herself in a difficult situation with limited options (Muzaffar 2011). These options include:

1. To accept the patient's will and decision and discharge the patient
2. To try to persuade and convince the patient to accept the treatment or the surgery

3. To approach close family members or friends to ask their help in persuading the patient to accept surgery
4. To delay the decision for surgery and keep the patient in the hospital for a few days to give him/her further opportunity to reconsider the decision and possibly ask other service for help, like the clinical ethics team, or one of the surgeon's partners as an "internally generated second opinion"

4.4.2.2 Illustrative Case (Refusal of Urgent Surgery)

A 52 year-old man was admitted through the emergency room, suffering from paraplegia, severe back pain, and sensory loss, and imaging showed a large mid-thoracic tumor compressing the spinal cord and involving the bodies, transverse processes, and the laminae. Although he had stated emphatically on admission that he did not wish to receive any surgical intervention, it was clear that the patient's condition required it. Family and friends, although convinced of the necessity, also failed to persuade the patient to consent to surgery. The patient remained in the hospital for a few days. As the patient's neurological condition deteriorated, many members of his family shared in further discussion with him and he ultimately agreed to laminectomy and tumor removal and instrumented fusion. Postoperatively, the patient showed immediate signs of improvement. The tumor was a metastatic adenocarcinoma. The patient received adjuvant radiation and made a reasonable recovery and was able to walk, until his death 18 months later.

4.4.2.3 Approach to the Case

It would appear that the patient was unaware of the seriousness of his condition, possibly due to ignorance or simplicity. The participation of the family members was very helpful in order to convince the patient to be operated. This case demonstrates conflict between autonomy (as the patient has the right to refuse treatment), beneficence (as everything should be done in the best interest of the patient), and non-maleficence (as the patient should be protected from harm). Simple patience and understanding on the part of the health-care team and a positive contribution of the family resulted in a satisfactory solution for all parties.

Some ethics scholars would find it difficult to accept the surgeon or treating team's right to doubt a patient's decision or his mental abilities. They would consider that attempting to persuade a patient to change his/her mind about refusing treatment, when he/she is in an already vulnerable state, to be unethical. Many medical practitioners and surgeons however do not agree with this way of thinking as they consider the patient's life and well-being as the highest value that should be considered. Especially utilitarians would say "The end justifies the means."

4.4.2.4 Illustrative Case (Refusal of Blood Transfusion)

A patient was admitted through the ER with his 18 year-old daughter, victims of a car accident. The man was fully conscious with GCS 15, fully oriented, and had no neurological deficit. The daughter was drowsy with a GCS of 9. CT scan showed right parietal depressed fracture over the superior sagittal sinus and epidural hematoma. The patient was scheduled for urgent surgery to evacuate the hematoma and elevate the depressed fracture. Her father was asked to sign the consent form. The father stated that they were Jehovah's witnesses and that blood transfusion is not permitted in their faith. He clarified that the daughter was "a believer" and would have agreed to such terms. The operation was uneventful, and the patient did not require a blood transfusion. She made a full recovery.

4.4.2.5 Approach to the Case

The father was the legal substitute decision-maker for the girl, but if she had been 8 years old, another dimension to this case would be raised – can an adult make a decision on behalf of an incompetent minor which could result in harm (Catlin 1996)? Such cases have been tested in court and generally the child has been ruled to receive a blood transfusion if it is needed. In our case, the treating team honored the patient's (i.e., surrogate's) stipulation that no blood transfusion be given, but fortunately, it was not tested. If the girl was exsanguinating and the surgeon gave a blood transfusion, it is unlikely a court of law would find him/her negligent because of the surrogate consent. But if the father who could give primary consent was undergoing surgery and received a blood transfusion against his will, a court of law would rule against the surgeon.

4.4.2.6 Illustrative Case (Patient's Right to Choose His/Her Surgeon and Decline Another)

A patient was admitted to a public hospital through the ER with a subacute myelopathy. She was admitted by the on-call neurosurgeon and was scheduled for surgery for anterior cervical discectomy. The patient decided that she would prefer a different neurosurgeon. After a discussion attended by both neurosurgeons, the patient was told that she should continue to be seen by the original, admitting consultant. The patient agreed that both neurosurgeons were capable of performing the surgery with the same care and degree of expertise but insisted that she wanted to switch to the second neurosurgeon. She claimed that it was her right to choose which surgeon she preferred. She was refused her request. The next day, the patient was discharged against medical advice.

4.4.2.7 Approach to the Case

Is it an absolute right for any patient to choose his/her surgeon in a public hospital where the treatment is free? Switching to another neurosurgeon could create conflict within the department and would represent a "corruption" of a system which has worked well for the department for thousands of previous patients. When both neurosurgeons are equally capable of carrying out the procedure, is it right to refuse the patient in order to maintain the system and the peaceful atmosphere within the department? There is a delicate balance between answering the patient's wish and respecting the department's policy and intradepartmental relationships. When should the decision be in favor of the patient and when in favor of good relations within the department?

Pearl
According to the principles of autonomy, patients have the right to choose or to refuse suggested methods of medical management. In cases where the patient initially refuses the medical treatment, time has to be spent to explain to the patient the consequences of his/her decision. If the patient's mental state, age, or culture casts doubts on the validity of the patient's decision, the patient's first-degree relatives should be brought into the discussion and should share in the decision, the patient should be given extra time to think about it, and/or additional help should be sought.

4.4.3   Patients' Families' Rights

4.4.3.1   Introduction
The nature of neurosurgical problems forces neurosurgeons to face their patients' families in difficult emotional situations, anxious over the seriousness of the situation, anxious to see a good result, disappointed with a poor outcome, and confused, denying, or angry. Neurosurgeons should learn the skill to absorb the first reaction of the patient's family and work with them as members of the team to help their loved one. The patient's family can also play a very positive part in the care of the patient.

Four widely accepted ethical imperatives (respect for autonomy, beneficence, non-maleficence, and justice) guide medical relationships in the conventional triad of patient, family, and health-care team. The patient has the ultimate authority, based on the ethical imperative of autonomy and the right of self-determination. While the capable and legally competent individual remains the protagonist, ideally, relatives and loved ones should be allowed to meaningfully participate in all aspects of the patient's experience. The expertise of medical and nursing teams should facilitate shared decision-making based on information, comprehension, and voluntariness.

Patients' families have the right to information about the patient's condition, treatment, and prognosis insofar as the patient consents to it. If it is a spouse or an adult child of the patient, consent is usually implied, although the treating team must be vigilant about intrafamilial conflicts, divorce with ex-spouses, recomposed families, and the like. The family members also do not have the inherent right to each speak to the surgeon – they should appoint one or two spokespeople so that the surgeon's time is protected and respected. Nowadays, it is common for the surgeon to receive an e-mail from someone in another distant city identifying himself/herself as a child of the patient and generally neurosurgeons take this on faith and respond, but care must be taken, and if the surgeon agrees to respond, he/she should at minimum inform the patient: "Your son John e-mailed me asking for information and I responded – I hope this was OK."

4.4.3.2 Illustrative Case (Helpful Family)

A 75 year-old lady is the wife of a terminal 75 year-old patient with recurrent glio-blastoma multiforme which left him obtunded and densely hemiplegic. He is on oxygen by mask. She requested the treating team to let her take her husband home, as she knows that he wanted to pass away in his bed. The team was initially concerned about her ability to do this, but agreed, and sat with her to teach her how to take care of her husband and the inevitable course of deterioration and how to deal with each stage. She received as well several phone numbers to reach the treating team at any time and some home-care visits by a palliative nurse were organized. Six weeks later, the wife came to thank the medical staff for giving her the chance to take care of her husband in his last days.

4.4.3.3 Approach to the Case

Families have a major role in end-of-life situations, participating in shared decision-making, as advocates or substitutes for the patient's wishes. When clinical procedures or treatments offer no significant benefit to the patient, they are considered futile. Complex ethical challenges are raised concerning the medical futility of various interventions. The expected quality of life must be considered in view of the balance between burden and perceived benefit for patients and their relatives. This patient's wife's wish was honored and facilitated and resulted in several positive outcomes: (1) honoring the patient's wishes, (2) honoring the wife's wishes and allowing her to make a huge contribution to her dying spouse, and (3) saving precious health-care resources (beds, nursing, and drugs that can be used for another patient).

4.4.3.4 Illustrative Case (Challenging Family)

A young woman who has been multiply treated for brain metastases from melanoma is progressing with several new tumors. There are about 15, including several radiation necrosis lesions from pervious radiosurgery. She is ataxic and mildly cognitively impaired but understands her situation; her mother demands another course of whole-brain radiation, but the treating team feels palliative care should be offered. The patient keeps wagging her head "no" but her mother forcefully and consistently says: "Just give her the radiation." The conversation is conducted through an interpreter as the mother's English is poor.

4.4.3.5 Approach to the Case

The family, in this case, her mother, is demanding treatment for her daughter which is highly unlikely to help and actually more likely to hasten her deterioration, and the latter seems to understand and wishes not to have further treatment. However, she cannot strenuously state her case, while her mother can. The mother's wishes should not trump the patient's autonomy, even though the daughter might be considered technically incompetent to sign her own consent. The principle of non-maleficence is also at stake. The treating radiation oncologist talks to the mother and daughter at length and finally the daughter nods "yes." In fact, the radiation oncologist then engages the patient's medical oncologist who offers an experimental drug which will be easier to handle for the infirm patient than radiation. A referral is also made to palliative care which is acceptable to the mother.

4.4.3.6 Dealing with/Preventing the Problem of Difficult Families

Spontaneously warm relations develop easily when individuals are well-intentioned and good natured. But in clinical relationships, medical staff can be stressed and tired and tend to be dismissive of "minor" complaints. These attitudes do not necessarily mesh with the needs for compassion and empathy of a patient's family members. When family clashes with the neurosurgeon, an attempt at rectifying the situation should be made and the family must be gently and kindly reminded that it is the patient that is paramount, and the family secondary. If a family member is obviously disruptive especially if he/she is upsetting to the patient, they must be forcefully told that they are exceeding their rights. The commonest source of major disagreement between family and neurosurgeon relates to unrealistic expectations such as not allowing withdrawal of care after the patient has been declared brain dead and requesting heroic treatment on a family member who is beyond help.

Although it may require specific attention and efforts of health-care workers, taking the needs and rights of patients' families into account is quite feasible. In this way, they can be constructive helpers of their loved one's medical experience, which will not only help the patient but will help the involved family members to feel useful and valued. Involving loved ones in various aspects of medical care, in particular, taking into account the concerns and interests of relevant others in medical decision-making, could be a policy, not dependent on solely the good will of the leading physicians. Centralizing input from patients and their relatives, proactively reaching out to patients' families, presenting ethical dilemmas and interests involved, discussing the various decision options and their implications, allowing contradictions and real debate, and justifying interventions in a transparent and understandable way can be better achieved when it is formalized with the participation of the entire surgical and nursing team.

> **Pearl**
> The patient's family has the right to know the details about the nature of the medical problem and the options of treatment and should participate in the medical decisions, if the patient consents to this. They should help the patient and the health-care team in any way they can.

4.4.3.7 The Family's Duties

Families must interact positively and constructively with the health-care team and advocate for the patient. They must treat the surgeon and others with respect and courtesy. They may be called upon to help a patient come to a good medical decision as described above. They may of course be called upon to be a surrogate decision-maker in the case of an incapable patient – many families may not welcome this difficult task, but they must at least be asked. They may also be asked to help with discharge planning like helping facilitate the return of the patient to his/her home or to that of a family member. Family members may also be called upon to help defray the financial costs of a patient's care, in a private health-care system.

Conclusion

Respecting patients' right is at the center of value-based medicine. The patient has the right to receive the best possible and available treatment; know the details and natural history of the disease; know the different methods and options for treatment and the anticipated outcome of each; confidentiality, the right to be respected and the right of preservation of dignity; know who is going to operate on him/her; choose, or at least to agree upon, the treating team and the surgeon; choose the method of treatment; refuse treatment; and others. Patients also have a duty to themselves to advocate on behalf of their own rights. Similarly, families have rights and duties, all of which should be focused toward the best interests of the patient.

References

AANS Board of Directors. AANS Code of Ethics (2007) Available at: http://www.aans.org/en/About%20AANS/~/media/4A6862BB037742FF99B833D609D23B1E.ashx

AMA Code of Ethics (2006) Editorially revised 2006. Available at: https://ama.com.au/codeofethics

Ammar A (1997) Influence of different cultures on neurosurgical practice. Childs Nerv Syst 13:91–94

Bahus MK, Steen PA, Førde R (2012) Law, ethics and clinical judgment in end-of-life decisions-how do Norwegian doctors think? Resuscitation 83(11):1369–1373

Bernstein M, Upshur REG (2008) The challenge of difficult patients. Parkhurst Exch 16:74–75

Bramall A, Bernstein M (2014) Improving information provision for neurosurgical patients: a qualitative study. Can J Neurol Sci 41(1):66–73

Catlin A (1996) The dilemma of Jehovah's Witness children who need blood to survive. HEC Forum 8(4):195–207

Diekema DS (2011) Adolescent refusal of lifesaving treatment: are we asking the right questions? Adolesc Med State Art Rev 22(2):213–228

World Federation of Neurological Societies, European Association of Neurological Societies (2000) Good practice: a guide for neurosurgeons. Br J Neurosurg 14:400–406

Glod W (2010) Conditional preferences and refusal of treatment. HEC Forum 22(4):299–309

Guven T, Sert G (2010) Advance directives in Turkey's cultural context: examining the potential benefits for the implementation of patient rights. Bioethics 24(3):127–133

Hebert PC, Hoffmaster B, Glass KC et al (1997) Bioethics for clinicians: 8. Confidentiality. CMAJ 158:521–524

Johnson AG, Johnson PRV (2007) Making sense of medical ethics. Oxford University Press, New York, pp 111–123

Jotkowitz AB, Glick S (2009) The Israeli terminally ill patient law of 2005. J Palliat Care 25:284–288

Knifed E, July J, Bernstein M (2008a) Neurosurgery patients' feelings about the role of residents in their care: a qualitative case study. J Neurosurg 108:287–291

Knifed E, Taylor B, Bernstein M (2008b) What surgeons tell their patients about the intra-operative role of residents: a qualitative study. Am J Surg 196:788–794

Marks R (2009) Ethics and patient education: health literacy and cultural dilemmas. Health Promot Pract 10(3):328–332

Muzaffar (2011) 'To treat or not to treat'. Kerrie Wooltorton, lessons to learn. Emerg Med J 28(9):741–744

Panico ML, Jenq GY, Brewster UC (2011) When a patient refuses life-saving care: issues raised when treating a Jehovah's Witness. Am J Kidney Dis 58(4):647–653

Pope TM (2010) Legal briefing: conscience clauses and conscientious refusal. J Clin Ethics 21(2):163–176

Redman B (2011) Ethics of patient education and how make it everyone's ethics. Nurs Clin N Am 46(3):283–289

Sine DM, Sharpe VA (2011) Ethics, risk, and patient-centered care: how collaboration between clinical ethicists and risk management leads to respectful patient care. J Healthc Risk Manag 31(1):32–37

Spike JP (2012) Care versus treatment at the end of life for profoundly disabled persons. J Clin Ethics 23(1):79–83

Cheshire Dignity Assessment Tool (2009) Available at: http://www.dignityincare.org.uk/_library/Resources/Dignity/CSIPComment/Cheshire_Dignity_Assessment_Tool_2.pdf

Weijer C, Singer PA, Dickens BM et al (1998) Bioethics for clinicians: 16. Dealing with demands for inappropriate treatment. CMAJ 159:960–965

White DB, Wicclair M (2012) Limits on clinicians' discretion to unilaterally refuse treatment. Am J Crit Care 21(5):361–364

World Federation of Neurosurgical Societies. Statement of ethics in neurosurgery (2007) Available at: http://www.wfns.org/filebin/WFNS%20Statement%20of%20Ethics%20in%20NS%20Mar%202008.pdf

Yu JJ, Bernstein M (2011) Brain tumor patients' views on deception: a qualitative study. J Neurooncol 104:331–337

Zanchetta C, Bernstein M (2004) The nursing role in patient education regarding outpatient neurosurgical procedures. Axone 25:18–21

Informed Consent

5

Patrick McDonald

5.1 Introduction

The requirement to obtain informed consent before a therapeutic intervention or participation in research is a relatively new phenomenon and is part of a more general shift over the last century from physician-centered care to patient-centered care. Consent is at the very center of value-based medicine. The modern concept of consent came about largely in response to atrocities committed by Nazi physicians in the Second World War and is articulated in the Nuremberg Code. Although initially designed to address medical research, the aspects of the Code that speak to consent apply equally to therapeutic interventions. The consent must be voluntary, the patient must have capacity, there must be sufficient knowledge and comprehension, and the decision to consent must be free from coercion and potential hazards are outlined (Annas and Grodin 1992; Etchells et al. 1996a, b and c).

Informed consent can be given for an intervention if and perhaps only if one is competent to act, receives a thorough disclosure, comprehends the disclosure, acts voluntarily, and consents to the intervention. Thus, five elements in the process of informed consent are required: (1) competence, (2) disclosure, (3) understanding, (4) voluntariness, and (5) authorization. To this, we would add the importance of appropriate documentation of the consent process (Etchells et al. 1996a, b and c). Although not an ethical requirement, most legal jurisdictions require such documentation in a contemporaneous note.

The bioethical foundation of informed consent is the principle of respect for autonomy. Autonomy, in relation to the health-care setting, allows persons to make decisions regarding their care "without controlling interference from others and

P. McDonald, MD, MHSc, FRCSC
Section of Neurosurgery, Department of Surgery, Manitoba Institute of Child Health,
Winnipeg Children's Hospital, University of Manitoba, GB-138, 820 Sherbrook Street,
R3A 1R9 Winnipeg, MB, Canada
e-mail: pmcdonald@hsc.mb.ca

A. Ammar, M. Bernstein (eds.), *Neurosurgical Ethics in Practice: Value-based Medicine*,
DOI 10.1007/978-3-642-54980-9_5, © Springer-Verlag Berlin Heidelberg 2014

from limitations, such as inadequate understanding, that prevent meaningful choice." The ability to make an autonomous decision requires both liberty (independence from controlling influences) and agency (capacity for intentional action).

Obtaining informed consent from neurosurgical patients can pose particular challenges. Diseases of the brain are far more likely to alter a patient's capacity or competence thus their ability to provide consent. The stakes are higher in neurosurgery, with the risk of permanent significant morbidity or death higher than in other illnesses. "Neurosurgical manipulations of the CNS usually have some irreversibility and always at least run a significant risk of irreversibility" (Ford 2009). Many patients and families still perceive the brain to be a mysterious almost mystical organ that is poorly understood. By their very nature, neurosurgical patients may be considered a vulnerable population (Ford 2009).

This chapter deals primarily with the ethical issues involved with informed consent, but informed consent also has legal implications and definitions that may vary depending on jurisdiction. The legal standard must be considered specifically in the jurisdiction an individual neurosurgeon practices, especially as it relates to standards of disclosure and statutory ages of consent for young adults.

> **Pearl**
> The ethical basis for informed consent is respect for autonomy. Informed consent requires competence, disclosure, understanding, voluntariness, and authorization.

5.2 Illustrative Case (Family Requests to Withhold Information from a Patient)

A 68-year-old male widower is admitted to the neurosurgical service with a right frontal enhancing mass, consistent with a glioblastoma multiforme. His imaging shows a significant amount of edema and midline shift. He is intermittently confused and drowsy with headache and a left hemiparesis. His family arrives for a discussion regarding management options and surgery is proposed. When you tell them that the mass is likely malignant, they ask you not to tell their father this.

5.3 Approach to the Case

This case poses a number of challenges to the usual consent process. First, the patient's capacity to make autonomous decisions is in question because of the effects of his tumor. A determination must be made as to whether the patient has capacity and if not, whether he will regain capacity with therapy such as dexamethasone to reduce peritumoral edema and ultimately be able to participate in the consent process. A number of tools are available to assess capacity in a patient with cognitive impairment (Appelbaum and Grisso 1988; Marson et al. 1995) and will be detailed further in the chapter.

If the patient is incapable of decision-making independently, then a surrogate decision maker, in this case, a member of the family, is asked to make a decision for the patient, and not necessarily what they themselves would do, but what they think, knowing the patient, they would request to have done if they had the capacity. Second, the family has asked that information be withheld from the patient. In a patient with competence or capacity, the withholding of information does not allow the patient to make an informed decision. Disclosure cannot occur, and as such, consent would be ethically and legally invalid. Certain cultural preferences or norms may allow for limits to disclosure. Where a patient lacks capacity, it may also be reasonable to withhold certain information.

The elements required in the informed consent for patients are considered a right for patients but not necessarily a duty, that is, physicians are obligated to disclose information regarding risks and benefits, but a patient may indicate that they do not wish to have this information. Surgeons should take extra caution to ensure it is truly what the patient wants when the right to consent is waived, and this situation should be well documented.

5.4   Discussion

5.4.1   Elements of Informed Consent

5.4.1.1 Capacity

At present, there are no universally accepted guidelines on assessment or definition of capacity (Etchells et al. 1996c; Johnson-Greene 2010) and no instruments specific to neurosurgery. The definition of competence and determinations of competence are legal decisions, whereas a determination of capacity is one made regularly by physicians. A lack of capacity can be permanent or temporary. Neurosurgeons commonly encounter patients whose capacity to consent to therapy is in question because of their underlying condition, be it a traumatic brain injury, malignancy, hydrocephalus, or infection. A person with the capacity to consent to therapy has the ability to (1) communicate choices, (2) understand relevant information, (3) appreciate the situation they are in and its consequences, and (4) reach rational conclusions (Appelbaum and Grisso 1988). A specific instrument to assess capacity has been developed, and although validated for patients with Alzheimer's disease, it has been widely used in the traumatic brain injury population and could be used in other neurosurgical patients where capacity is in question (Johnson-Greene 2010; Marson et al. 1995). In this instrument, patients are presented with a clinical vignette that either they read or is read to them, and then they are asked a series of questions regarding the scenario. The instrument tests the ability to make a reasonable treatment choice, appreciate the consequences of that choice, provide reasons for the choice, and understand the clinical situation.

When a patient does not have the capacity to consent to treatment and no previously made directives, written or otherwise, exist, decisions are left to a surrogate. Usually a spouse, partner, or close family member is asked to serve as a surrogate and make a decision that, given their knowledge of the patient, they believe the patient would make if they were to regain capacity.

Pearl
Capacity or competence requires the ability to communicate choices, understand relevant information, appreciate the consequences of action or inaction, and make rational decisions.

5.4.1.2 Disclosure of Information
The standard required for disclosure of relevant information to patients, both in the therapeutic and research setting, has evolved over time (Bock 2008; Etchells et al. 1996a; Samuels 2003). The "professional practice" standard, sometimes known as the "reasonable doctor" standard, requires disclosure of information that most other physicians would provide in a similar situation. This standard has been largely replaced or augmented by the "reasonable person" standard – the physician must disclose all information that a hypothetical "reasonable person" would want to know under the circumstances. Unfortunately, what constitutes a "reasonable" person has never been well defined and is dependent on cultural, religious, and other factors. As a minimum, the following information should be provided to the patient or their surrogate decision maker: (1) the diagnosis or likely diagnosis, (2) the proposed intervention or options for intervention, (3) the risks and benefits of the proposed treatment and risks and benefits of not undergoing treatment, and (4) reasonable alternatives to the proposed treatment and the risks and benefits of the alternatives.

There is good evidence that patient retention of disclosed information is poor. In a study of neurosurgical patients' recall of a perioperative discussion, an average of only 4 of 32 risks for cranial surgery and 25 for spinal neurosurgery was remembered. Sixty-five percent of patients could recall only two of six major risks (Krupp et al. 2000). Similarly, a qualitative study of the informed consent process in neuro-oncology clinical trials demonstrated that recall of risks by participants was low (Knifed et al. 2008).

Although recall of disclosed information can be poor, it remains important to explain and ensure patients understand the risks, benefits, and alternatives to surgical intervention. A study of patients with high-grade gliomas demonstrated lower anxiety levels in patients who had a higher degree of comprehension of the information presented and those who showed a desire to receive information regarding their illness (Diaz et al. 2009). Some have argued that full disclosure for a surgical procedure is an unrealistic and unattainable expectation in either the clinical or research context (Bernstein 2005; Schmitz and Reinacher 2006) given the number of potential complications of a procedure, both foreseen and unanticipated.

> **Pearl**
> Patients' recollection of risks of surgical procedures is consistently low. Neurosurgeons should be mindful of this and make extra efforts to make sure the patient understands the important risks.

5.4.1.3 Understanding

As illustrated above, patient retention of disclosed information in the informed consent process is often poor, in both the clinical and research context (Knifed et al. 2007; Krupp et al. 2000). Understanding or comprehension is related to many factors, including age, educational level, intelligence, cognitive function, and anxiety level (Etchells et al. 1996c; Hall et al. 2012). It is important that the neurosurgical clinician or researcher ensure that an adequate amount of information has been received and understood. Simple checks such as asking the patient to repeat what they heard and understand and asking if they have any questions related to the procedure can be effective (Diaz et al. 2009; Schmitz and Reinacher 2006). Other tools that have been shown to be of some benefit to increasing understanding of disclosed information include patient educational curricula, multimedia decision aids such as videos, repeat consent discussions, and test-feedback techniques (Hall et al. 2012).

Most studies of the adequacy of the consent process have focused on the relaying back of specific information given (Krupp et al. 2000). It may be, however, that not recalling every last detail given by a physician is not as important as a general understanding of the process. A qualitative study of the consent process in neuro-oncology trials showed that while recall of risks was poor, general understanding of the purpose of the trial was good, and patients were generally satisfied with the informed consent process (Knifed et al. 2008).

A challenge to both capacity and understanding is the patient who is simple and unsophisticated and overwhelmed by even the simplest language from the surgeon. These patients are vulnerable, and the surgeon must try to judge just how much information to give. He/she must give enough information so that the patient understands enough to make a reasonable decision but not so much to overload them and frighten them unduly. In these situations, it is often appropriate to give the "extra information" to a loved one like a spouse.

5.4.1.4 Voluntariness

An action such as consenting to a neurosurgical procedure is considered voluntary if it is undertaken freely, without undue influence or coercion from others (Etchells et al. 1996b). Human beings, however, do not live in isolation, and philosophers have argued that there may be no such thing as a truly autonomous act. Indeed, medical decision-making is almost always influenced by multiple factors – the opinion of family and friends, past experience, the media, and not least importantly, the recommendation of their neurosurgeon. The very nature of having a life-threatening illness cannot help but change one's outlook on things compared to before the illness.

The difference between persuasion, which can be allowable and under certain circumstance perhaps even obligatory, and coercion can be simply illustrated. It is coercive if a neurosurgeon threatens to no longer care for a patient with a ruptured intracranial aneurysm if they choose to have it treated endovascularly rather than clipped through open surgery. In contrast, it is reasonable for that same neurosurgeon to try to convince a patient that open clipping is preferable because of the location and configuration of the aneurysm or the age of the patient.

5.4.1.5 Authorization

The final act of the consent process is the patient authorizing, usually both verbally and in writing, that they consent for the procedure to occur. The actual patient signing of a consent form is usually an administrative requirement and protects one from a claim of battery. Informed consent is a process, the final act of which, for the purposes of a neurosurgical procedure, is the signing of a form.

As stated previously, although not a moral or ethical requirement, it is desirable to document the nature of the consent process, either in a dictated letter or a contemporaneous note in the patient's chart.

> **Pearl**
> The discussion about consent for a surgical procedure should be documented in the patient's chart, and/or with a separate dictated note, and in the note describing the operation.

5.4.2 Special Considerations

There are a number of circumstances or considerations that may alter the elements of the consent process that are commonly encountered in neurosurgical practice. Although not an exhaustive list, they are reviewed below.

5.4.2.1 Children

Historically, children have been thought to lack capacity and are hence unable to provide consent on their own. Typically, decisions were made by their surrogate, usually a parent or guardian, and often without the input of the child. More recently, with new understanding of developmental psychology and evidence that children as young as 14 can make rational and appropriate medical decisions (Harrison et al. 1997; Leiken 1983), it has been proposed that developmentally capable minors be allowed to consent on their own, and those without the developmental capacity still participate in the process of decision-making through assent (Lee et al. 2006). The American Academy of Pediatrics issued a policy statement in 1995 on assent that should be followed for pediatric neurosurgery patients. The process of assent involves (1) helping the child achieve a developmentally appropriate awareness of the nature of his/her condition, (2) telling the child what they can expect from tests and treatments, (3) assessing the child's understanding of the situation and the factors influencing how they are responding, and (4) soliciting an expression of the child's willingness to accept the proposed care (American Academy of Pediatrics 1995).

5.4.2.2 Surrogate Consent

As alluded to above, there are situations in which the patient is not mentally competent to give consent either due to age or cognitive impairment (Lazar et al. 1996). In these cases, consent can be provided by a substitute decision maker or surrogate, usually a family member but sometimes by someone not related to the patient by blood or marriage. The substitute decision maker may be known about in advance or be identified when consent is needed. The hierarchy of who can be a substitute decision maker is contained in law, and different jurisdictions may have slightly different hierarchies, but generally it starts with a spouse or partner of the patient and progresses through family and to a court-appointed guardian if no family is available (Substitute Decision Maker 2014).

5.4.2.3 Cultural Differences

The provision of information or disclosure in the consent process is considered a right, but patients do not have a duty to receive this information. In other words, a patient may waive the right to receive any or all information. Certain cultural groups can react to information regarding risk in a negative way, resulting in the refusal of treatment they might otherwise accept if the consent process was different from the one outlined above. A fascinating example of this is illustrated by the Navajo people, the largest federally recognized Native American tribe in the United States. Traditional Navajo believe that "both thought and language have the ability to control future events without the intercession of an agent" (Taylor 2004). Thus, talking of the possibility of future harm will "either bring about the negative result that is discussed or will make it more likely to occur" (Carrese and Rhodes 1995). In this instance, telling a Navajo that there is a risk of stroke during carotid endarterectomy may lead them to refuse the procedure, even if their risk of stroke is significantly higher without surgery.

Similarly, a study of elderly persons from different ethnic backgrounds in California showed that Korean Americans and Mexican Americans were significantly less likely than African Americans or European Americans to believe that a patient should be told of the diagnosis of cancer (Blackhall et al. 1995). In the neurosurgical literature, a survey of Japanese neuro-oncologists found that only 44 % disclosed the diagnosis of glioblastoma multiforme to patients (Yamamoto et al. 2011). These examples underscore the importance of tailoring the consent process to the individual patient and that cultural considerations should be taken into account.

Pearl
The informed consent process is not uniform across cultures. When dealing with a patient from an ethnic minority, the neurosurgeon should seek advice if he/she is not well informed about the customs of that ethnic group.

5.4.2.4 Novel Neurosurgical Therapies

The history of neurosurgical innovation has often lacked both the methodological and ethical rigor that is a requirement of the development of pharmaceutical therapies. Progress occurs largely by trial and error, with case reports, eventual retrospective reviews of case series, and occasionally a randomized clinical trial. This has often resulted in surgical treatments becoming widely used without proper evaluation. More and more, however, surgeons are calling for increased vigilance and evaluation prior to novel surgical treatments becoming accepted practice (McCulloch et al. 2009).

The consent process must be necessarily different when providing an innovative neurosurgical procedure. There can be little or no track record to discuss the likelihood of success or adverse outcomes. Often, neurosurgical advances or novel procedures are attempted as a last resort on patients where conventional treatment has failed (Lipsman et al. 2012). These patients are often a vulnerable group, "since the most interesting and important advancements occur using patients with diminished abilities to fully appreciate and adjudicate risk" (Ford 2009). If anything, the consent process for novel neurosurgical procedures should be more rigorous, with special efforts to ensure the patient understands the risk involved and the unknown likelihood of success. It has been suggested that completely new procedures or ones that have undergone a major modification undergo review by a research ethics board or an institutional review board and be sanctioned by a more senior peer or the surgeon-in-chief (Bernstein and Bampoe 2004).

With novel therapies for typically treatment-resistant disorders such as depression or obsessive-compulsive disorder, "referral to a neurosurgeon typically constitutes the crossing of an invisible border, from treatment to research" (Lipsman et al. 2012). Patients who undergo novel procedures, whether as a "one-off" or part of a trial, are particularly prone to the therapeutic misconception, where a research subject does not appreciate the distinction between the research and clinical paradigm and attributes therapeutic intent to a research procedure (Lidz and Appelbaum 2002). Special care must be taken to ensure that patients are fully aware that a novel treatment may be of no benefit to them.

Conclusion

Informed consent is a process and when done properly, often a time-consuming one. Its ethical foundation rests on respect for autonomy. Neurosurgical patients, by virtue of the severity of their illnesses, the risks involved in many neurosurgical procedures, and their often diminished capacity, represent a challenging patient population in ensuring that all elements of the informed consent process are met.

References

American Academy of Pediatrics, Committee on Bioethics (1995) Informed consent, parental permission, and assent in pediatric practice. J Pediatr 102:169–176

Annas GJ, Grodin MA (1992) The Nazi doctors and the Nuremberg code – human rights in human experimentation. Oxford University Press, Oxford

Appelbaum PS, Grisso T (1988) Assessing patient's capacity to consent to treatment. N Engl J Med 319:1635–1638

Bernstein M, Bampoe J (2004) Surgical innovation or surgical evolution: an ethical and practical guide to handling novel neurosurgical procedures. J Neurosurg 100:2–7

Bernstein M (2005) Fully informed consent is impossible in surgical clinical trials. Can J Surg 48:271–272

Blackhall LJ, Murphy ST, Frank G (1995) Ethnicity and attitudes towards patient autonomy. JAMA 274:820–825

Bock DW (2008) Philosophical justifications of informed consent in research. Oxford textbook of clinical research ethics. Oxford University Press, Oxford

Carrese JA, Rhodes LA (1995) Western bioethics on the Navajo reservation: benefit or harm? JAMA 274:826–829

Diaz JL, Barreto P, Gallego JM et al (2009) Proper information during the surgical decision-making process lowers the anxiety of patients with high-grade gliomas. Acta Neurochir 151:357–362

Etchells E, Sharpe G, Burgess MM et al (1996a) Bioethics for clinicians: 2. Disclosure. CMAJ 155:387–391

Etchells E, Sharpe G, Dykeman MJ et al (1996b) Bioethics for clinicians: 4. Voluntariness. CMAJ 155:1083–1086

Etchells E, Sharpe G, Elliott C et al (1996c) Bioethics for clinicians: 3. Capacity. CMAJ 155:657–661

Ford PJ (2009) Vulnerable brains: research ethics and neurosurgical patients. J Law Med Ethics 37:73–82

Hall DE, Prochazka AV, Fink AS (2012) Informed consent for clinical treatment. CMAJ 184:533–540

Harrison C, Kenny NP, Sidarous M et al (1997) Bioethics for clinicians: 9. Involving children in medical decisions. CMAJ 156:825–828

Johnson-Greene D (2010) Informed consent issues in traumatic brain injury research: current status of capacity assessment and recommendations for safeguards. J Head Trauma Rehabil 25:145–150

Knifed E, Lipsman N, Mason W et al (2008) Patients' perception of the informed consent process for neurooncology clinical trials. Neurooncology 10:348–354

Krupp W, Spanehl O, Laubach W et al (2000) Informed consent in neurosurgery: patients' recall of preoperative discussion. Acta Neurochir 142:233–239

Lazar NM, Greiner GG, Robertson G et al (1996) Bioethics for clinicians: 5. Substitute decision-making. CMAJ 155:1435–1437

Lee KJ, Havens PL, Sato TT et al (2006) Assent for treatment: clinical knowledge, attitudes and practice. Pediatrics 118:723–730

Leiken SL (1983) Minors' assent or dissent to medical treatment. J Pediatr 102:169–176

Lidz CW, Appelbaum PS (2002) The therapeutic misconception: problems and solutions. Med Care 40:S55–S63

Lipsman N, Giacobbe P, Bernstein M et al (2012) Informed consent for clinical trials of deep brain stimulation in psychiatric disease: challenges and implications for trial design. J Med Ethics 38:107–111

Marson DC, Ingram KK, Cody HA et al (1995) Assessing the competency of patients with Alzheimer's disease under different legal standards. Arch Neurol 52:949–954

McCulloch P, Altman DG, Campbell WB et al (2009) No surgical innovation without evaluation: the IDEAL recommendations. Lancet 374:1105–1112

Samuels A (2003) Did the neurosurgeon warn the patient of the risks? Br J Neurosurg 17:117–120

Schmitz D, Reinacher PC (2006) Informed consent in neurosurgery-translating ethical theory into action. J Med Ethics 32:497–498

Substitute Decision Maker (2014) Available at: http://www.lco-cdo.org/en/older-adults-lco-funded-papers-margaret-hall-sectionIV

Taylor JS (2004) Autonomy and informed consent on the Navajo Reservation. J Soc Philos 35:506–516

Yamamoto F, Hashimoto N, Kagawa N et al (2011) A survey of disclosure of diagnosis to patients with glioma in Japan. Int J Clin Oncol 16:230–237

Privacy and Confidentiality

6

Ta-Chih Tan and Ahmed Ammar

6.1 Introduction

> Whatever, in connection with my professional service, or not in connection with it, I see or hear, in the life of men, which ought not to be spoken of abroad, I will not divulge, as reckoning that all such should be kept secret. (Hippocrates)

A patient's right to privacy and confidentiality is a well-known medical concept, already incorporated in the Hippocratic Oath, as well as in numerous medical professional codes (Higgins 1989; Patient's Bill of Rights; Thompson 1979; Umansky et al. 2011). As easy at it seems to protect a patient's privacy and confidentiality, in reality, there are many situations in clinical daily life where both aspects are at risk, and we healthcare providers are not always fully aware of it. Clearly, patients expect their privacy to be protected (Akyüz and Erdemir 2013), and this is central to value-based medicine.

In certain well-studied cases, the known facts a doctor has about a patient concern a physical threat to other people (Stone 1976). In these cases, a conflict arises – who (the patient) or what (the principle of justice) should we protect? Less egregious and less visible but more common examples of privacy breaches include everyday conversations between colleagues in public places and the way patients' files are kept (Howe and Bernstein 2014).

T.-C. Tan, MD (✉)
Division of Pediatric Neurosurgery, Department of Pediatrics,
HSK-Wiesbaden, Ludwig-Erhard-Strasse 100, Wiesbaden 65199, Germany
e-mail: ta-chih.tan@hsk-wiesbaden.de

A. Ammar, MBChB, DMSc, FICS, FACS, FAANS
Department of Neurosurgery, King Fahd University Hospital,
Dammam University, 40121, Al Khobar 31952, Saudi Arabia
e-mail: ahmed@ahmedammar.com

A. Ammar, M. Bernstein (eds.), *Neurosurgical Ethics in Practice: Value-based Medicine*, 63
DOI 10.1007/978-3-642-54980-9_6, © Springer-Verlag Berlin Heidelberg 2014

Furthermore, privacy and confidentiality are ever-changing concepts, subject to technological advances, culture, society, legislation, and, last but not least, autonomy of a patient, which has actually increased over time, thanks to the law and patients' easier access to medical information (Ammar 1997; Higgins 1989; Thompson 1979). Examples of new issues which have evolved include the acquisition and securing of molecular information in surgical patients (Bernstein et al. 2004). In order to ensure a patients' autonomy, they must be certain that privacy and confidentiality of their information is safeguarded.

> **Pearl**
> A patient's right to privacy and confidentiality is an ever-changing concept, based on culture, society, and legislation, but it derives directly from a patient's right to autonomy. The awareness in daily clinical practice about protecting a patient's privacy and confidentiality is not yet optimal.

6.2   Illustrative Cases

Case 1 (Speaking About a Patient in a Public Place)
Two colleagues talk jokingly about an upcoming procedure on a patient in an elevator. The daughter of the patient is standing behind them in the elevator. She finds out that these colleagues are the surgeons of her father and she files a complaint. How to avoid these situations?

Case 2 (Family's Request to Withhold Information from Another Doctor)
A mother asks you not to reveal any information concerning her son's condition or planned procedures to the previous surgeon, because she is dissatisfied with that first surgeons' treatment. The first surgeon calls you to inquire about the wellbeing of his former patient. How do you proceed?

Case 3 (Family's Request to Withhold Information from the Patient)
A mother does not want her son, a 12-year-old bright good athlete without neurological deficits, to know that his cerebellar astrocytoma has only been partially removed (Figs. 6.1 and 6.2). She thinks that knowing this fact would place her son in emotional jeopardy, because a second procedure could diminish his sporting abilities. Over time, the follow-up MRI showed a slow but clear progress of the tumor requiring further treatment (Fig. 6.3). What are the issues and how does one solve this dilemma?

Fig. 6.1 The preoperative
MRI

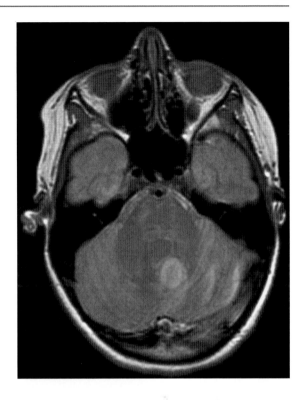

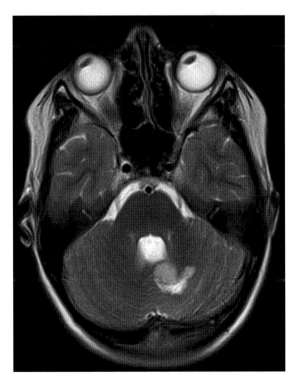

Fig. 6.2 The postoperative
MRI at 7 months

Fig. 6.3 The postoperative
MRI at 12 months

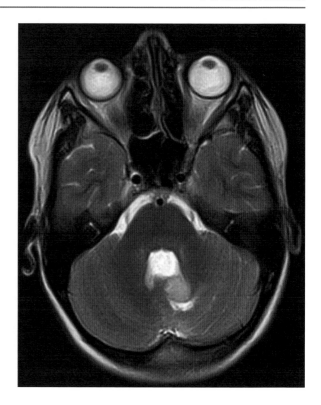

Case 4 (Patient Shares Criminal Intent with the Psychiatrist)

A paranoid patient tells his psychiatrist he is going to murder his wife.
The psychiatrist deems the threat idle and does not take action (i.e., informing the
police or forcing a hospital admission of the patient). The patient actually tries to
kill his wife and harms her severely. What would have been the
wisest thing to do?

Case 5 (Lack of Privacy in the Surgeon's Waiting Room)

A man accompanies his wife for a consultation with the neurosurgeon about spinal stenosis. In the waiting room, he hears the secretary call out, "Mr. Bob Smith,
Dr. Cushing will see you now." He looks over to see that the man is the same Bob
Smith who works under him at the office and is currently up for a promotion. He
also recognizes Dr. Cushing's name as a leading malignant brain tumor surgeon
and wonders whether Smith's recent promotion at work should perhaps be
reconsidered.

6.3   Approach to the Cases

The first case is an example of a breach in privacy of the patient with no benefit to anyone but just harm, an egregious violation of the patient's autonomy.

In the second case, confidentiality is demanded from the physician, which brings him into an awkward situation concerning his colleague. If he violates the family's request and speaks to the first surgeon, there are no disadvantages to the patient so the violation might be justifiable.

In the third case, there is a conflict between the patient's universal, ethical right to autonomy, the legal local law, and the physician's personal decision, which derives from beneficence. To withhold the information from the boy and consequently limit his autonomy holds a great risk of maleficence. The son has the right to autonomy, being a bright young boy with the capacity to understand his situation and the consequences. Due to the legislation in his country, his mother has parental responsibility as well as the parental right to determine the course of treatment, although most Western societies recognize that there is no definitive age cutoff for determining competence and a mature 12-year-old might be deemed competent by the surgeon. The surgeon knows the tumor will require repeat surgery and/or radiation, so by following the mother's will, harm will be done to the boy.

In the fourth case, the patient's confidentiality is respected, but harm was done to a third party, which could have been prevented if dealt with differently. This case illustrates a clash between utilitarian ethics (do what produces the best outcome for the most people) and Kantian deontology (do what is deemed right irrespective of the consequences).

In the fifth case, imperfect systems have led to the disclosure of information about a patient to someone who can use this information in a way which may hurt the patient. The case highlights how much improvement is needed in everyday systems in our hospitals.

6.4   Discussion

6.4.1   Definition of Privacy and Confidentiality

The distinction between patient's privacy and a patient's confidentiality can be murky (Higgins 1989; Kleinman et al. 1997; Thompson 1979). In law, privacy has been described as "the right to be left alone." A broad but fitting description of the difference between both is that privacy relates to a person and confidentiality relates to the information and data about an individual. The distinction is not that important as practically speaking, there is a great overlap between privacy and confidentiality.

In medical practice, privacy is probably best described as the right of the patient to have his/her person and information kept confidential, as well as the right to transfer this information in confidential surroundings. For example, physical examinations are conducted in a closed room. During rounds on the ward, family members and friends are requested to leave temporarily. Results of medical examinations and treatment plans are discussed in a private area.

A patient's confidentiality is the right of the patient to nondisclosure of his/her information and data. This concerns verbally transferred information of the patient, as well as the security of the documented information, written or, nowadays ever more often, digital files. Exceptions are made when information is required by law, in the public interest. Clinical everyday examples are computers which are encrypted and have multiple password protection of patient files, and the storage of hard copies of patient files in separate, lockable spaces, not in open sight on counters or desks.

> **Pearl**
> Privacy is the right of the patient to transfer his/her personal information in a confidential surrounding, and confidentiality is the right of the patient to nondisclosure of his/her documentary information.

6.4.2   Privacy in Daily Clinical Life

The privacy of patients applies to many situations and is essentially an ever-present concern to the patient and to healthcare providers. The lack of privacy starts in the neurosurgery clinic waiting room. If ten patients are waiting in a common waiting room at any given time of the day, it is entirely possible that privacy could be lost by one patient recognizing another or one patient or family member recognizing a public figure or someone in their work life. Some corrective measures can be taken. Most psychiatrists have offices with separate entrance and exit doors so no two patients ever come face to face. Medical history-taking and physical examination should always take place in a private room with a door, although in many parts of the word, especially resource-poor settings, two or three patients often share one examining room. The patients' hard copy files should be kept in a separate room where only limited people have access and should even be stored in a space, which can be locked, to ensure the utmost possible privacy. To follow these guidelines is unfortunately not always possible, due to the ever more limited time we have for the growing workload and logistic issues like limitations of space.

Modern systems provide the possibility to have a digital patient file. Even without a patient file, many patients' data are accessible online in a hospital. The digitizing of the patients' data facilitates our work and under the contemporary progressive strain in healthcare it saves time. At the same time, it is a liability concerning the patient's privacy, because all digital data can be accessed both inadvertently and maliciously (i.e., hacking).

Conversations about patients between colleagues are often held in the hallway or elevators and can easily be overheard unnoticed – these behaviors should be avoided.

> **Pearl**
> Patient data should be kept confined in a safe space as much as possible. Conversations about patients should be held behind closed doors. Healthcare providers must always be aware of the public place they are in.

6.4.3   Confidentiality in Daily Clinical Life

Not to disclose the patient's information seems a straightforward rule, even when one takes into account the exceptions, when disclosure is demanded for the public good or by law. Still, breaching confidentiality occurs more often than we think. Most of the time, we do not talk to the patient openly about whom we may disclose his/her medical information to, but it is understood that whenever we talk of a patient's condition, consent is implicit (e.g., speaking to the patient's spouse) or we must obtain verbal or written consent to do so. Confidentiality of patient data has become more complex and problematic as the medical profession progresses closer toward electronic records, which are subject to many abuses, both accidental and intentional (Graves 2013).

A very common example is when a neurosurgeon is called on the phone or e-mailed by a distressed, unknown family member of a recently operated patient inquiring about the condition of the patient (Weiss 2004). Most clinicians are trusting empathetic people, and we generally trust that the person is who they say they are and we provide some general information without checking the identity of the caller. If we do this, which is strictly speaking ill-advised, we should at minimum inform the patient as soon as possible of the conversation. Sometimes, sharing information can be very problematic in, for example, a situation where there is marital discord and a girlfriend presents herself as the person to communicate with, as opposed to the patient's legal wife. In these situations, the surgeon must be extremely careful not only to protect the patient but also to protect himself/herself. As long as no harm is done to the patient, his/her confidentiality must be categorically and unconditionally respected.

> **Pearl**
> Clinicians should get consent upfront as to whom medical information may be disclosed. A patients' confidentiality is to be completely respected, as long as no harm is done to the patient or anyone else.

6.4.4   Confidentiality and Minors

Parental responsibility and right, according to local law, can turn already intricate matters of privacy and confidentiality into even more complex situations, as in the third case above. The age at which a minor receives legal autonomy differs, according to different local legislation; often it is not measured by numerical age but whether it is deemed that the child is mature enough to be considered competent. When parents request information to be kept from their children, it may be legally the right thing to do, but at the same time, the universal, ethical right of the child to autonomy is compromised (Baskin 1974; Bennett 1976; Fan 2011; Friedrichsen vs Niemotka 1962; Gillon 1994; Goldstein 1997; Wheeler 2006). Therefore, a careful assessment of the following aspects is obligatory: (1) the ability of the minor to fully understand the situation and to anticipate and evaluate future consequences. The capability of a child or adolescent to comprehend the situation depends largely on the maturity and intelligence of a child, which makes a clear cutoff age for all individuals impossible to define (Baskin 1974; Bennett 1976; Fan 2011; Friedrichsen vs Niemotka 1962; Gillon 1994; Goldstein 1997; Wheeler 2006). (2) Is the parental surrogate decision-making in the best interest of the child or does it obstruct beneficence? After assessment of these aspects, it is the duty of the physician to form a personal opinion (with help from ombudsmen or other authoritative persons or bodies, as needed), based on the concept of beneficence, and to try to act accordingly to work with the parents to take the right course of action.

> **Pearl**
> Confidentiality and privacy derived from parental responsibility and right or parental surrogate decision-making should not compromise the ethical right of a minor to autonomy. Careful assessment of the competence of the minor to fully understand the situation and the consequences of his/her decisions is obligatory.

6.4.5   Confidentiality and the Mentally Ill

Confidentiality and especially the "allowed" breaches of it concerning the mentally ill are a much discussed and challenging subject especially when a patient is assessed violent or suicidal (Higgins 1989; Thompson 1979). Assessing the violent nature of a patient differs from predicting the risk of a violent act. A patient's violence toward others has shown low specificity over time (Simon and Shuman 2009). Acting on the announcement of planned violence by warning the third party, the police or forced hospitalization of the patient can lead to victimizing the patient, due to psychological stress, or discontinuation of the physician-patient relationship, which is often already tenuous, leaving the patient uncared for. It can also cause aggression toward the physician, coming from the patient, or even the warned third party (Simon and Shuman 2009). Additionally, it could lead to unnecessary hospitalization, due to the rarity of an actual violent act (Simon and Shuman 2009; Stone 1976).

Different advice has been given how to handle such situations. One approach is to warn the third party in the presence of the patient as a form of informed consent. This could be dangerous for the physician. Another approach includes more frequent follow-up to monitor the patient.

Overall, there is no gold standard under these circumstances. Important is an assessment according to reasonable degree of skill, knowledge, and reasonable care with complementing careful documentation. In the fourth case above, the psychiatrist can be held not liable if his documentation shows reasonable care, skill, and knowledge, as well as continued frequent follow-up of the patient (Simon and Shuman 2009; Stone 1976).

6.4.6 Confidentiality and Clinical Research

Special issues of privacy and confidentiality of patient data are raised when one considers clinical research. Patient data bases are inherent to every type of clinical research – randomized phase III trials, phase I and II studies, qualitative research, and others, as patient identification is required, for example, to relate demographic data to outcomes (Gilkes et al. 2003). Often, patients are assigned numbers on the paperwork and e-files but ultimately any patient's identity is traceable. Similarly, more and more molecular information is being secured on patients for diagnostic, therapeutic, and research purposes, and these data could compromise patients if it were discovered by the wrong people (Bernstein et al. 2004; Lunshof et al. 2008).

Conclusion

Medical ethical conduct concerning patient's privacy and confidentiality is a substantial and ever-present part of daily clinical life. We should make ourselves aware of it, notwithstanding the increasing time pressure we are all under. It is important to find a workable balance between protecting privacy and confidentiality and an efficient daily routine. Patients' information and files should be kept in separate spaces as much as possible, away from public pathways. Conversations about patients should be kept behind closed doors. Digitalization of patient's data will streamline our work, but it creates an extra liability, taking into account the risk of inadvertent sharing this information or malicious hacking. Computers should be locked when left unattended. Common sense is required so that we always act in a way that we would want our privacy and confidentiality protected. We should also help create systems which will help safeguard patients' privacy and confidentiality.

In conflict situations, it is sometimes difficult to find the right course of action. In the end, justice is our main goal and our actions should be based on the patient's right to autonomy, beneficence, and nonmaleficence.

Acknowledgment We would like to thank Professor Norbert Paul of the Medical Ethics Department of the Johannes Gutenberg University of Mainz for his patience and help.

References

Akyüz E, Erdemir F (2013) Surgical patients' and nurses' opinions and expectations about privacy in care. Nurs Ethics 20(6):660–671

Ammar A (1997) The influence of different cultures on neurosurgical practice. Childs Nerv Syst 13:91–94

Baskin SJ (1974) State intrusion into family affairs: justifications and limitations. Stanf Law Rev 26:1383–1409

Bennett R (1976) Allocation of child medical care decision-making authority: a suggested interest analysis. Virginia Law Rev 62(2):285–330

Bernstein M, Bampoe J, Daar AS (2004) Ethical issues in molecular medicine of relevance to surgeons. Can J Surg 47:414–421

Fan R (2011) The Confucian bioethics of surrogate decision making: its communitarian roots. Theor Med Bioeth 32(5):301–313

Friedrichsen v. Niemotka (1962) 71N.J. Super. 398, 177 A.2d 58. Accessible at http://www.leagle.com/decision/196246971NJSuper398_1423

Gilkes CE, Casimiro M, McEvoy AW et al (2003) Clinical databases and data protection: are they compatible? Br J Neurosurg 17(5):426–431

Gillon R (1994) Medical ethics: four principles plus attention to scope. BMJ 309:184–188

Goldstein J (1997) Medical care for the child at risk: on state supervention of parental autonomy. Yale Law J 86:645–670

Graves S (2013) Confidentiality, electronic health records, and the clinician. Perspect Biol Med 56(1):105–125

Higgins GL (1989) The history of confidentiality in medicine: the physician-patient relationship. Can Fam Physician 35:921–926

Howe K, Bernstein (2014) Privacy concerns in the surgical environment. J Clin Res Bioeth 4:3

Kleinman I, Baylis F, Rodgers S et al (1997) Bioethics for clinicians: 8. Confidentiality. CMAJ 156:521–524

Lunshof JE, Chadwick R, Vorhaus DB et al (2008) From genetic privacy to open consent. Nat Rev Genet 9(5):406–411

Patient's bill of rights, Public Health Law (PHL)2803 (1)(g) Patient's Rights, 10NYCRR, 405.7,405.7(a)(1),405.7(c). Accessible at http://www.health.ny.gov/publications/1449/section_2.htm

Simon IR, Shuman DW (2009) Therapeutic risk management of clinical-legal dilemmas: should it be a core competency? J Am Acad Psychiatry Law 37(2):155–161

Stone AA (1976) The Tarasoff decisions: suing psychotherapists to safeguard society. Harv Law Rev 90:358–378

Thompson IE (1979) The nature of confidentiality. J Med Ethics 5:57–64

Umansky F, Black PL, DiRocco C et al (2011) Statement of ethics in neurosurgery of the World Federation of Neurosurgical Societies. World Neurosurg 76(3–4):239–247

Weiss N (2004) E-mail consultation: clinical, financial, legal, and ethical implications. Surg Neurol 61:455–459

Wheeler R (2006) Gillick or Fraser? A plea for consistency over competence in children. BMJ 332:807

Severe Neurosurgical Conditions in Children

7

T.H.R. de Jong and Erwin J.O. Kompanje

7.1 Introduction

Neonates may be afflicted with severe congenital anomalies, and young children may present with severe acquired neurosurgical diseases. The treatment of vulnerable patients or populations is a vital challenge in value-based medicine. Whether or not treatment should be started can be a difficult decision, especially when severe and permanent neurological deficits can be expected. What in such cases is in the best interest of the child? To what extent are parents responsible for their child in such circumstances? What guidelines can be used by the responsible physician in order to ensure proper reasoning and correct decision making?

In order to discuss these questions, a discussion based around three pediatric patients with severe neurological conditions is presented. All three were surgically treated by their neurosurgeon after continued insistence of the parents. Two patients survived with severe lifelong handicaps. The third patient died within 1 year after the initial diagnosis.

Some will argue that patients should not be treated with neurosurgical interventions if their anticipated handicaps are too severe for an acceptable quality of life and will state that it is ethically sound and merciful to let these newborns die, or eventually deliberately end their lives (Klotzko 1997; Verhagen and Sauer 2005a, b; Verhagen 2013). What are their arguments? What are the arguments against? Is it in the best interests of these newborns to die? When is a neurosurgical intervention "futile," "inappropriate," or "disproportionate"?

T.H.R. de Jong, MD (✉)
Department of Neurosurgery, Erasmus MC University Medical Center, 2040, 3000 CA Rotterdam, The Netherlands
e-mail: t.h.r.dejong@erasmusmc.nl

E.J.O. Kompanje, PhD
Intensive Care Medicine, Erasmus MC University Medical Center, Rotterdam, The Netherlands
e-mail: erwinkompanje@me.com; e.j.o.kompanje@erasmusmc.nl

A. Ammar, M. Bernstein (eds.), *Neurosurgical Ethics in Practice: Value-based Medicine*,
DOI 10.1007/978-3-642-54980-9_7, © Springer-Verlag Berlin Heidelberg 2014

7.2   Illustrative Cases

7.2.1   Case 1 (A Newborn with a Large Thoracic Myelomeningocele)

A girl was born with a very large thoracic myelomeningocele accompanied by massive hydrocephalus (Figs. 7.1 and 7.2). Despite these severe malformations, she appeared vital and there was no need for admission to a neonatology intensive care unit. The multidisciplinary myelomeningocele (MMC) team was uncertain whether neurosurgical treatment was technically possible and medically appropriate. The parents of the girl consistently asked the team to do everything possible. After thorough consideration and deliberation, it was decided to honor the parents' request and on the third day of life, the girl was operated. The dural defect was closed, and extensive rotation flaps and split skin grafts were used to close the large dorsal defect (Fig. 7.3). The hydrocephalus was treated 5 days later with a ventriculoperitoneal shunt. Two months later, the shunt had to be removed because of an infection, which was treated adequately, and 2 weeks later, a new shunt was inserted.

Seven years later, she is living with her family (Fig. 7.4). Although she is a cooperative and attentive girl, she is cognitively very challenged, needing special school. She can speak words and short sentences and is wheelchair dependent, but can play by herself. Concerning transfers, she is almost completely dependent and she also needs to be catheterized six times a day. Up till now, she has needed ten operations.

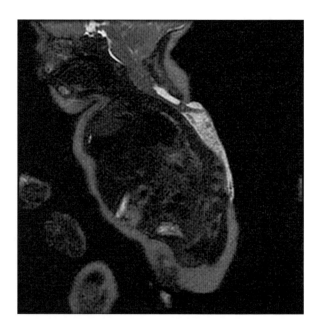

Fig. 7.1 MRI of high thoracic myelomeningocele

Fig. 7.2 MRI showing massive hydrocephalus

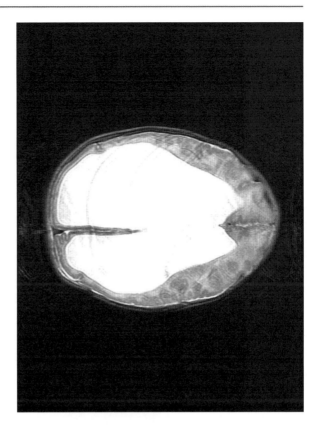

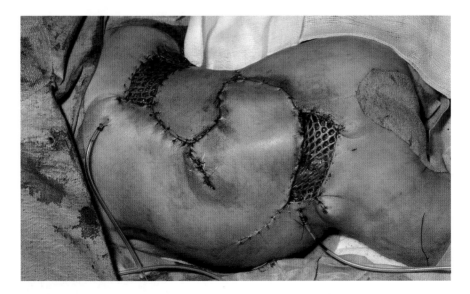

Fig. 7.3 Closure of the defect with rotation flaps and split skin techniques

Fig. 7.4 The girl at the age of 7 at home (printed with permission of her parents)

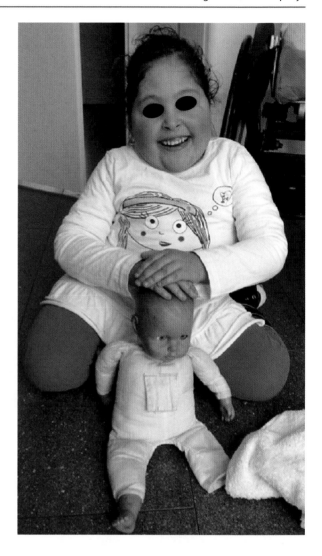

7.2.2 Case 2 (A Boy with a Huge Intramedullary Tumor)

At birth, this boy appeared to have paraplegia at a high thoracic level. MRI revealed a huge intramedullary tumor extending from the upper thoracic region down to the sacral region (Fig. 7.5). Biopsy revealed a malignant peripheral nerve sheath tumor. Six months after birth and after many multidisciplinary deliberations and following consistent requests of the parents, it was decided to operate the boy and remove the tumor en bloc by a spinal cord transection just below the normal cervical spinal cord and a resection of the distal cord together with the dural sac and all the roots

Fig. 7.5 MRI of large intramedullary tumor extending from the upper thoracic level

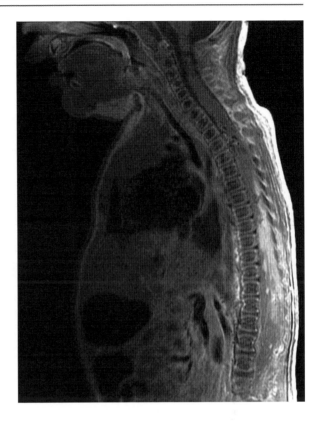

(Fig. 7.6). Surgical removal was followed by systemic chemotherapy (three cycles of vincristine, actinomycin, and cyclophosphamide).

At the age of 7, he remains in remission. He grew up as a short-statured wheelchair-dependent boy. He has feeding problems, which necessitate PEG tube feeding. Arm function is normal, but he is completely paraplegic. Because of a neurogenic bladder, he needs to be catheterized four times a day. He is attending normal school, and despite his physical condition and dependency, up till now, he is seldom frustrated by his handicaps.

7.2.3   Case 3 (A Young Girl with an Anaplastic Glioma)

At the age of 4½ years, this girl was admitted to the hospital with progressive right-sided hemiparesis. MRI scan revealed a large thalamic tumor (Fig. 7.7). Biopsy revealed a highly malignant glioma. Subsequently, the girl was operated. A transcallosal approach was performed which resulted in a partial resection of the tumor. Postoperatively she was aphasic but cognitively preserved. Systemic chemotherapy

Fig. 7.6 MRI after en bloc
resection of the tumor below
the cervical spinal cord

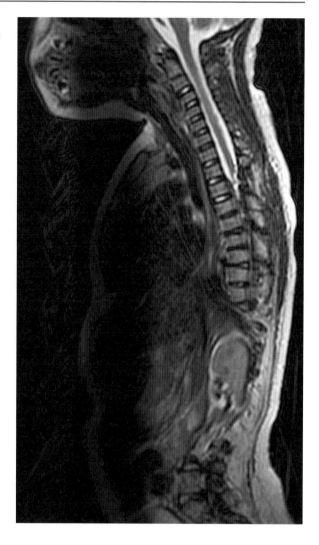

was started (VP16 and carboplatin), but follow-up MRI showed again an aggressive tumor growth. A second operation was considered to be disproportionate by the medical team, but the parents urgently requested to do anything to prolong her life. Two months after the initial operation, the young girl underwent partial resection of the recurrent malignant glioma. The occurrence of progressive hydrocephalus required a ventriculoperitoneal shunt. After the second operation, 30 days of radiation therapy followed, each time under general anesthesia because of her young age.

For a few months, she did moderately well, but gradually, she developed severe neurological deficits. MRI revealed a huge recurrence of the tumor (Fig. 7.8). Palliative treatment was started and she died at the age of almost 5½ years.

Fig. 7.7 MRI of diffuse
thalamic anaplastic glioma

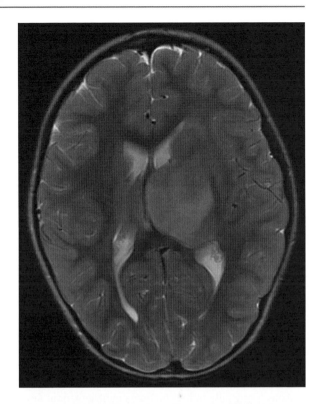

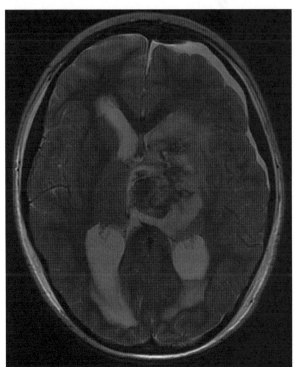

Fig. 7.8 MRI showing
regrowth of the tumor after
surgical debulking and
chemotherapy

7.3   Discussion

7.3.1   "Inappropriate" Neurosurgical Interventions

An appropriate neurosurgical intervention is adequate, timely, and proper following moral standards and codes of the profession. Inappropriate neurosurgical interventions therefore can be defined as "not proper or untimely" use of neurosurgery. Inappropriate neurosurgical interventions include disproportionate neurosurgical interventions such as "excessive, too much, or more than enough" but also as "not enough" and even "futile use of neurosurgical interventions."

7.3.2   "Disproportionate" Neurosurgical Interventions

Proportionate neurosurgical interventions could be defined as interventions that reduce patient's risk of death in acute and life-threatening conditions or improve or restore the quality of life by avoiding long-term physical or mental sequelae. Disproportionate neurosurgical interventions are perceived by most healthcare providers, patients and their relatives, and/or society as disproportionate and/or out of balance, in relation to the condition of the patient or the expected outcome or reduction in risk of death of the patient or quality of life.

Neurosurgical treatment can be "not enough" in terms of inadequate treatment. Inadequate treatment can take place due to inadequacy of the physician, for financial reasons (especially in low-income countries), or at the explicit request of the patient or caretakers. More prevalent, disproportionate neurosurgical interventions are judged by physicians, nurses, patients, relatives, or society as "too much" or "more than enough." In a small proportion of the cases, the inappropriate neurosurgical treatment can be judged as futile, in the sense of being ineffective or pointless.

> **Pearl**
> Converse to earlier bioethical writings, the use of the terms inappropriate or disproportionate neurosurgical treatment would be better than futile treatment as a reflection of the actual situation.

7.3.3   Medical Futility

Medical futility as a concept and the use of the term "futile care" are controversial and troublesome. Futile care can be defined as the initiation or prolongation of "ineffective, pointless, or hopeless" use of neurosurgical treatments. Therefore, medical futility is by definition inappropriate care. However, the inappropriate or disproportionate uses of neurosurgical interventions do not necessarily need to be futile. An example of medical futility would be the use of mechanical ventilation in a brain-dead patient who has declined to be a donor. Medical futility by this definition is rather rare in neurosurgery.

7.3.4   Disproportionate Use of ICU Resources in the Sense of "More than Enough"

Other than the patient her/his relatives can judge the use of neurosurgical interventions to be "more than enough" if it is not in the patient's best interest. Physicians involved in the care of patients with severe neurological conditions should question themselves if there are medical interventions used in these patients that they can label as disproportionate because they, the nurses, or relatives of the patients are sufficiently confident that the interventions will not be beneficial. Excessive resources are sometimes used to provide life-sustaining medical care in debilitating conditions. Especially in older patients and in patients with multiple comorbidities, this could be labeled as "too much" or "more than enough." Because we have the possibility and the resources to postpone and orchestrate death for a sometimes indefinite time, we have the moral responsibility to deliberate with all professionals involved and the patient and/or relatives, whether the continued care is still in the best interest of the patient. Alternatively, we should question ourselves whether initial institution of neurosurgical care is in the patient's interest.

7.3.5   Disproportionate Use of Neurosurgical Interventions in the Sense of "Too Much"

When the initiation or prolongation of neurosurgical interventions is not anymore in the patient's best interests, "too much" and thus disproportionate care is delivered. This occurs when the condition of the patient is irreversible or has become irreversible during the course of neurosurgical intervention according to current knowledge, as in the following circumstances:

(a) No effective treatment is available or the prolonged treatment has no real pathophysiologic rationale anymore.
(b) Effective treatment is available; however, the patient is not responding to therapy ("a nonresponder"), even when treatment is at its maximal level and it is not plausible anymore to assume that cure will occur.
(c) Effective treatment has already been given to the patient with no or only minimal response ("a minimal responder"; marginally effective interventions).
(d) It is certain or nearly certain that the treatment will not achieve the goals that the patient or the parents have specified or is against the patient's or parents' will (e.g., in patients with advanced directives).

7.4   Analysis of the Three Cases

7.4.1   Case 1 (Is Surgical Treatment Appropriate in a Large Thoracic Myelomeningocele?)

Directly after birth, the multidisciplinary MMC team was uncertain concerning what to do. Some members considered closing of such a large defect as disproportionate in the sense of "too much." Furthermore, before the birth of the girl, the parents were told that their child would be stillborn or would die soon after birth. So why not let the baby die? Was not that perhaps in her best interests? But the girl was not stillborn and did not die soon after birth resulting in the situation in which the parents urged consistently and repeatedly to do everything possible to save the life of their child. The child herself appeared to be in a reasonable state, as no intensive care was necessary and the Comfort and VAS scores were most of the time below threshold. Finally, closing the defect was considered as an appropriate treatment to achieve two goals: to diminish the discomfort being caused by the huge MMC and to prevent a possible life-threatening complication (i.e., a fulminant meningitis). The decision was also made following the assumption that the parents loved their child and would be able to offer competent care should the girl survive. The operation itself would only harm the patient by causing wound pain for a limited period of time which was expected to be treatable effectively using standard pain medication.

Seven years later, this girl lives at home with her parents and her brothers in quite good health. Nevertheless, she is physically severely handicapped and mentally retarded and this will not change very much (Fig. 7.4). Is she really better off alive or would it have been better to have let her die just after birth? Could perhaps active termination of life have been a better option at the time? The age-old question looms: how do we measure the value of a human life and who has the right to decide if a life is not worth preserving?

Is the intervention appropriate? The unexpected birth of a child with a MMC constitutes a shock for parents. A prediction regarding physical handicaps and intellect would possibly help parents to plan for the future. Clinical hydrocephalus at birth is not a solid prediction of poor outcome (Beeker et al. 2005). They also found that shunt infections do not cause low IQ. In our case, it was presumed that the girl should have a bad outcome. Although her IQ was not high, it is not reasonable to state that her life is a misery (Freeman 1998; Wilkinson 2006, 2008). Prognostication is unavoidable in medicine and elicits potent and troubling attitudes and behaviors in physicians (Christakis 1999). Physicians who routinely tell pregnant women that their fetus with MMC will be mentally retarded, never will be able to walk, and will suffer lifelong bowel and bladder incontinence are ignoring a body of literature that contradicts this stereotype (Bruner and Tulipan 2004). MMC results in a spectrum of disabilities, but most children will grow into adulthood with acceptable disabilities. For these reasons, it was reasonable enough to treat the vital newborn girl in our case. The first intention in treatment of such a child is "to do everything we can to save and prolong her life." It seems appropriate. MMC in itself is not a terminal disease when treated actively and the majority of cases, even the more severely affected as in the illustrative case, will survive to develop into adults who are satisfied with their lives (Beeker et al. 2005).

> **Pearl**
> MMC results in a spectrum of disabilities, but most children will grow into adulthood with acceptable disabilities.

Some will state that we can prognosticate with great certainty that the life of a child born with MMC will be a life of suffering. The prognostication is of such a certainty that they state that active termination of life is the only option to relief the child; this has been reported in the Netherlands (Verhagen and Sauer 2005a, b; Verhagen 2013). This report was made in the context of a new protocol for termination of newborns, the so-called Groningen Protocol. The single most important reason that necessitated life termination was "unbearable and hopeless suffering which could not be dealt with in any other way." This suffering consisted not only of acute pain but also of the prospects of a miserable life with no possibility to communicate at all, either verbally or nonverbally, extensive dependency on medical care, and untreatable chronic pain.

However, the Groningen Protocol is in the case of MMC controversial. The criteria used in the Groningen Protocol, especially "unbearable suffering" and the "expected quality of life," have been questioned (Jotkowitz and Glick 2006; De Jong 2008; Barry 2010). Some have addressed the poor quality and the insufficiency of the offered palliative care and questioned whether legalization of active termination of life might not lead to the abuse of it (Feudtner 2005a, b). Others warned that neonatologists must be careful not to start on the slippery slope ending in the practice of euthanasia of newborns (Saugstad 2005). Others articulated that an important line has been crossed if the international medical community consents to the active euthanasia of severely ill infants and are concerned about the extension of the policy to other groups at risk (Jotkowitz and Glick 2006). Other commentators have voiced similar concerns (Bondi et al. 2006; Chervenak et al. 2006; Kodish 2008; Manninen 2006).

Suffering which cannot be relieved is an important argument for deliberate termination of life in newborns with MMC. But do these newborns suffer? An assessment of the degree of discomfort and pain in 28 newborns with MMC concluded that during their initial treatment, newborns with MMC had low levels of discomfort and pain (Ottenhoff et al. 2012). Even in untreated MMC patients who are discharged to their parents at home, severe suffering was seldom seen (Delight and Goodall 1988, 1990).

> **Pearl**
> Prognostication in medicine is never inconsequential or insignificant. Judgments must be based on the best available evidence. In cases of doubt, one must search for more evidence to the greatest extent possible – only then can care be considered as proportionate and appropriate.

7.4.2 Case 2 (Is Surgical Treatment of a Large Intramedullary Tumor Appropriate Care?)

After the diagnosis of malignant peripheral nerve sheath tumor had been made, the oncologists asked the neurosurgeon whether it would be possible to perform a radical resection to achieve long-term tumor control. The operation itself should be regarded as severely mutilating (e.g., causing spinal dysmorphism or instability) and also putting the patient at risk of increasing neurological deficits by compromising the cervical spinal cord. Perhaps it could be regarded as disproportionate?

However, after consistent requests of the parents, it was decided to operate the child and the tumor was resected en bloc. After adjuvant chemotherapy, the child is a long survivor and therefore the operation could therefore be regarded as proportionate. But, if severe complications would have been the sequelae of the operation, could it then still be regarded as proportionate?

After 7 years, this boy is living at home with his family and attending normal school. Most of the time, he is happy enough with his life, as are the parents, in spite of severe neurological compromise. His treatment at the time therefore is felt to be appropriate and proportionate.

In this case, it is also clear that prognostication is a difficult task. If the parents had not insisted on radical treatment, the responsible doctors would likely have agreed with nontreatment and then this boy would have died. Would that have been in his best interests? The answer is presumably not. So, although it was a major operation, this surgical treatment followed by chemotherapy is considered to be appropriate because it did save his life and provided an acceptable quality of life.

7.4.3 Case 3 (Is Aggressive and Recurrent Treatment in the Case of a Highly Malignant Cerebral Tumor Appropriate Care?)

After the diagnosis had been made of a highly malignant anaplastic glioma, the initial treatment modality of choice was gross total resection, which is considered to help provide long-term survival, albeit based on Class 2 and 3 data (Cage et al. 2012). So, although a transcallosal resection could cause harm to the child, the first operation should be regarded as appropriate. Aggressive chemotherapy was also instituted.

Six weeks later, however, on the next MRI, a significant recurrence of the malignant tumor was noted. At this point of disease, one should conclude that the prognosis was dismal and that the girl would die because of uncontrollable tumor growth. The parents however insisted on a second operation followed by radiotherapy (30 fractions each requiring general anesthesia), hoping this would extend the life of their daughter for some months. They insisted to do everything possible for their daughter. After much discussion, the second operation was performed and the radiotherapy was administered. Some months later she died. This extensive adjuvant treatment could be considered to be "too much," as disproportionate, as aggressive treatment would extend her life for perhaps only a few months. It appears to be difficult to withhold a patient from disproportionate therapy when parents insist to continue. One could also raise the question whether the costs for this adjuvant treatment can be considered appropriate, although most clinicians are appropriately loathe to bring discussions of cost to the bedside.

The first surgical approach of the tumor and the following chemotherapy can be morally defendable and were appropriate and proportionate. Based on the interests of the child, the second debulking of the anaplastic tumor and the radiation treatment under general anesthesia could certainly be judged as disproportional and inappropriate. At this point, palliative care might have been more appropriate for the child (Feudtner et al. 2007).

> **Pearl**
> When the prognosis is considered hopeless in the setting of an incurable disease and when death is inevitable, continuing major treatment modalities should be regarded as disproportionate and inappropriate as this will only prolong the suffering of the patient. In such situations, palliative care should be offered.

Conclusion

Prognostication in severe cases of congenital anomalies or acquired diseases may be difficult. However, doctors are obliged to counsel the parents in an objective way and give a picture of the child's future as realistically as possible. Even in the most severe cases, starting treatment can be considered as proportionate and appropriate, and acquiescing to parents' wishes should be always be strived for, within reason. However, when cure is no longer possible and death is inevitable, major treatment modalities should be reconsidered and palliative care should be discussed with families. The single most important guideline in this decision making is: "What is in the best interest of this child?"

References

Barry S (2010) Quality of life and myelomeningocele: an ethical and evidence-based analysis of the Groningen protocol. Pediatr Neurosurg 46:409–414

Beeker TW, Scheers MM, Faber JAJ et al (2005) Prediction of independence and intelligence at birth in meningomyelocele. Childs Nerv Syst 22:33–37

Bondi SA, Gries D, Faucette K (2006) Neonatal euthanasia? Pediatrics 117:983–984

Bruner JP, Tulipan N (2004) Tell the truth about spina bifida. Ultrasound Obstet Gynecol 24:595–596

Cage TA, Mueller S, Haas-Kogan D et al (2012) High-grade gliomas in children. Neurosurg Clin N Am 23:515–523

Chervenak FA, McCullough LB, Arabin B (2006) Why the Groningen protocol should be rejected. Hast Cent Rep 36:30–33

Christakis NA (1999) Death foretold. Prophecy and prognosis in medical care. The University of Chicago Press, Chicago

De Jong THR (2008) Deliberatie termination of life of newborns with spina bifida, a critical reappraisal. Childs Nerv Syst 24:13–28

Delight E, Goodall J (1988) Babies with spina bifida treated without surgery: parents' views on home versus hospital care. BMJ 297:1230–1233

Delight E, Goodall J (1990) Love and loss. Conversations with parents of babies with spina bifida managed without surgery 1971–1981. Dev Med Child Neurol Suppl 61:1–58

Feudtner C (2005a) Hope and the prospects of healing at the end of life. J Alternat Complement Med 11:S23–S30

Feudtner C (2005b) Control of suffering on the slippery slope of care. Lancet 365:1284–1286

Feudtner C, Santucci G, Feinstein JA et al (2007) Hopeful thinking and level of comfort regarding providing pediatric palliative care: a survey of hospital nurses. Pediatrics 119:e186–e192

Freeman JM (1998) Changing ethical issues in the treatment of spina bifida: a personal odyssey. Ment Retard Dev Dis Res Rev 4:302–307

Jotkowitz AB, Glick S (2006) The Groningen protocol: another perspective. J Med Ethics 32:157–158

Klotzko AJ (1997) What kind of life? What kind of death? An interveiew with Dr Henk Prins. Bioethics 11:24–42

Kodish E (2008) The art of medicine. Paediatric ethics: a repudiation of the Groningen protocol. Lancet 371:892–893

Manninen BA (2006) A case for justified non-voluntary active euthanasia: exploring the ethics of the Groningen protocol. J Med Ethics 32:643–651

Ottenhoff MJ, Dammers R, Kompanje EJO et al (2012) Discomfort and pain in newborns with myelomeningocele: a prosepctive evaluation. Pediatrics 129:e741–e747

Saugstad OD (2005) When newborn infants are bound to die. Acta Paediatr 94:1435–1537

Verhagen AAE (2013) The Groningen protocol for newborn euthanasia; which way did the slippery slope tilt? J Med Ethics 39:293–295

Verhagen AAE, Sauer PJJ (2005a) The Groningen protocol – euthanasia in severly ill newborns. NEJM 352:959–962

Verhagen AAE, Sauer PJJ (2005b) End-of-life decisions in newborns: an appraoch from the Netherlands. Pediatrics 116:736–739

Wilkinson D (2006) Is it in the best interests of an intellectually disabled infant to die? J Med Ethics 32:454–459

Wilkinson R, Harris J (2008) Moral and legal reasons for altruism in the case of brainstem biopsy in diffuse glioma. Br J Neurosurg 22:617–618

Part III

End of Life Issues

End-of-Life Care

8

James Downar and Mark Bernstein

8.1 Introduction

End-of-life (EOL) decisions are relatively common in neurosurgical practice and a vital issue in value-based medicine. EOL decisions can take many forms in this context: (1) a decision to not perform an intervention for a patient who is terminally ill or has a grave prognosis; (2) a decision to limit the escalation or addition of certain life-sustaining treatments for a patient who is already under the care of the neurosurgeon (also known as withholding life-sustaining treatments (WHLS)); (3) a decision to stop certain life-sustaining treatments for a patient under the care of the neurosurgeon (also known as withdrawing life-sustaining treatments (WDLS)); (4) a decision to actively assist or cause the death of the patient (also known as active euthanasia or physician-assisted death (PAD), which is illegal in most countries); and (5) a decision to continue to offer all available treatments as they are indicated, with no limitations until the point of death.

EOL decisions may be common but they are never straightforward or easy. They involve a combination of medical considerations (e.g., prognosis), cultural or religious considerations, patient values, and legal obligations. Each one of these considerations may be sufficient to tell the surgeon what he/she should not do, but they rarely tell the surgeon what he/she should do. As with all ethical

J. Downar, MD, MHSc, FRCPC (✉)
Division of Respirology/Critical Care, Toronto General Hospital,
200 Elizabeth Street 9N-926, Toronto, ON M5G 2C4, Canada

Divisions of Critical Care and Palliative Care, University of Toronto,
200 Elizabeth Street 9N-926, Toronto, ON M5G 2C4, Canada
e-mail: james.downar@utoronto.ca

M. Bernstein, MD, MHSc, FRCSC
Division of Neurosugery, Toronto Western Hospital, University of Toronto,
399 Bathurst Street, Toronto, ON M5T 2S8, Canada
e-mail: mark.bernstein@uhn.ca

A. Ammar, M. Bernstein (eds.), *Neurosurgical Ethics in Practice: Value-based Medicine*,
DOI 10.1007/978-3-642-54980-9_8, © Springer-Verlag Berlin Heidelberg 2014

decisions, there is often no "right" answer. The physician must rely on an ethically sound decision-making process and be open to input from the patient, family, and members of the interdisciplinary care team.

> **Pearl**
> There is often no right or wrong answer when faced with an end-of-life decision. The physician must rely on an ethically sound decision-making process.

8.2   Illustrative Case

A 42 year-old married mother of three young children is referred for surgical management of a subarachnoid hemorrhage due to a middle cerebral artery aneurysm. The operation is successful and she is transferred to the intensive care unit for postoperative management. The following day, she develops bradycardia, hypertension, and asymmetrically dilated pupils. CT shows a large subdural hematoma and she is taken back to the OR for evacuation and decompressive craniectomy, but the patient has already suffered a significant ischemic injury to the cortex. Follow-up CT scans reveal diffuse bilateral cortical ischemic findings.

Three weeks after the hemorrhage, she remains in the Intensive Care Unit and continues to require intermittent mechanical ventilator support. Her brainstem reflexes remain intact, and she opens her eyes intermittently but does not track or respond to voice. She has developed infectious complications, including a central venous catheter-related infection, and two ventilator-associated pneumonias. These have all resolved with antibiotic therapy. Her neurological status is unchanged, and she is diagnosed with persistent vegetative state. The healthcare team approaches her husband to discuss withdrawal of life support and initiation of comfort measures. Her husband reacts angrily to this suggestion, demands ongoing aggressive care, and demands a trial of stem cell transplantation, a deep brain stimulator, and high-dose vitamins to promote neurological recovery.

8.3   Approach to the Case

In this case and in general, EOL decisions are often prompted by a specific trigger – either a new diagnosis, a complication, or a change in clinical status. This prompts the patient, family, or healthcare team to ask whether or not to add specific therapies in response to the trigger. If the issue is not raised, or a decision is not made, care typically follows a default pathway of aggressive care with no prescribed limitations. Thus, if someone raises a question about limiting escalation of care, this implies that there is a poor prognosis, and he/she feels that it might not be appropriate to escalate care.

Table 8.1 Relationship between coded physician behaviors and shared decision-making

Dimension of shared decision-making	Coded physician behaviors
Providing medical information	(1) Discuss the nature of the decision. *What is the essential clinical issue we are addressing?*
	(2) Describe treatment alternatives. *What are the clinically reasonable choices?*
	(3) Discuss the pros and cons of the choices. *What are the pros and cons of the treatment choices?*
	(4) Discuss uncertainty. *What is the likelihood of success of treatment?*
	(5) Assess family understanding. *Is the family now an informed participant with a working understanding of the decision?*
Eliciting patient values and preferences	(6) Elicit patient values and preferences. *What is known about the patient's medical preferences or values?*
Exploring the family's preferred role in decision-making	(7) Discuss the family's role in decision-making. *What role should the family play in making the decision? Families should be offered a role in decision-making even if some will decline, preferring to defer to the physician.*
	(8) Assess the need for input from others. *Is there anyone else the family would like to consult?*
Deliberation and decision-making	(9) Explore the context of the decision. *How will the decision affect the patient's life?*
	(10) Elicit the family's opinion about the treatment decision. *What does the family think is the most appropriate decision for the patient?*

Adapted from White et al. (2007)

Decision-making typically follows one of four models (Emanuel and Emanuel 1992; Cook 2001). In the parental model, the physician will decide the plan of treatment and present the patient or surrogate decision-maker (SDM) with enough information to consent to the plan. In the informative or consumer model, the physician will present a list of potential plans and allow the patient/SDM to choose among them. In the interpretive model, the physician works to understand the patient's values and helps the patient/SDM choose a plan of care that is most consistent with those values. Finally, in the deliberative model, the physician works to understand the patient's values, while simultaneously teaching the patient/SDM about the medical situation, in the hope that each party comes to a shared understanding of facts and values that will lead to a decision.

In practice, most critical care societies endorse a model of "shared decision-making" (Table 8.1), which includes a sharing of medical information, an exploration of the patient's values and the patient/SDM's preferred role in decision-making, and a process of deliberation that ideally arrives at a decision (White et al. 2007).

8.4   Discussion

8.4.1   EOL Decisions in the Intensive Care Unit

Although neurosurgeons and intensivists are confronted by similar clinical scenarios in many parts of the world, their approach to EOL decisions is highly variable. In European ICUs, decisions to WHLS vary from 16 to 70 % of deaths, depending on the country, while decisions to provide all therapies including CPR up to the point of death vary from 5 to 48 % (Wunsch et al. 2005; Sprung et al. 2003). In the United States, there is similar variability in EOL decisions among ICUs, with rates of CPR at the time of death ranging from 4 to 75 % and some ICUs never performing WDLS at all (Prendergast et al. 1998).

Clearly, this degree of variability in practice cannot be explained by local variability in case mix and illness severity. The fact is that patients, SDMs, and healthcare teams all interpret medical information differently and have different ethical norms that guide behavior. One study found that Canadian neurosurgeons, neurologists, and intensivists used highly variable approaches to prognosticate for patients with traumatic brain injury (Turgeon et al. 2013). In this study, when presented with a hypothetical case and asked if the 1-year prognosis was poor, one third agreed, one third disagreed, and one third were neutral; only 10 % were comfortable recommending WDLS. In another famous study, an international audience of healthcare practitioners was asked how they would manage a patient with a probable advanced cancer and an acute subarachnoid hemorrhage due to a ruptured aneurysm, whose family was divided over whether to continue aggressive life-sustaining measures or to WDLS (Kritek et al. 2009). Regional responses varied greatly; 24–68 % said they would WDLS, 15–30 % would continue aggressive care and consult an ethicist, and 16–49 % would write a Do Not Resuscitate order and transfer the patient to a skilled nursing facility.

Religion can also be an important consideration in EOL decision-making (Bulow et al. 2008). Jewish, Muslim, or Greek Orthodox patients who die in the ICU tend to have life support withheld (WHLS) rather than withdrawn (WDLS), whereas Catholic or Protestant patients have equal proportions of WHLS and WDLS (Sprung et al. 2007). Of note, the religion of the physician was as important as that of the patient for predicting whether life support would be withheld or withdrawn. There are many other demographic and system-related factors that are also associated with EOL decisions in the ICU, including race, socioeconomic status, insurance coverage, and bed availability (Muni et al. 2011; Barnato et al. 2007; Fowler et al. 2010; Stelfox et al. 2012).

The fact that physicians interpret clinical information inconsistently and that EOL decisions appear to be influenced by a host of nonmedical considerations should remind all clinicians of the need for humility and open-mindedness when discussing EOL decisions. This does not mean that physicians should refrain from providing an opinion or recommending an EOL decision when they feel it is appropriate, but physicians need to recognize the importance of an ethically sound approach to decision-making and conflict resolution.

> **Pearl**
> Physicians interpret clinical information inconsistently, and their decisions are often influenced by a host of nonmedical considerations. This speaks to the importance of humility and open-mindedness when recommending an EOL decision.

8.4.2   Autonomy

Autonomy is a core bioethical principle that underpins most of modern western medicine. Our respect for autonomy is manifest in the importance we attach to informed consent, disclosure, and other everyday occurrences. Respecting autonomy is complicated when making EOL decisions in the ICU, because most ICU patients are incapable of participating in decisions about their care. We then rely on substitute decision-making to provide the perspective of the patient. Ideally, SDMs would make decisions on behalf of the patient using the patient's values. In reality, SDMs find it difficult to make decisions without applying their own values and interests (Vig et al. 2006), and their predictions of patient preferences are often inaccurate (Shalowitz et al. 2006). Sometimes, patients have recorded their preferences in a document such as a living will or an advance directive. Unfortunately, such documents are often difficult to apply at the bedside because they do not contain instructions that can be applied in the present clinical situation (Teno et al. 1997).

Despite these limitations we should still strive to obtain a clear picture of a patient's preferences when making decisions on their behalf. In neurosurgical patients, EOL decisions often hinge on a consideration of functional outcome and quality of life. These are highly subjective concepts, and a quality of life that would not appeal to a young, highly functional healthcare worker may be perfectly acceptable to other people, particularly when the alternative is death.

8.4.3   Non-maleficence

Non-maleficence is a principle rooted in the Hippocratic tradition and is a major driver behind EOL decision-making. Aggressive medical care, surgical procedures, life support, and cardiopulmonary resuscitation can all be associated with harms, such as pain, suffering, and loss of dignity for both the patient and the family. We accept the risk of harm when there is a reasonable prospect of benefit, but as the prospect of benefit decreases, the risk of harm is hard to justify.

On the other hand, some would argue that we have a duty to prolong life in any condition, regardless of the potential for harm or the prospects for recovery. According to this principle ("vitalism"), all life is of infinite value, and death is the ultimate harm that should be avoided. Although vitalism is not endorsed by any professional society, it is a principle that is sometimes invoked by SDMs to justify ongoing aggressive care for patients with profound neurological impairment (e.g., persistent vegetative state).

> **Pearl**
> Aggressive medical care, surgical procedures, life support, and cardiopulmonary resuscitation can all be associated with harms, such as pain, suffering, and loss of dignity for both the patient and the family. The risk of harm is acceptable when there is a reasonable prospect of benefit, but as the prospect of benefit decreases, the risk of harm is hard to justify.

8.4.4 Beneficence

EOL decisions are typically motivated by a desire to avoid harm, but our illustrative case also emphasizes the importance of trying to do good. Family members will sometimes advocate for unproven or experimental therapies in the hope that these will restore health and function to patients with severe incurable illness. At times, healthcare workers may agree, simply because they feel that the patient has nothing to lose. But the condition of the patient does not override the principle of ensuring that all therapies offered to patients have a reasonable likelihood of being beneficial. This does not mean that a physician cannot offer off-label, unproven, or experimental therapies; he/she must be convinced that there is a realistic prospect that these therapies will be beneficial, either because of published reports, previous experience, or biological plausibility. But the principle of beneficence is as valid for incurable patients as it is for healthy ones.

8.4.5 Justice

Justice is arguably the most challenging principle to apply in EOL decisions, simply because there are so many concepts of justice. From a simplistic perspective, a physician should always try to make EOL decisions and recommendations based on purely clinical considerations, viewed in the context of the patient's values. In other words, treat like cases alike. However, this is a naïve exercise. Physicians cannot avoid considering nonclinical factors and applying their own culture and values to a given decision. So to ensure that EOL decisions are made consistently, it may be necessary to create explicit standards of care (Umansky et al. 2011) or even use interdisciplinary committees to review challenging cases (Ford and Kubu 2006).

At a higher level, physicians must also consider the importance of "fairness" in making EOL decisions, and how "fairness" can be defined when allocating a scare resource such as a neurosurgical ICU bed to a patient with little or no hope of recovery. On one hand, a physician might consider Rawls' argument that the greatest proportion of resources should be allocated to those who are most disadvantaged (Rawls 1999). Given our patient's condition, this would suggest that she ought to receive a commensurately high level of resources. On the other hand, a physician could take the position that if every person in a persistent vegetative state were kept alive in a neurosurgical ICU bed, these resources would not be available to other patients seeking to have the same surgery as our patient.

In other words, future patients would be denied the opportunity that was given to this patient, which would be manifestly unfair.

8.4.6   Approach to Resolution

The approach described above does not always yield agreement between the patient, SDM, and healthcare team. Conflict is common in the ICU setting and often involves disagreements about the intensity of care provided for patients with a poor prognosis (Azoulay et al. 2009). In situations like our case, a common response to conflict is disengagement on the part of the healthcare team and continuation of aggressive care. This approach may avoid angry confrontations and medicolegal consequences, but it may ultimately be harmful for all concerned. The patient will continue to receive aggressive care without a realistic prospect of benefit. The medical team will lose the ability to provide support to the husband at a time when he clearly needs it. The ongoing care will consume a large quantity of healthcare resources, and it may contribute to burnout and distress among the ICU staff (Poncet et al. 2007).

The optimal approach would be to use an ethically sound decision-making process to develop a plan of care that is acceptable to all parties, demonstrated in a published checklist for meeting the ethical and legal obligations (Sibbald et al. 2011). This checklist is shown in Table 8.2 and can be applied in many other jurisdictions as well. If conflict escalates, physicians should attempt to use conflict resolution techniques shown in Table 8.3 (Knickle et al. 2012) or mediation by a third party. Mediated solutions are usually preferable to arbitrated solutions, because in mediated solutions the two parties to the conflict are able to craft the resolution themselves. In arbitrated solutions, the resolution is created by a third party and may be unacceptable to both the healthcare team and the SDM. It is often useful to consult one's hospital Ethics Committee and/or the bioethics consult service which is usually staffed by appropriately ethics-trained physicians, social workers, PhDs, theologians, or others (Bernstein and Bowman 2003).

> **Pearl**
> In cases of conflict, many physicians disengage from the interaction with the SDM. This approach may avoid angry confrontations and medicolegal consequences, but it may ultimately be harmful for all concerned.

8.4.7   Illustrative Case Revisited

After further discussion and exploration with the patient's husband and family, the healthcare team determined that the patient had made clear statements prior to the operation that she would not want to remain on life support if she were in a "vegetative state." After multiple meetings with patient relations and the bioethics consultation team, her husband consented to withdrawal of life support, in accordance with the patient's prior capable wish.

Table 8.2 Checklist for meeting ethical and legal obligations at the end of life

Step	Dialogue and documentation
1. Ask the capable patient about wishes and beliefs	(a) "What is your understanding of your condition?"
	(b) "What worries you about your situation?"
	(c) "How do you make decisions in your family?"
	(d) "What is important to you right now when making decisions?"
	(e) If the patient is not capable, document this before proceeding to step 2
2. Identify the legally correct SDM	(a) See hierarchy of decision-makers (HCCA, Sec. 20; Government of Ontario 1996)
	(b) Document decision-maker(s)
3. Ask questions of the SDM	(a) "Is there a living will?"
	(b) "Do you know your role?" (e.g., to act on prior expressed wishes or best interests)
	(c) "Do you know what the patient would have wanted in this situation and what was important to this person?" (share beliefs or stories)
	(d) Document what you learn
4. If there is no prior applicable wish, inform the SDM about "best interests"	"If there are no prior expressed wishes, we then have to consider what is in the best interests of the patient – this means we can propose treatments that will change or improve the condition of the patient for the better, while taking into account this individual's goals, values, and beliefs"
5. Propose an indicated treatment plan	(a) "We are going to do what will benefit your loved one, and we will continue the treatments that are indicated and in [his/her] best interests"
	(b) "[Patient's name] is really sick. We will provide treatment that improves or changes [his/her] condition for the better, so that leaves us with the following options: palliative care, comfort care …"
	(c) "When a treatment is no longer indicated, we will let you know that we are no longer providing it"
6. If no consent is obtained, state the following	(a) "It is a challenge when we cannot reach agreement; however, we have a resource that can help us, called the Consent and Capacity Board. It is a neutral third party that will come into the hospital and listen to both sides of the story. The board will then decide what is in the best interests of the patient." "The patient would be appointing a lawyer, and the physician may have a lawyer as well. You personally are entitled to have one also (refer to www.ccboard.on.ca)"
	(b) Document that you have explained the role of CCB. Give the family time to ask questions

CCB Consent and Capacity Board, *HCCA* Health Care Consent Act, *SDM* substitute decision-maker
Adapted from Sibbald et al. (2011)

8.4.8 Withdrawal of Life Support, Assisted Death, and the Doctrine of Double Effect

Even after the decision is taken to WHLS/WDLS, patient management can be highly variable. There are no published guidelines for the clinical management of WDLS, although some groups have developed standardized order forms (Treece et al. 2004). As life support is withdrawn, physicians have a clear duty to provide adequate symptom management. Although some comfort medications (e.g., opioids) have the potential to shorten life if given in inappropriate doses, studies have

Table 8.3 Conflict resolution techniques

Technique/skill	Function	Example
Validating: support and acknowledgement of the parties' feelings	Acknowledges the feeling of hurt and conveys respect and acceptance. Allows understanding of feelings and other perspectives.	"You're feeling overwhelmed by having to make these decisions… where do you begin?"
Reflecting (in the form of a question): checking in and interpreting what you have heard	Similar to clarifying, reflecting provides an opening for a richer and more thorough response. Allow an opportunity to expand upon and clarify a perspective. An opportunity to confirm and acknowledge feelings.	"You're feeling like your efforts aren't being recognized or respected by the intensive care unit staff or by me… am I accurate?"
Paraphrasing: using your own words to interpret your colleagues' thoughts and feelings	Lets the speaker know that you hear the message they are sending. Gives the receiver (perceiver) the same opportunity. Slows down the pace of the conversation.	"You feel like we have been disrespectful and neglectful in your mother's care"
Questioning: appropriate use of open- and close-ended questions	Opens up discussion. Allows exchange of information. Encourages expression. Obtains information about facts and feelings. Confirms understanding. Provides insight about who, what, where, why, and how.	Open: "Can you help me understand more about…?" Closed: "When did you decide to…?"
Clarifying: checking to verify facts, information, or feelings that have been expressed	Proof positive that you are listening closely. Helps elucidate or disarms conflict issues.	"You're finding this hard because you're not sure if it's what your mother would have really wanted… Would that be fair to say?"
Summarizing: brief verbal reviews throughout your conversation and a final summary moving to settlement	Helps to maintain a mutual and accurate understanding of facts, interests, needs, and positions. Keeps the discussion on track (i.e., "where we are"). Helps focus the parties. A final summary of your mutual agreement enhances the resolution process.	"You think we don't respect your efforts and goals, so you have been unwilling to engage in any more discussion with us"

Adapted from Knickle et al. (2012)

shown that comfort medications do not shorten life when given in appropriate dose (Chan et al. 2004; Gallagher 2010).

Nevertheless, some physicians may undertreat symptoms in an attempt to ensure that they do cross the line between symptom control and assisted death, which is illegal in most parts of the world. Indeed, doses of opioids and sedatives used for symptom management during WDLS are similar to those used for many cases of assisted death in the ICU, suggesting that the distinction cannot be made on the basis of medication dose alone (Sprung et al. 2008).

The Doctrine of Double Effect holds that it is acceptable for a physician to inadvertently shorten life by administering a dose of comfort medication, provided that the intent of the physician was to provide comfort rather than shorten life. The "Double Effect" refers to the effect that is intended (comfort) as well as the effect that is foreseen but not intended (shortening of life). Provided that the physician is administering reasonable doses of medication, the key distinction between comfort care and assisted death is the intent of the physician.

Conclusion

EOL decisions are common among neurosurgical patients, especially in the ICU. In order to make good EOL decisions, physicians must engage in an ethically sound process of shared decision-making, with mediation and conflict resolution as needed to ensure that the decisions are acceptable to patients, SDMs, and the healthcare team alike.

References

Azoulay E, Timsit JF, Sprung CL et al (2009) Prevalence and factors of intensive care unit conflicts: the conflicus study. Am J Respir Crit Care Med 180:853–860

Barnato AE, Chang C-CH, Saynina O et al (2007) Influence of race on inpatient treatment intensity at the end of life. J Gen Intern Med 22:338–345

Bernstein M, Bowman K (2003) Should a medical/surgical specialist with formal training in bioethics provide health care ethics consultation in his/her own area of specialty? HEC Forum 15:274–286

Bulow HH, Sprung CL, Reinhart K et al (2008) The world's major religions' points of view on end-of-life decisions in the intensive care unit. Intensive Care Med 34:423–430

Chan JD, Treece PD, Engelberg RA et al (2004) Narcotic and benzodiazepine use after withdrawal of life support: association with time to death? Chest 126:286–293

Cook D (2001) Patient autonomy versus parentalism. Crit Care Med 29(2 Suppl):N24–N25

Emanuel EJ, Emanuel LL (1992) Four models of the physician-patient relationship. JAMA 267:2221–2226

Ford PJ, Kubu CS (2006) Stimulating debate: ethics in a multidisciplinary functional neurosurgery committee. J Med Ethics 32:106–109

Fowler RA, Noyahr L-A, Thornton JD et al (2010) An official American Thoracic Society systematic review: the association between health insurance status and access, care, delivery, and outcomes for patients who are critically ill. Am J Respir Crit Care Med 181:1003–1011

Gallagher R (2010) Killing the symptom without killing the patient. Can Fam Physician 56(6): 544–546, e210–512

Knickle K, McNaughton N, Downar J (2012) Beyond winning: mediation, conflict resolution, and non-rational sources of conflict in the ICU. Crit Care 16:308

Kritek PA, Slutsky AS, Hudson LD (2009) Clinical decisions. Care of an unresponsive patient with a poor prognosis – polling results. NEJM 360:e15

Muni S, Engelberg RA, Treece PD et al (2011) The Influence of race/ethnicity and socioeconomic status on end-of-life care in the ICU. Chest 139:1025–1033

Poncet MC, Toullic P, Papazian L et al (2007) Burnout syndrome in critical care nursing staff. Am J Respir Crit Care Med 175:698–704

Prendergast TJ, Claessens MT, Luce JM (1998) A national survey of end-of-life care for critically ill patients. Am J Respir Crit Care Med 158:1163–1167

Rawls J (1999) A theory of justice revised. Oxford University Press, Oxford

Shalowitz DI, Garrett-Mayer E, Wendler D (2006) The accuracy of surrogate decision makers: a systematic review. Arch Intern Med 166:493–497

Sibbald RW, Chidwick P, Handelman M et al (2011) Checklist to meet ethical and legal obligations to critically ill patients at the end of life. Healthc Q 14:60–66

Sprung CL, Cohen SL, Sjokvist P et al (2003) End-of-life practices in European intensive care units: the Ethicus Study. JAMA 290:790–797

Sprung CL, Ledoux D, Bulow HH et al (2008) Relieving suffering or intentionally hastening death: where do you draw the line? Crit Care Med 36:8–13

Sprung CL, Maia P, Bulow HH et al (2007) The importance of religious affiliation and culture on end-of-life decisions in European intensive care units. Intensive Care Med 33:1732–1739

Stelfox HT, Hemmelgarn BR, Bagshaw SM et al (2012) Intensive care unit bed availability and outcomes for hospitalized patients with sudden clinical deterioration. Arch Intern Med 172:467–474

Teno JM, Licks S, Lynn J et al (1997) Do advance directives provide instructions that direct care? SUPPORT Investigators. Study to understand prognoses and preferences for outcomes and risks of treatment. J Am Geriatr Soc 45:508–512

Treece PD, Engelberg RA, Crowley L et al (2004) Evaluation of a standardized order form for the withdrawal of life support in the intensive care unit. Crit Care Med 32:1141–1148

Turgeon AF, Lauzier F, Burns KEA et al (2013) Determination of neurologic prognosis and clinical decision making in adult patients with severe traumatic brain injury: a survey of Canadian intensivists, neurosurgeons, and neurologists. Crit Care Med 41:1086–1093

Umansky F, Black PL, DiRocco C et al (2011) Statement of ethics in neurosurgery of the world federation of neurosurgical societies. World Neurosurg 76:239–247

Vig EK, Taylor JS, Starks H et al (2006) Beyond substituted judgment: how surrogates navigate end-of-life decision-making. J Am Geriatr Soc 54:1688–1693

White DB, Braddock CH, Bereknyei S et al (2007) Toward shared decision making at the end of life in intensive care units: opportunities for improvement. Arch Intern Med 167:461–467

Wunsch H, Harrison DA, Harvey S et al (2005) End-of-life decisions: a cohort study of the withdrawal of all active treatment in intensive care units in the United Kingdom. Intensive Care Med 31:823–831

Dying with Dignity

9

Yoko Kato and Michael Reid

9.1 Introduction

Over the last decade end-of-life care has made a transition from a passive to an active discipline in order to allow patients a dignified death. The patient's last days and eventual death can have a profound effect on the patient, his/her family and those involved in his/her healthcare. Care of this period in every patient's journey is a vital element of value-based medicine. It is crucial that doctors understand the ethical and moral concepts surrounding this topic.

Most people would choose to die at home if given the option (Department of Health UK 2008), though opinions are likely to vary due to different cultural and religious beliefs, and suffering at home for dying patient can be substantial (Ruijs et al. 2013). A minority die in hospice care (Sexauer et al. 2014), but it is more likely that they will die in hospital (Gomes and Higginson 2008). This disparity is likely to continue to grow as medical technologies advance giving us the ability to prolong life further. Accompanying this development is a growing debate around the removal of life support and an increasing emphasis on the quality of patients' lives as they near death. Central to this debate is the ability to allow patients to die with dignity, that is, to be able to die without undue or prolonged suffering (in accordance with article 3 of the Human Rights Act 1998) but just as importantly to die in a place and manner in accordance with the patient's wishes.

Y. Kato, MD, PhD (✉)
Department of Neurosurgery, Fujita Health University, 1-98 Dengakugakubo,
Kutsukake-choToyoake, Aichi, 470-1192, Japan
e-mail: neuron1@fujita-hu.ac.jp

M. Reid
Addenbrooke's Hospital, University of Cambridge School of Clinical Medicine,
Box 111, Hills Road, Cambridge, CB2 0SP, UK
e-mail: mdr47@cam.ac.uk

A. Ammar, M. Bernstein (eds.), *Neurosurgical Ethics in Practice: Value-based Medicine*, 101
DOI 10.1007/978-3-642-54980-9_9, © Springer-Verlag Berlin Heidelberg 2014

A thorough understanding of these aspects is crucial in providing appropriate and sensitive end-of-life care (Vincent 2001). This is especially relevant in neurosurgery where patients may often lack autonomy, for example, when cognitively impaired, intubated or paralysed. This is further complicated by unclear and potentially debilitating prognoses. However, it should be noted that dying with dignity should not be reserved solely for complicated patients. Instead, it should be omnipresent in every doctor's mind when faced with a patient at the end of life (Singer and MacDonald 1998).

As these issues become more prevalent, it is our duty as doctors and healthcare professionals to review our practice and each individual must form their own opinions as well as develop appropriate strategies for dealing with these complex cases at a departmental and societal level. This chapter will display the different views and objective data around the care at the end of patients' lives and aims to provide a framework for future decision-making in order to facilitate dying with dignity.

9.2 Illustrative Case (Withdrawal of Life Support When All Hope Is Lost)

A 72 year-old man presents with sudden loss of consciousness. CT demonstrates a subarachnoid haemorrhage. Despite best efforts, he suffers extensive brain injury leaving him ventilator dependent. He has no advanced directive to refuse treatment or written record of his wishes and he is not well known to his family physician. After 2 weeks with no sign of neurological recovery, the medical team begins to consider the withdrawal of intensive care. However, his wife is keen to continue ventilatory support in the hope that her husband will recover. The nursing staff have raised concerns that they feel uncomfortable continuing the patient's treatment and are uneasy answering his wife's questions.

When should life-sustaining treatment be withdrawn? Who has the right to make this decision? What strategies can be used to avoid conflict? How can the teams concerns be alleviated? What further steps should be taken once life-sustaining treatment has ceased?

9.3 Approach to the Case

In the absence of any legally binding document stating the patient's wishes, it falls to the doctor to make a decision that they believe would be in the patient's best interest – including when it is appropriate to withdraw life-sustaining treatment and begin palliative care. To make this decision a thorough understanding of the literature and current opinions around the patient's condition and possible avenues of treatment is needed. This knowledge provides the basis from which decisions can be made.

The first port of call should then be the patient's family, both to explore the patient's wife's wishes and to better understand what the patient may have wanted. If the patient engaged in advanced care planning with his loved ones, the process is smoother for family and healthcare providers (Singer et al. 1996). It is also imperative that the family fully understand the nature of the patient's terminal condition and the futility of continuing treatment. Taking time to talk through these issues with the family can often save time and avoid unnecessary conflict (Oppenheim et al. 2004). Furthermore, these conflicts have the potential to compromise patient care (Prendergast and Puntillo 2002). The case should also be discussed with everyone involved in the patient's care and everyone should have an opportunity to voice their opinions.

Pearl
Documentation is important in all cases, but especially where decisions around end-of-life care are involved and/or the patient lacks autonomy.

If both the patient's family and healthcare professionals agree on the decision to withdraw life-sustaining treatment, it is essential that a discussion takes place where the reasoning behind the decision is explained and the family has the chance to ask any questions that they may still have. Once again it is important that this discussion is documented. It is often appropriate to provide support services for the family such as the option to meet a faith leader, ethicist or counsellor.

It must be emphasized that the withdrawal of life-sustaining treatment is not the end of the doctor's duty of care but rather the start of a new phase of treatment with an aim to ease the transition from life to death. Before, throughout and after the removal of ventilation, a careful plan should be used to provide symptomatic relief for the patient, for example, pain relief and anti-emetics.

Formal integrated care pathways have also been used to provide a guide to end-of-life care where there are no longer any treatment options, for example, the National End of Life Care Programme in the United Kingdom (Department of Health 2008).

Pearl
The opinion of other colleagues not directly involved in the patient's care can provide an objective view in complex cases.

9.4 Discussion

When making decisions about end-of-life care and the removal of life-sustaining treatment, it is useful to refer to the principles of biomedical ethics (Beauchmap and Childress 1979).

9.4.1   Autonomy

Autonomy is often compromised in neurosurgical patients and ultimately this is the source of many of the difficulties discussed above. In order to avoid such difficulties, decisions concerning end-of-life care should be discussed with the patient before any procedure is undertaken and their wishes recorded in an advanced directive or equivalent document. These legal documents ensure that the patient is treated in accordance with their wishes even when they are no longer able to communicate them. Unfortunately, the opportunity to discuss these decisions with patients and their families is not often taken (Bosshard et al. 2005).

In cases where advanced directives have not been completed, the families' wishes will often mirror that of the patient and their views should be held in high regard. However, care must be taken and ultimately it is the doctor's decision when treatment should be withdrawn. In instances where the patient's family and doctor disagree, it is wise for the doctor to seek support from others, including the legal and bioethics services.

9.4.2   Justice

At an individual level, all patients deserve to be treated with the same high level of respect, care and professionalism regardless of their individual choices or background. This should extend up to and beyond the end of their lives.

At a population level, the needs of a patient should be taken in the context of the needs of others. This presents a tricky ethical issue where it is hard to reconcile non-maleficence and the fair allocation of resources. This contention is likely to continue as the expected level of care at the end of life increases in line with its cost. Demands on cost savings may then begin to compromise ethical principles (Bernat 1997).

9.4.3   Beneficence and Non-maleficence

Beneficence and non-maleficence should be guiding principles, both in the decision process and in the institution of palliative treatment. It is often uncomfortable for doctors when the aim of their treatment is no longer curative but instead purely palliative. This does not just refer to the removal of life support but also to the cessation or withholding of futile treatments. It might be considered that this contradicts the principle of non-maleficence and ignores beneficence. However, when there is no hope of recovery to a meaningful quality of life for the patient, the doctor's role changes to one solely of care rather than cure. The wishes of patients may also be unfamiliar or opposed to the doctor's own way of thinking, but nevertheless it is the doctor's duty to enact them to the best of his/her ability. In doing so they should not impeach any other patients' rights nor their own ethical code.

> **Pearl**
> The doctor's role does not end when life-sustaining treatment is removed.
> Instead care becomes purely palliative but is of no less importance. This is the
> essence of dying with dignity.

Many doctors struggle with the concept of withdrawing life-sustaining treatment
as it seems to create conflict between beneficence and non-maleficence. However,
as most patients in neurological intensive care die from the removal of life support
(Varelas et al. 2009), doctors must be clear on the ethical basis of this judgement.
The argument in favour of the removal of life support states that to continue this
treatment puts the patient through unnecessary suffering with no clear positive outcome, thus contravening non-maleficence and beneficence, respectively. The
removal of endotracheal tubes has also been shown to allow more effective communication at the end of life, which may provide 'moral clarity' for both the doctor
and family (Reynolds et al. 2005).

The counterargument is that the withdrawal of life-sustaining treatment is an act
of maleficence since it hastens death. It has also been argued that continuing ventilation allows for better prognostication and management of the dying patient by the
family, though this is only ethically defensible when the patient's wishes do not
oppose it (De Lora and Blanco 2013).

Formal integrated care pathways, such as the National End of Life Care
Programme in the UK, have attracted much attention from the media who incorrectly
infer that they encourage doctors to start palliative care inappropriately. However,
when used responsibly these pathways can provide a useful tool in managing patients
and ensure that measures are taken to allow as many patients as possible to die with
dignity. They have been shown not to be harmful but have yet to show any clinically
significant benefit, though they are still considered the gold standard by many physicians (Chan and Webster 2010). It has been suggested that this lack of evidence is
due to the ethical and practical issues involved with performing randomized control
trials among palliative patients (Fowell et al. 2004; Karlawish 2003).

9.4.4   The Role of the Team

The duty of a patient's care is not solely the responsibility of the doctor and working
as a team in complex cases is needed to achieve a good outcome. A discussion of
complex cases not only allows the team to make a more informed decision (Vincent
2001) but also ensures that each member of the team understands the objective of
any treatment. Establishing these meetings as a precedent is important since the
most common hurdles facing satisfactory end-of-life care are a lack of communication among decision makers, no agreement on a course of end-of-life care and failure to implement a timely end-of-life plan of care (Travis et al. 2002). Even when
patients choose to die at home, multidisciplinary team management is needed to
provide effective symptomatic relief (Pace et al. 2009).

> **Pearl**
> Multidisciplinary team meetings can provide an opportunity for ideas and concerns to be expressed by any member of the healthcare team, ultimately leading to improved patient care.

9.5 Recommendations

The National End of Life Care Programme is an example of a formalized collection of pathways that 'aims to ensure that high quality, person-centred care is provided which is well planned, coordinated and monitored, while being responsive to the individual's needs and wishes'. It proposes six steps as outlined in Fig. 9.1.

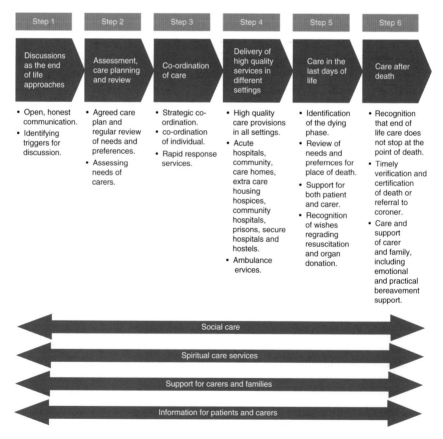

Fig. 9.1 The six steps of the National End of Life Care Pathway (Reprinted courtesy of the Department of Health, England)

These integrated care pathways can provide a useful guide for doctors with patients approaching the end of life but may need to be adapted dependent on availability of resources and cultural variability. As mentioned above, there is currently not sufficient evidence to prove the efficacy of these pathways. However, it is likely that in the future quantitative evidence will be available and that further refinement will consolidate these pathways' central role in patient care.

Algorithms that have a focus on a particular aspect of end-of-life care have been proposed. An example algorithm has been proposed (Szalados 2007) which approaches the issues from an ethical and legal perspective but provides a practical step-by-step guide for the removal of ventilation. This algorithm is split into three phases:
1. During the determination of directives and delineation of end-of-life care
2. Prior to discontinuation of life support or ventilator withdrawal
3. During and after ventilation removal

There are many tools available to help healthcare professionals deal with the difficulties of end-of-life care, but ultimately they share the common but often complicated aim of allowing patients to die with dignity. Whatever approaches are used, it is important that they are sustainable, practical and agreed upon by the healthcare team.

Conclusion

'Dying with Dignity' is a complex and expanding topic that is particularly relevant in neurosurgery. It is likely to become more prominent in the future as technology advances, the population ages and expectations of healthcare rise. A useful approach to the ethical problems is to follow the four principles of biomedical ethics. The role of the team is essential in both the decision-making process and in the provision of care. Formal integrated pathways can provide a pragmatic structure for care at the end of life.

Acknowledgement The authors thank Mr. Jeremy Sharma for his invaluable help with the manuscript.

References

Beauchmap TL, Childress JF (1979) Principles of biomedical ethics. Oxford University Press, New York

Bernat JL (1997) Quality of neurological care: balancing cost control and ethics. Arch Neurol 54(11):1341–1345

Bosshard G, Nilstun T, Bilsen J, European End-of-Life Consortium et al (2005) Forgoing treatment at the end of life in 6 European countries. Arch Intern Med 165(4):401–407

Chan R, Webster J (2010) End-of-life care pathways for improving outcomes in caring for the dying (Review). Cochrane Database Syst Rev 1:1–16. doi:10.1002/14651858.CD008006.pub2

De Lora P, Blanco AP (2013) Dignifying death and the morality of elective ventilation. J Med Ethics 39(3):145–148

Department of Health (2008) End of life care strategy – promoting high quality care for all adults at the end of life. www.dh.gov.uk/publications

Fowell A, Russell I, Johnstone R et al (2004) Randomisation or randomised consent as an appropriate methodology for trials in palliative care: a feasibility study. BMC Palliat Care 3(1):1

Gomes B, Higginson I (2008) Where people die (1974–2030): past trends, future projections and implications for care. Palliat Med 22:33

Karlawish JH (2003) Conducting research that involves subjects at the end of life who are unable to give consent. J Pain Symptom Manage 25(4):S14–S24

Oppenheim D, Brugières L, Corradini N et al (2004) An ethics dilemma: when parents and doctors disagree on the best treatment for the child. Bull Cancer 91:735–738

Pace A, Di Lorenzo C, Guariglia L et al (2009) End of life issues in brain tumor patients. J Neurooncol 91(1):39–43

Prendergast TJ, Puntillo KA (2002) Withdrawal of life support: intensive caring at the end of life. JAMA 288(2):2732–2740

Reynolds S, Cooper AB, McKneally M (2005) Withdrawing life-sustaining treatment: ethical considerations. Thorac Surg Clin 15(4):469–480

Ruijs CD, Kerkhof AJ, van der Wal G et al (2013) Symptoms, unbearability and the nature of suffering in terminal cancer patients dying at home: a prospective primary care study. BMC Fam Pract 14:201

Sexauer A, Cheng MJ, Knight L et al (2014) Patterns of hospice use in patients dying from hematologic malignancies. J Palliat Med 17(2):195–9

Singer PA, MacDonald N (1998) Bioethics for clinicians: 15. Quality end-of-life care. CMAJ 159:159–162

Singer PA, Robertson G, Roy DJ (1996) Bioethics for clinicians: 6. Advance care planning. CMAJ 155:1689–1692

Szalados JE (2007) Discontinuation of mechanical ventilation at end-of-life: the ethical and legal boundaries of physician conduct in termination of life support. Crit Care Clin 23(2):317–337

Travis S, Bernard M, Dixon S et al (2002) Obstacles to palliation and end-of-life care in a long-term care facility. Gerontologist 42(3):342–349

Varelas PN, Hacein-Bey L, Schultz L et al (2009) Withdrawal of life support in critically ill neurosurgical patients and in-hospital death after discharge from the neurosurgical intensive care unit. Clinical article. J Neurosurg 11(2):396–404

Vincent JL (2001) Cultural differences in end-of-life care. Crit Care Med 292(2):n52–n55

Brain Death

10

Jeffrey M. Singh and Mark Bernstein

10.1 Introduction

Brain death is the determination of death by neurological criteria, in contrast to the traditional determination of death by assessing a lack of circulation and respiration. Brain death is only relevant in patients who have suffered severe brain injuries, many of which are due to neurosurgical conditions, and who are receiving modern critical care, such that they have complete and irreversible loss of all brain function, but their other vital organs are supported and continue to function. Many jurisdictions have equated brain death with death determined by cardiopulmonary arrest, as brain death reflects the notion of irreversibly lost personhood due to the irreversible loss of brain function.

Brain death is important because the concept of brain death exposes a diversity of beliefs in society, and frequently becomes the flashpoint for ethical dilemmas for healthcare teams, or conflicts between healthcare teams and families (Lazar et al. 2001). These conflicts can be a source of anxiety and stress to surgeons and can undermine trust between physicians and families. It is important that all practicing neurosurgeons have a strong understanding of the clinical and ethical framework for the determination of brain death, as well as the specific legal statutes and legal framework supporting brain death in their practice jurisdiction. It is a core issue in the practice of value-based medicine.

J.M. Singh, MD, FRCPC (✉)
Division of Respirology, Interdepartmental Division of Critical Care Medicine,
Toronto Western Hospital, University of Toronto, 399 Bathurst Street 2 McLaughlin
PavillioN 411K, Toronto, ON M5T 2S8, Canada
e-mail: jeff.singh@uhn.ca

M. Bernstein, MD, MHSc, FRCSC
Division of Neurosurgery, Toronto Western Hospital, University of Toronto,
399 Bathurst Street, Toronto, ON M5T 2S8, Canada
e-mail: mark.bernstein@uhn.ca

A. Ammar, M. Bernstein (eds.), *Neurosurgical Ethics in Practice: Value-based Medicine*, 109
DOI 10.1007/978-3-642-54980-9_10, © Springer-Verlag Berlin Heidelberg 2014

> **Pearl**
> Skillful communication surrounding brain death may allow families to start the grieving and closure process earlier, and help them navigate this emotionally and culturally charged issue.

10.2 Illustrative Case (Family's Refusal of Withdrawal of Care After Brain Death Declared)

A 30-year-old woman is brought to the emergency department after a witnessed collapse following which she was found to have a cardiac arrest. Following EMS response and 30 min of resuscitative efforts, she has return of spontaneous circulation and is brought to the emergency department, where she is found on computed tomography to have a large subarachnoid haemorrhage secondary to a ruptured basilar aneurysm. Despite insertion of a ventricular drain, she never recovers motor responses or brainstem reflexes. On the third day in the neurosurgical intensive care unit, she has no response to pain, no brainstem reflexes, and has no respiratory efforts on apnea testing. There are no metabolic or pharmacologic confounders, and she has never received sedatives or paralytic agents. In accordance with local medical guidelines and law, she is declared brain dead.

When the family is informed that she has been declared brain dead, they refuse to accept this determination and are adamant in their belief that she is alive. They refuse to allow discontinuation of the mechanical ventilator, stating that in their eyes she is still alive while her heart is still beating and she is warm. They demand ongoing interventions and care including tracheostomy, enteral nutrition, and mechanical ventilation.

10.3 Approach to the Case

Death is a universal life event which is deeply founded in cultural, religious, and spiritual beliefs. The impact of pronouncing someone dead has immense personal, legal, and social implications. Indeed, death is simultaneously a medical, social, and legal event.

Until the twentieth century, death was determined by medical practitioners by the irreversible interruption of one of the three vital functions: respiration, circulation, and brain function. When an individual had cessation of any of respiration, circulation, or brain function, the termination of the remaining functions quickly followed. This determination was relatively simple and highly valid given the inability of practitioners to intervene and support vital functions. The development of modern life support, specifically positive pressure mechanical ventilation and haemodynamic support, has complicated the determination of death by allowing temporary uncoupling of these three vital functions. Indeed, the circulatory and respiratory systems can be supported for some time despite the irreversible destruction of the entire brain and brainstem. This requires a novel method for determination of death in these patients, thus the inception of brain death.

In this case, the approach is simply to talk to the family, have others talk to them like their spiritual leader and/or the ethics consultation team, and hope things get resolved favourably. In the uncommon situation of an absolute impasse happening, the healthcare team generally honours the family's wishes as opposed to taking the issue to the legal system. In extreme situations cases have gone to the courts, and in these cases the family is generally ruled against (Life support for pregnant woman ordered removed by Texas judge 2014).

Pearl
When an impasse occurs between a family and the healthcare team over brain death, a number of simple strategies may help: (1) talk at length to the family in simple but informative terms, (2) engage help from ethics teams and/or spiritual leaders, (3) invite the family to witness a brain death test on their loved one, and (4) be as patient and compassionate as possible.

10.4   Discussion

10.4.1   History of Brain Death

As outlined above, the evolution of critical care and life-sustaining therapies required the development of a novel method for determining death in patients with severe and irreversible injuries to the entire brain. Critics of brain death determination have often used the tight temporal association of the development of formal brain death criteria and the advent of organ donation as proof that the concept of brain death was developed to serve a utilitarian purpose of organ donation (Parker and Shemie 2002; Truog and Robinson 2003). This is not entirely correct, as the concept of brain death was already evolving within the medical community prior to the first successful organ transplants.

Medicine had recognized by the mid-twentieth century that brain function was necessary for life, and the irreversible cessation of brain function was sufficient in and of itself for death. There were initially multiple publications of observations that patients who had severe brain injury, persistent unresponsive coma, and apnea had absence of intracranial blood flow on angiography (Riishede and Ethelberg 1953; Wertheimer et al. 1960). Further reports confirmed that such patients also had absence of electroencephalographic activity and uniformly had cardiac arrest upon withdrawal of mechanical ventilation or haemodynamic support. Finally, the term 'coma dépassé' was coined; this later became the foundation for the modern conceptual framework of brain death (Mollaret and Goulon 1959).

Following this seminal paper the concept that patients on respiratory and haemo-dynamic support could be determined dead by neurological criteria evolved slowly. In the United States, the advent of organ donation precipitated the creation of the Ad Hoc Committee of the Harvard Medical School in 1968 that published the first cri-teria for the determination of brain death (A definition of irreversible coma 1968). Since then medical associations in countries around the globe have produced guidelines for the diagnosis of brain death (Diagnosis of brain death 1976).

10.4.2   Clinical Determination of Brain Death

The requirement that brain function is necessary for life is justified by the fact that the brain conducts the critical functions of the body as a whole and coordinates the various vital organs to maintain homeostasis. Most medical societies and countries have adopted either the whole-brain (Shemie et al. 2006; American Academy of Neurology 1995) or brainstem formulations of brain death (Diagnosis of brain death 1976).

The majority of jurisdictions require demonstration of whole-brain death, mean-ing all functions of the brain, including the brainstem, diencephalon, and both cerebral hemispheres, have irreversibly ceased. The pathophysiology of whole-brain death usually involves the progression of severe brain injury to elevated intracranial pressure, critical reduction of cerebral perfusion, and infarction of all brain structures. Consequently, the determination of death under this formulation requires the demonstration of the irreversible cessation of all brain functions. Some jurisdic-tions, notably the United Kingdom, have adopted a formulation of brain death requiring only irreversible and complete injury to the brainstem (brainstem death), on the rationale that the brainstem is required for arousal and maintenance of respi-ration and circulation. Consequently, this formulation does not require the irreversible loss of all brain functions but only those required for the integrated functioning of the organism as a whole.

The clinical process of brain death declaration usually includes several compo-nents: (1) determination of a mechanism of injury compatible with brain death, e.g. imaging evidence of cerebral herniation; (2) the ruling out of any metabolic or pharmacologic confounders; (3) evaluation of brainstem functions including apnea testing; and (4) confirmatory testing if required (e.g. electroencephalography or transcranial Doppler assessment of blood flow). Some jurisdictions also allow for ancillary testing, which replaces the clinical examination in situations where confounders preclude reliable clinical examination (e.g. barbiturate coma) or when clinical examination is impossible. These are usually imaging examinations which evaluate the presence of intracranial blood flow, with death being confirmed when no cerebral blood flow is evident. It should be noted that brain death declaration should be conducted with the purpose of proving death, with the base assumption that the individual is not dead. Consequently, one of the core principles in the clinical determination of brain death is that the well-being of the patient should not be jeopardized during the determination itself. For example, apnea testing should be aborted if cardiorespiratory instability develops, and caloric testing should be deferred if there is significant ear or tympanic membrane trauma and irrigation is contraindicated.

Critics have voiced the obvious concern that the two formulations of brain death (whole-brain death and brainstem death) allow for inherent inconsistencies. For example, the whole-brain formulation would require loss of all brain functions, even though neuroendocrine function is observed to persist in some patients (e.g. not all brain-dead patients develop diabetes insipidus from a lack of antidiuretic hormone), and not all patients become poikilothermic (Truog and Miller 2012). This apparent contradiction is sidestepped, however, with the brainstem death formulation. The application of confirmatory or ancillary tests is also problematic, as the whole-brain death formulation would require complete infarction and intracranial circulatory arrest, while this would not be necessarily required in the brainstem formulation. These inconsistencies have led to a call for a global consensus and definition of death to ensure consistent determination across jurisdictions (Smith 2012).

It is important to recognize that the criteria for declaring brain death in neonates and children may be slightly different than that for adults, and especially paediatric neurosurgeons need to be clear on this issue (Nakagawa et al. 2012).

> **Pearl**
> Determination of brain death usually includes (1) determination of a mechanism of injury compatible with brain death, e.g. imaging evidence of cerebral herniation; (2) the ruling out of any metabolic or pharmacologic confounders; (3) evaluation of brainstem functions including apnea testing; and (4) confirmatory testing if required (e.g. EEG or transcranial Doppler assessment of blood flow).

10.4.3 Prognostic Implications of Brain Death

A key tenet of brain death is the irreversibility of the neurological injury. One retrospective review included over one thousand patients, reported in the literature, who were ventilated until asystole after meeting clinical criteria for brain death and found no survivors (Pallis 1983). A systematic review that was part of an update to the 1995 American Academy of Neurology statement found no reports of neurological recovery after brain death using modern brain death criteria (Wijdicks et al. 2010). Case reports of improvement following determination of brain death are often refuted based on failure to adhere to standard procedures and guidelines, resulting in misdiagnosis of brain death (Gardiner et al. 2012).

For decades, it had been recognized that brain death heralds inevitable cardiovascular collapse. With modern critical care there are now increasing reports of prolonged somatic or physiological support of individuals following determination of brain death, usually involving the physiological support of pregnant women who were declared brain dead until the baby could be delivered. There is one reported case of a child supported for many years, although the diagnosis of brain death was made in retrospect and was never strictly confirmed according to modern criteria (Repertinger et al. 2006). One retrospective case series found 175 cases of brain death in which the patient was maintained on physiological support for greater than 1 week and found seven patients survived to 6 months. Unfortunately, the rigour of the brain death declarations could not be ascertained retrospectively, and the study included cases of diagnostic controversy (Shewmon 1998). Finally, it should be noted that in these cases of prolonged physiological support, there was no improvement in neurological function, despite the prolonged period of observation, supporting the belief that both the neurological injuries were irreversible and permanent (Gardiner et al. 2012).

10.4.4 Adoption of Brain Death Across Jurisdictions and Cultures

There is broad acceptance of the concept of brain death across medical communities, jurisdictions, religions, and countries. Medical societies in several countries have published consensus statements and guidelines both defining and outlining the clinical determination of brain death (American Academy of Neurology 1995; Australian and New Zealand Intensive Care Society 1993; Shemie et al. 2006). In the United States the concept of brain death was also validated by a Presidential Commission in 1981 that published *A Report on the Medical, Legal and Ethical Issues in the Determination of Death*. This report embraced the concept that the irreversible loss of whole-brain function was death and gave it equivalent footing to death determined by cardiopulmonary criteria. These statements were affirmed in 2008 after the US President's Council on Bioethics performed a detailed review on all of the ethical and philosophical arguments that defined brain death as death and concluded that the definition was still valid (Controversies in the determination of death 2008).

Many jurisdictions do not have a definition of death codified into law. Although death has significant legal implications, there are no legal statutes to support or refute determination of death by cardiopulmonary, neurological, or other criteria. From a legal point of view, a person is considered dead when a qualified person pronounces that no further medical care is appropriate and that a patient should be considered dead under the law. The specific criteria by which a patient is declared dead may vary somewhat across jurisdictions, but it is important for healthcare providers to note that statutory law in most countries does not specifically outline the explicit clinical criteria with which a person is declared dead – the practice and clinical standards of declaring death are usually deferred to the medical profession.

There are several jurisdictions in which brain death has been codified into statutory law. In the United States, the Uniform Determination of Death Act gave statutory recognition to brain death as a concept and equated it with the more widely recognized concept of death determined by cardiorespiratory arrest (e.g. brain death is death in the eyes of the law) (National Conference of Commissioners on Uniform State Laws 1980). Similar legislation has been passed in Australia and the United Kingdom and supported by the Canadian provincial case law.

Pearl

Brain death has been accepted broadly in ethics, medicine, and law, but some surgeons and societies still have not embraced and adopted it. Furthermore, some individuals do not accept brain death, even though they live within jurisdictions that accept brain death as a group.

10.4.5 Criticism of Brain Death and Accommodation

Despite this widespread acceptance, there remain some populations in which there are strong criticisms of brain death and occasionally rejection of the concept as a whole. For example, in Japan (Lock 1999) and Germany (Schöne-Seifert 1999), there has been gradual acceptance of brain death by the medical and legal communities, but the concept still faces criticism from a significant proportion of the public. Strong religious opposition also exists within certain segments of the Muslim, Buddhist, Native American, and Orthodox Jewish communities globally. Rejection of brain death and insistence on the traditional cardiopulmonary determination of death have been based on ethical or religious arguments (Truog and Robinson 2003).

Accommodation of religious and moral dissent to the concept of brain death varies across jurisdictions. This ranges from non-acceptance and reliance on the traditional cardiopulmonary determination of death in some countries, to conditional acceptance, to accommodation on an individual basis. In Japan, where the traditional Buddhist and Shinto concepts of death require cessation of heartbeat and respiration, brain death is still recognized but is only acknowledged as human death when a transplant is to be performed.

Perhaps the most confusing and variable example of such variability is in the United States, where such legislation falls not under federal law, but to the individual states. New York and New Jersey have enacted legislation to require healthcare providers and hospitals to either accommodate the refusal of the determination of brain death by families or prevent the determination of brain death itself based on the objection of the family. This may lead to the confusing scenario where an individual is dead in one state but not in another or may be conditionally dead depending on their religious or expressed beliefs.

Even within countries in which there is strong support for the concept of brain death within the medical and legal communities, healthcare providers may meet significant objection or disagreement with the determination of death due to misunderstanding, misinterpretation, of other experiences with coma, or personal, cultural, or religious beliefs about death.

When families disagree with the determination of brain death, there have been legal disputes in which families had sought to prevent the withdrawal of nontherapeutic mechanical ventilation from these patients. Very few of these cases have reached resolution in the courts because either the patients progress to cardiorespiratory arrest or the parties find an out-of-court settlement, such as discharging the patient home with nontherapeutic mechanical ventilation.

10.4.6 Ethical Considerations in Conflicts Regarding Acceptance of Brain Death

With the complete and irreversible loss of all cognition in brain death, autonomy (which is fundamentally grounded in cognition) is also permanently lost. An individual, once dead, ceases to be a patient, no further healthcare can be provided, and their physical body is a corpse. This distinction is reflected legally in many jurisdictions by the distinction between a power of attorney for personal care (who is the substitute decision-maker for healthcare decisions) and the estate executor (who carries out the instruction of a will and manages the remaining estate after death). Although physicians may choose to continue providing care to brain-dead patients after the determination, it is an important distinction that this is done out of a sense of caring to the family, rather than a duty of care to, or a fiduciary relationship with the now deceased individual.

Even in considering the scenario that the capable wishes of the patient were to continue nontherapeutic mechanical ventilation and haemodynamic support following brain death, it has been suggested given the societal, legal, and medical implications of brain death that this is one of the few scenarios in which the autonomy of the individual patient or substitute decision-maker should be trumped by that of the physician or by societal consensus (Sprung et al. 1995).

With respect to non-maleficence, a brain-dead patient lacks any cognition or interpretation of the external environment and is insensate. The discontinuation of mechanical ventilation will not be felt by the patient, because in effect it is the discontinuation of medical treatments on a corpse. It is for this reason that anaesthesia is not required for organ procurement. Non-maleficence is a consideration in the provision of nontherapeutic physiological support to brain-dead individuals and includes the indignity of invasive care in an intensive care unit with no benefit to the patient, providing false hope to families, and prolonging the grieving process, including delayed burial or cremation and psychological closure.

Finally, although accommodation of an individual's or group's rejection of brain death respects autonomy, these accommodations must be just and must not infringe on the rights of others. Consequently, the determination of brain death must be consistent across individuals in a jurisdiction, and the provision of nontherapeutic critical care to a brain-dead patient must not deny scarce resources from others.

10.4.7   Brain Death and Organ Donation

Although the concept that the irreversible loss of brain function represents death of the person had been evolving for some time, it was the need for a method to determine death by neurological criteria to allow organ donation to occur that drove the widespread development of consensus definitions. The requirement is driven by the dead donor rule which is an ethical principle of organ donation and transplantation which has at its core two tenets: (1) vital organs should be taken only from dead patients; and (2) living patients should not be killed for or by organ procurement. Consequently, organ procurement can only occur if the patient is declared dead by neurological criteria prior to organ procurement.

If one accepts that brain death is death and as such represents the irreversible loss of personhood and consciousness, the patient (i.e. corpse) is neither harmed nor wronged when vital organs are procured. A dilemma arises, however, if one rejects the construct of brain death itself, in which case the dead donor rule would traditionally preclude organ donation in the absence of brain death, and vital organs would be seen to be procured from a living patient. This conundrum coupled with the modern realities of organ donation from living donors has led several leaders to question the requirement for the dead donor rule, suggesting that it should be replaced by an ethical foundation based on autonomy, consent, and non-maleficence (Truog et al. 2013). In this framework the overriding principles would be autonomy (that the patient consents to organ donation) and non-maleficence (that the patient is neither harmed nor wronged with the organ procurement and dies from the withdrawal of life support and not from the procurement of organs).

> **Pearl**
> Brain death is important in the procurement of organs, so other patients can benefit and be saved from death. However the first priority is always the patient who is critically ill, and no treatment should conflict with the duty of care to the patient. This is why nontherapeutic ventilation is very controversial, and it exemplifies a conflict between utilitarian and deontological ethics.

10.4.8   Approach to Conflict Resolution

Conflicts involving brain death and requests for physiological support in brain-dead patients can be extremely distressing for both families and healthcare teams. The sudden and unexpected death of a love one is a traumatic event for families, and the acceptance of death may be made even more challenging by the complexities of brain death as a concept, difficulties in communication, and assimilating these concepts with personal, spiritual, and religious views. Physicians may help avoid these stressful conflicts by carefully ensuring impeccable practice in the determination of brain death, communication and knowledge of their specific legal rights, and responsibilities in their local jurisdiction.

It is essential that the declaration of brain death is performed with strict adherence to local standards and guidelines. Repeated determinations by independent physicians are advised and in fact required in some jurisdictions. One recent survey demonstrated a disturbing lack of consistency in determination of brain death despite guidelines being disseminated for over a decade (Greer et al. 2008). Family presence during brain death determination may also be helpful at improving family acceptance of brain death, as witnessing the apnea test and the prolonged lack of respiratory efforts over 8–10 min has considerable face validity for individuals whose understanding of death is rooted in the traditional cardiopulmonary criteria (Kompanje et al. 2012). One study found that witnessing brain death determination did help families understand that their family member was dead, but increased emotional distress for the family (Ormrod et al. 2005).

The language conventionally used in communications with families may also contribute to misunderstandings (Molinari 1982). It has been suggested that the term brain death not be used as it implies a distinction from traditional death and replaced by terms such as 'neurological determination of death' (Shemie et al. 2006). Irrespective of language, physicians must be consistent in their communication that the individual is medically (and legally if appropriate) dead. In discussions regarding requests for and discontinuation of physiological support, the use of the term 'life support' is inappropriate and confusing to families and should be avoided. Many families may infer that the discontinuation of these therapies in the brain-dead patient is in fact the proximal cause of death. It is important that physicians patiently and consistently explain (1) the determination of death, (2) the inappropriateness of providing ongoing physiological support in the dead patient, and (3) the timeline for discontinuation of such therapies.

Finally, it is also important that physicians understand their legal rights and responsibilities in their local practice jurisdiction. Where brain death is codified into law, physicians may not have a legal duty to continue to provide treatment to a dead person. However, in jurisdictions in which there is legislation allowing conscientious accommodation, the situation is more complicated: the physician may not be able to proceed with determination without consent of the family or be tasked with providing nontherapeutic ventilation or support to a patient declared brain dead. Many physicians might continue to provide mechanical ventilation and existing therapies but not escalate treatments or treat new conditions while they provide more time for discussion and education of families.

10.5   Illustrative Case Revisited

The family of the 30-year-old woman continues to refuse that their loved one is dead, despite two independent determinations at different time points. They accepted the opportunity to witness the second brain death determination and were tearful at its conclusion. The physicians know that the local law supports brain death as death and that they are not compelled to the family's request for nontherapeutic ventilation. Nevertheless, they continue with physiological support for an additional 48 h while they continue to have conversations with the family and explain the situation. After the witnessed apnea test and further discussions with the primary team, their church leader, and the hospital bioethicist, the family accepts the diagnosis and assents to discontinuation of physiological support. After this they are approached by the local organ procurement organization they consent to organ donation, leaving a lasting legacy for the memory of their loved one.

Conclusion

Brain death is the neurological determination of death and is widely accepted and equated with death by traditional cardiovascular criteria. Rejection of the concept of brain death on religious or personal beliefs, however, can lead to stressful conflicts between surgeons and families and ethical dilemmas for healthcare providers. Strict adherence to clinical practice guidelines, superlative and patient communication, and thorough knowledge of the specific legal rights and responsibilities of physicians are all important in diffusing conflicts and finding mutually agreeable resolutions to these stressful and tragic scenarios.

References

A definition of irreversible coma (1968) Report of the Ad Hoc Committee of the Harvard Medical School to examine the definition of brain death JAMA 205:85–88

American Academy of Neurology (1995) Practice parameters for determining brain death in adults (summary statement). The Quality Standards Subcommittee of the American Academy of Neurology. Neurology 45(5):1012–1014

Australian and New Zealand Intensive Care Society (2010) The ANZICS statement on death and organ donation. Australian and New Zealand Intensive Care Society, Melbourne Available at: http://www.donatelife.gov.au/Media/docs/Prereading%20-%20ANZICS%20 Statement%20on%20Death%20and%20Organ%20Donation-227a9f86-0602-4712-948c-b423ac255500-0.pdf

Controversies in the determination of death: a white paper by the President's Council on Bioethics (2008), Washington, DC. Available at: http://bioethics.georgetown.edu/pcbe/reports/death/Controversies%20in%20the%20Determination%20of%20Death%20for%20 the%20Web%20(2).pdf

Diagnosis of brain death (1976) Statement issued by the honorary secretary of the Conference of Medical Royal Colleges and their faculties in the United Kingdom on 11 October 1976. BMJ;2(6045)1187–1188

Gardiner D, Shemie S, Manara A et al (2012) International perspective on the diagnosis of death. Br J Anaesth 108(Suppl 1):i14–i28

Greer DM, Varelas PN, Haque S et al (2008) Variability of brain death determination guidelines in leading US neurologic institutions. Neurology 70(4):284–289

Kompanje EJ, de Groot YJ, Bakker J et al (2012) A national multicenter trial on family presence during brain death determination: the FABRA study. Neurocrit Care 17(2):301–308

Lazar NM, Shemie S, Webster GC et al (2001) Bioethics for clinicians. 24. Brain death. Can Med Assoc J 164:833–836

Life support for pregnant woman ordered removed by Texas judge (2014) Available at: http://www.cbc.ca/news/world/life-support-for-pregnant-woman-ordered-removed-by-texas-judge-1.2510614

Lock M (1999) The problem of brain death: Japanese disputes about bodies and modernity. In: Youngner SJ, Arnold RM, Schapiro R (eds) The definition of death: contemporary controversies. Johns Hopkins University Press, Baltimore, pp 239–256

Molinari GF (1982) Brain death, irreversible coma, and words doctors use. Neurology 32(4):400–402

Mollaret P, Goulon M (1959) Le coma depasse. Rev Neurol (Paris) 101:5–15

Nakagawa TA, Ashwal S, Mathur M, Mysore M, Committee For Determination Of Brain Death In Infants Children (2012) Guidelines for the determination of brain death in infants and children: an update of the 1987 task force recommendations-executive summary. Ann Neurol 71(4):573–785

Ormrod JA, Ryder T, Chadwick RJ et al (2005) Experiences of families when a relative is diagnosed brain stem dead: understanding of death, observation of brain stem death testing and attitudes to organ donation. Anaesthesia 60(10):1002–1008

Pallis C (1983) ABC of brain stem death. Prognostic significance of a dead brain stem. Br Med J (Clin Res Ed) 286(6359):123–124

Parker M, Shemie SD (2002) Pro/con ethics debate: should mechanical ventilation be continued to allow for progression to brain death so that organs can be donated? Crit Care 6(5):399–402

Repertinger S, Fitzgibbons WP, Omojola MF et al (2006) Long survival following bacterial meningitis-associated brain destruction. J Child Neurol 21(7):591–595

Riishede J, Ethelberg S (1953) Angiographic changes in sudden and severe herniation of brainstem through tentorial incisura. Arch Neurol Psychiatry 70:399–409

Schöne-Seifert B (1999) Defining death in Germany: brain death and its discontents. In: Youngner SJ, Arnold RM, Schapiro R (eds) The definition of death: contemporary controversies. Johns Hopkins University Press, Baltimore, pp 257–271

Shemie SD, Doig C, Dickens B et al (2006) Severe brain injury to neurological determination of death: Canadian forum recommendations. Can Med Assoc J 174(6):S1–S13

Shewmon DA (1998) Chronic 'brain death' meta-analysis and conceptual consequences. Neurology 51:1538–1545

Smith M (2012) Brain death: time for an international consensus. Br J Anaesth 108 (Suppl 1):i6–i9

Sprung CL, Eidelman LA, Steinberg A (1995) Is the physician's duty to the individual patient or to society? Crit Care Med 23(4):618–620

Truog RD, Miller FG (2012) Brain death: justifications and critiques. Clin Ethics 7(3):128–132

Truog RD, Robinson WM (2003) Role of brain death and the dead-donor rule in the ethics of organ transplantation. Crit Care Med 31(9):2391–2396

Truog RD, Miller FG, Halpern SD (2013) The dead-donor rule and the future of organ donation. N Engl J Med 369(14):1287–1289

Uniform Determination of Death Act. National Conference of Commissioners on Uniform State Laws (1980) Chicago Available at: http://pntb.org/wordpress/wp-content/uploads/Uniform-Determination-of-Death-1980_5c.pdf

Wertheimer P, de Descotes R, Jouvet M (1960) Angiographical data concerning the death of the brain during comas with respiratory arrest (so-called protracted coma). Lyon Chir 56:641–648

Wijdicks EF, Varelas PN, Gronseth GS et al (2010) Evidence-based guideline update: determining brain death in adults: report of the Quality Standards Subcommittee of the American Academy of Neurology. Neurology 74(23):1911–1918

Part IV

Neurosurgeons' Duties

Neurosurgeons' Duties

11

Ahmed Ammar and Mark Bernstein

11.1 Introduction

There is general agreement about the tasks and duties of neurosurgeons as stated in several neurosurgical codes, guides for practice, and job descriptions (AANS Code of Ethics 2007; AANS Professional Conduct Program 2001; World Federation of Neurosurgical Societies and European Association for Neurosurgical societies 1999). Most neurosurgeons know their duties and responsibilities, but their articulation herein is pivotal to developing the practice of value-based medicine.

A neurosurgeon should provide the best possible care to his patients. It is vital for every neurosurgeon to update his knowledge and gain new skills. Within the field of neurosurgery, it is known and accepted that following evidence-based medicine guides is the way to assist the patient in choosing the best treatment plan. To a certain extent, modern medicine judges and weighs the different approaches according to, or in reference to, evidence-based medicine results. The importance of finding and following evidence cannot be overstated especially to a young neurosurgeon or to a neurosurgeon who may find he/she is working alone in a remote area with less expert colleagues to ask advice. Neurosurgeons are also obliged to adhere to medical ethics principles. These and other issues are elaborated in this chapter.

A. Ammar (✉)
Department of Neurosurgery, King Fahd University Hospital,
Dammam University, 40121, Al Khobar 31952, Saudi Arabia
e-mail: ahmed@ahmedammar.com

M. Bernstein, MD, MHSc, FRCSC
Division of Neurosurgery, Toronto Western Hospital, University of Toronto,
399 Bathurst Street, Toronto, ON M5T 2S8, Canada
e-mail: mark.bernstein@uhn.ca

A. Ammar, M. Bernstein (eds.), *Neurosurgical Ethics in Practice: Value-based Medicine*,   123
DOI 10.1007/978-3-642-54980-9_11, © Springer-Verlag Berlin Heidelberg 2014

11.2   Illustrative Case (Surgeon's Duty to Communicate Adequately with Family)

A patient was admitted to the hospital unconscious, GCS 4, intubated, with evidence of a comminuted depressed fracture of the left temporoparietal area. Following CT scan the patient underwent emergency surgery to elevate the depressed fracture and remove the associated ICH. The patient was kept in ICU for 32 days. He never made good progress. He developed posttraumatic hydrocephalus; therefore, a VP shunt was inserted. Several times his family asked the neurosurgeon to give e-mail updates to the patient's cousin who was a neurologist in another country, which the neurosurgeon did. Some weeks later the patient made limited progress and started to breathe via tracheostomy, and he was able to open his eyes spontaneously and showed grade 3 power on the left side. He received daily physiotherapy. The patient's father and family were repeatedly informed about the details of the case and about the expected unfavorable outcome. The consultant visited him once or twice a week and met the father several times. The father complained to the hospital administration that the consultant did not see his son every day.

11.3   Approach to the Case

Families of patients with a serious condition, particularly long term, are subject to an enormous amount of stress and grief. This may lead to posttraumatic stress disorder and certainly causes anxiety and an altered mental state. It is important for the treating team to show understanding and compassion and give special care to these families. It is important to be available for the family, as much as is feasible. The reaction and response of patients and their families to difficult life situations differ according to their cultural background, and the health-care team should be aware of these issues and as sensitive to them as possible (Ammar 1997). The neurosurgeon has the obligation to give adequate attention and care to these families.

In the case above, the neurosurgeon appears to have discharged his duties of caring and communication to the best of his ability and according to the standard of care. To the father it would have to be gently explained that his claim is unfair. The Patient Relations Department may be able to play a role in helping the neurosurgeon deal with this father.

11.4   Discussion

The main duties of neurosurgeons are shown in Fig. 11.1.

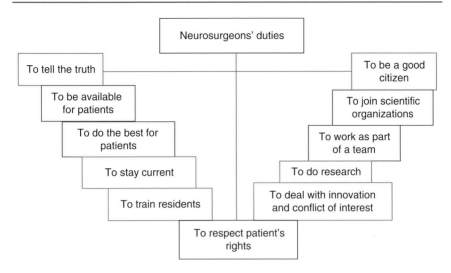

Fig. 11.1 Neurosurgeons' duties

11.4.1 Communication

The principle of beneficence dictates that the neurosurgeon should create good communication with the patient in order to appreciate and understand the patient's needs and act in the patient's best interests. This line of communication usually begins with the patient's first appearance in the neurosurgical service, either in the outpatient clinic or in the emergency department. Good communication should be enhanced during the patient's stay in the hospital. This communication is based on face-to-face communication. On discharge, the patient should always receive a follow-up appointment in the outpatient clinic to continue the care and the conversation.

It is impossible for any neurosurgeon to be available all the time to answer his/her patients' telephone calls, especially when multiple family members request information. It is important that the treating neurosurgeon spends enough time with the patient before his discharge explaining the possible course of recovery and any possible complications or new complaints, describing clearly what the patient should do in such situations. Many patient calls may be handled by the residents, nurse practitioner, or the neurosurgeon's secretary. The neurosurgeon should exercise his/her right to sign out to a colleague, like the neurosurgeon on call. A good neurosurgeon makes his/her patient feel all the time that he/she is available, always working for the best of the patient, and ready to help at any time. The neurosurgeon should establish, through communication, a professional relationship with the patient and his family.

Pearl

Good communication, including multiple paths of communication, forms a strong base of trust and partnership with the patient and family to help fight the patient's disease. The neurosurgeon should show compassion and understanding to the patient and families and make himself/herself as available as possible.

11.4.2 Truth Telling

A fundamental element that bridges all the four bioethics principles is that the surgeon should always be truthful with the patient (Hebert et al 1997). Basic medical ethics obliges every medical practitioner to be honest and inform their patients honestly about the details of their problem, the expected outcomes, the different options for treatment, and the recommended method of treatment. Telling the truth is very important to build up a strong bond of trust and confidence between the patients and their treating staff. It is not rare that the course of treatment of some patients does not go as wished and planned. Unavoidable or avoidable complications or unintended errors do occur in every neurosurgeon's practice, and they should openly discuss these adverse events with patients and should not try to hide such information.

11.4.3 Duty to Do the Very Best for the Patient

This of course goes without saying, but neurosurgeons should do their very best for their patients and not allow distractions or conflicts of interest get in the way of that. The patient's care and well-being should be the top priority of every neurosurgeon. The neurosurgeon should think carefully about the patient's medical condition, never take "simple" cases for granted, and build a strategy for management. In some cases, this may involve getting help from a colleague with more experience, and the surgeon's ego should never block doing the best for the patient. In fact the neurosurgeon should search for the best method to treat the patient, and if a technology or expertise is not available in the neurosurgeon's hospital, he/she should inform the patient about that and refer them to the right place.

11.4.4 Duty to Respect the Patient's Rights

The patients' rights should be respected and strictly observed all the time. Every neurosurgeon should follow an ethical code. The patient is at the center of the medical ethics and medical care. Therefore everything should be ethically and professionally done for the best of that patient. This includes "small" things like apologizing to patients if they have waited too long in the waiting room or their elective surgery has to be rescheduled due to circumstances beyond the surgeon's control. Every patient should receive excellent care, and they should perceive that they have received excellent, dignified, and professional care.

11.4.5 Duty to Work as Part of the Team

Modern neurosurgery is not a one-person show. Proper and efficient management of any neurosurgical problem is a complex multistep procedure which needs a fully trained team. Therefore, neurosurgeons should work always within teams, including specialists, residents, nurses, physiotherapists, radiologists, pathologists, lab staff, and other related services. The neurosurgeon is clearly the head of the team for a patient scheduled for surgery under his/her care, but the head of the team must listen to and incorporate all different opinions and share with the entire team to construct and execute a suitable management plan. For example, if the physiotherapist says the patient is not ready to go home on the fourth post-op day, the neurosurgeon must not react in anger but listen and discuss and ultimately respect the opinion of a fellow professional. The treatment plan should of course be discussed with the patient (and family) as well, as the patient in reality is the head of the team.

> **Pearl**
> Working as an integral team member is still difficult for some neurosurgeons, but it is the right thing to do and will ultimately improve team morale and, more importantly, patient care.

11.4.6 Duty to Ethically Deal with Innovation and Avoid Conflict of Interest

Industry is active in providing new innovation in the form of instruments, equipment, and medications. Often these innovations have been driven by neurosurgeons by either their expressed need or their intelligence and foresight. Innovation is welcomed and needed in order to refine neurosurgical practice and improve the outcomes for neurosurgical patients (Bernstein and Bampoe 2004). It is the duty of neurosurgeons to be aware of new innovations, and choose, and properly use what is the best for the patients. The proper use of new equipment or techniques requires proper training and possibly mentoring. Medical instruments are a huge market, and it is very important that neurosurgeons deal ethically with the industrial companies and avoid any conflict of interest, as medical companies do more and more to thank neurosurgeons for using their product, most of which is well intended (Morris and Taitsman 2009; Robertson 2008; White et al. 2007).

11.4.7 Duty to Teach Students and Train Residents

Neurosurgeons in university practice (which ranges from perhaps 10–90 % of neurosurgeons in any given country) have the duty and task to teach students and residents the art and science of neurosurgery. Therefore the trainees must have the opportunity to assist and operate under supervision in a graded responsibility model. It is the duty of neurosurgeons to ensure that their trainees are safe, able, and skillful enough to treat and operate patients independently once they are certified and qualified. Teaching of residents has a myriad of its own ethical tensions and challenges which neurosurgeons deal with every day (Bernstein and Knifed 2007).

11.4.8 Duty to Do Research

Research is the backbone and the source for many developments in medicine and neurosurgery. Neurosurgeons should be involved in different types of research – basic neuroscience investigation, clinical trials, outcomes research, and qualitative research. The laboratory benches may answer the questions which are seen in the patients' beds. Not every neurosurgeon should be involved in primary research, but it may be part of his/her job description to do so, and certainly most university-based neurosurgeons are also involved in some way. If a neurosurgeon is not primarily involved, he/she should at minimum support research such as by participating when asked by colleagues or by sharing financial resources to promote research in his/her university, hospital, or organizations. Any research involving patients should be ethically controlled.

11.4.9 Duty to Be a Good "Citizen" Including Membership in Professional Organizations

Every day in their hospitals, surgeons must be respectful to their own colleagues, to anesthetists, to nurses, and to all members of the hospital staff. They must respect and live by the rules of the Medical Advisory Committee and other in-hospital governing bodies. Good citizenship begins at home.

The main aims of all national and international neurosurgical societies and organizations all over the world are to regulate neurosurgical practice in that country, to provide a forum for continuous neurosurgical education, to promote research, to promote public outreach and education, and to promote international initiatives like global partnerships. Neurosurgeons should actively participate in such organizations so that they contribute to their local, country, subspecialty, and world communities of neurosurgeons.

> **Pearl**
> Neurosurgical practice is a noble job. Neurosurgical practice is guarded and regulated by strict ethical and professional codes. The duty of neurosurgeons should extend from treating individual patients to serving the whole of society and all of the world.

11.4.10 Duty to Undertake Continuous Medical Education (CME)

11.4.10.1 A Moral and Practical Necessity

The rapid progress and development in neurosurgery requires that neurosurgeons do their best to be current, learn the new developments, and gain new skills. The neurosurgeon has to be current in order to provide modern cutting-edge care for the patients. There is much to be done to improve the outcome of some serious and common neurosurgical problems like malignant brain tumors, severe brain and spinal cord injury, and congenital disease. Therefore, neurosurgeons must continuously educate themselves and participate in CME to stay current, update knowledge, and gain new skills in order to provide the best possible care for their patients. Not only is it essential to the continual improvement of the surgeon, but it is required by neurosurgeons' governing bodies and if not fulfilled can lead to consequences such as loss of membership in society or even license revocation. Most neurosurgical governing bodies clearly spell out the number of hours required often in 2- or 3-year cycles and what sorts of activities qualify and have online forms to fill out at the end of every evaluation period (Royal College of Physicians and Surgeons of Canada Maintenance of Competence).

11.4.10.2 Who Should Pay for CME?

Attending workshops, conferences, and seminars is costly. Most hospitals and universities do not have the budget to support their medical staff. Many neurosurgical groups have internal redistribution of portions of their income to be used specifically for academic and CME activities. The tax system in some countries (not all) may allow a certain amount of training to be offset against taxes paid.

Some neurosurgeons may see attending the conferences and workshops, to obtain CME and gain new skills, as an investment in their own career, so they are willing to cover the cost. However, others believe that obtaining CME has become very expensive and they cannot afford it. When continuous education is a requirement by the hospital, one could argue that the cost should be covered by the workplace. Ultimately, a staff with up-to-date skills reflects positively on the patient and on the image and quality of the workplace (Ahmed and Ashrafian 2009).

11.4.10.3 Duty to Avoid CME Conflict of Interest with Industry

Financial support of pharmaceutical and equipment industry companies has become commonplace. This particularly relates to meetings in which the company is offering training with a new piece of equipment they produce or a meeting sponsored by the company on a topic related to one of their products (e.g., a drug company sponsors a meeting about brain tumor research as the company produces a drug which is used to treat a type of brain tumor). These are extremely tempting to neurosurgeons who truly wish to learn about the subject but would probably not have gone if the company were not paying their expenses. Additional strong attractants for attendance include lovely locations and venues and high-profile neurosurgeons highlighted as keynote speakers.

The relationship between neurosurgeons and the companies should be very well regulated and handled with great transparency. In many countries, industry-sponsored CME programs are regulated by an independent body, such as ACCME in USA, which observes that all CME programs must be free from any commercial interest. However, some authors suggest that that regulation could be manipulated easily (Minter et al 2011). There should be a very clear line between commercially sponsored oriented CME programs and educational and scientifically oriented CME programs. The Accreditation Council for Continuing Medical Education published standards to ensure independence in CME activities in the USA (The Accreditation Requirements of the Accreditation Council for Continuing Medical Education 2012). The neurosurgeon must do his/her honest best to recognize that there is a conflict of interest and deal with it as ethically as possible.

While it is evident that the companies have an overwhelming commercial interest, they also claim an educational and scientific interest. The line between the commercial interest and educational and scientific interest is not always clear and may be overlapping; that is why some authors suggest excluding industry workshops from CME programs (Morris and Taitsman 2009; Robertson 2008; White et al. 2007). However, current financial realities may not permit excluding the companies' support from CME programs entirely.

> **Pearl**
> Continuous medical education programs are a vital part of modern neurosurgery. Every neurosurgeon should strive to obtain new skills and update his/her knowledge. Hospitals and universities should ideally support their employees by facilitating staff attendance at approved conferences, workshops, and courses. The industry may play a role in supporting CME programs. Transparency is the key to prevent and/or manage conflicts of interest.

11.4.11 Duty to Be a Good Doctor

What makes a great doctor? The concept of what constitutes a great doctor has long been studied and discussed both in the medical field and in the media. It seems that there is a difference between the patient's perspective and that of the clinicians. Definitely, the term good or great doctor goes beyond academic qualifications and training. One study showed that the general public considered knowledge and keeping updated as the most important factors, while the physicians considered honesty and responsibility to be the two most important factors (Fones et al. 1998). Other attributes of a great doctor include confidence, empathy, humanity, personality, forthrightness, respectfulness, and thoroughness. Other aphorisms have been handed down folklore style such as the three A's of a good doctor – affability, availability, and ability. A qualitative research study from a large tertiary academic hospital found that doctors who love patient care, have compassion for their patients, and put their patients first are the best doctors (Mahant et al 2012).

Neurosurgeons should be inherently trained to have true compassion for their patients, work in partnership to solve their problems, give time to listen carefully to complaints, and be honest enough to admit mistakes (Bernstein et al 2003; Parmar 2002; Wolpe 2002). The young trainee should be encouraged to adopt these characteristics and learn from the role models, the consultant neurosurgeons. Skills alone do not produce a great doctor.

11.4.12 Duty to Take Care of Oneself

Neurosurgeons work very hard in a high-stress profession; older generations of surgeons often work 90–100 h weeks and feel that they must always be available for their patients. Many give their cell phone numbers and e-mail addresses to their patients and respond even when they are far away on work-related or recreational travel. This is unnecessary as long as the surgeon makes provisions for complete coverage of his/her patients' needs in the surgeon's absence.

Sleep deprivation may negatively affect surgical performance (Woodrow et al. 2008), and there is a strong movement at present to limit work hours of both staff and resident neurosurgeons (Hochberg et al 2013; Miulli and Valcore 2010). Many consultants and trainees have concerns about the reduction in allowable work hours suggesting that it will compromise the training of competent neurosurgeons, which is weighed against the argument of the possibility of reduced patient safety because of overtired surgeons (Neurosurgery residents oppose restrictions on work hours 2011). Other sources of moral distress among neurosurgery residents have also been identified (Knifed et al. 2010).

Neurosurgeons and their residents have duty to attend to their physical and psychological welfare. The profession is an all-consuming passion for many, but an ill neurosurgeon cannot fulfill his/her family roles and certainly cannot help his/her patients. Even Kant emphasized that one must take care of himself/herself before taking care of others. Burnout is a very real occupational hazard for surgeons (Balch and Shanafelt 2011). Modern generations of neurosurgeons appear to have better balance than those currently in their last 10–15 years of practice, and obtaining balance is certainly not only possible but probable (Troppmann et al. 2009).

11.4.13 Duty to Role Model Ethics and Teach Ethics to Future Neurosurgeons

Some neurosurgeons and trainees are inherently of good character and good values, and some practice good characteristics and values as a duty or out of fear of consequences. Most evaluation forms of trainees include an item on ethics or professionalism. The difficulty is that one's ethics and behavior cannot be easily measured. From the earliest times in medicine, there has been a general belief or presumption that everyone wearing a white coat must have good values and ethics and be honest, caring, and trustful. Unfortunately this is not always true. Surgeons are well-meaning but pressures for perfection in a high-stress occupation, time constraints, and other pressures can lead to imperfect ethical behavior. The most practical method to assess the behavior and ethics of the trainee is by observing their relationship with their patients, colleagues, and paramedical staff. Perhaps patients should also be called upon to help evaluate the behavior and conduct of trainees. Neurosurgeons should take every opportunity to discuss the ethical dimension of cases by the bedside and in the operating room as well as the scientific and technical issues, to supplement the more formal ethics teaching surgical residents are increasingly receiving (Helft et al 2009; McKneally and Singer 2001).

11.4.14 Duty to Self-Monitor and Know One's Limitations

All neurosurgeons without exception have their own learning curve starting with the first day of training and continuing to the last day of their practice. There will always be a first time doing a certain operation and first use of an instrument or equipment. Measures should be taken in order to make this sizable learning curve safe and beneficial for the patient. As well, there will always be three categories of cases from a surgical competency and comfort perspective: (1) those the surgeon does a lot of and is very comfortable with; (2) those he/she feels competent to do but does not do a lot of and there is moderate comfort level; and (3) those he/she knows they should not be doing (and their partners know this as well). It is ultimately the responsibility of every neurosurgeon not do cases he/she feels others can do significantly better and refer those they know they should not even attempt to do, but there is some evidence that surgeons' insight into their own performance may be lacking (Warschkow et al. 2010). The profession and/or external bodies can police neurosurgeons, but it will be very delayed and only after serious harm is done to patients and to one's career. Neurosurgeons must be vigilant and proactive about monitoring their practice and their competencies. Neurosurgeons eventually will need to slow down with advancing years, and sometimes this transition is not handled as gracefully as it could be. Graceful retirement is the last duty of most neurosurgeons (Ausman 2009).

Conclusion

Neurosurgeons have many duties, but all can be reduced to giving the best care he/she possibly can to every patient while respecting all of the patient's rights to the best of his/her ability. All of the other duties highlighted in this chapter help the neurosurgeon to serve these overarching goals and provide the patient with impeccable value-based care.

References

AANS Board of Directors (2007, 13 April) AANS code of ethics. Available at: http://www.aans. org/en/About%20AANS/~/media/4A6862BB037742FF99B833D609D23B1E.ashx

Ahmed K, Ashrafian H (2009) Life-long learning for physicians. Science 326(5950):227

Ammar A (1997) The influence of different cultures on neurosurgical practice. Childs Nerv Syst 13:91–94

Ausman JI (2009) What will you do with the rest of your life? Surg Neurol 72(6):642

Balch CM, Shanafelt T (2011) Combating stress and burnout in surgical practice: a review. Thorac Surg Clin 21(3):417–430

Bernstein M, Bampoe J (2004) Surgical innovation or surgical evolution: an ethical and practical guide to handling novel neurosurgical procedures. J Neurosurg 100(1):2–7

Bernstein M, Knifed E (2007) Ethical challenges of in the field training: a surgical perspective. Learning Inquiry 1:169–174

Bernstein M, Hebert PC, Etchells E (2003) Patient safety in neurosurgery: detection of errors, prevention of errors, and disclosure of errors. Neurosurg Q 13(2):125–137

Fones CS, Kua EH, Goh LG (1998) What makes a good doctor? – views of medical profession and the public in setting priorities for medical education. Singapore Med J 39(12):537–542

Hebert PC, Hoffmaster B, Glass KC et al (1997) Bioethics for clinicians. 7. Truth telling. Can Med Assoc J 156:225–228

Helft PR, Eckles RE, Torbeck L (2009) Ethics education in surgical residency programs: a review of the literature. J Surg Educ 66(1):35–42

Hochberg MS, Berman RS, Kalet al et al (2013) The stress of residency: recognizing the signs of depression and suicide in you and your fellow residents. Am J Surg 205(2):141–146

Knifed E, Goyal A, Bernstein M (2010) Moral angst for surgical residents: a qualitative study. Am J Surg 199(4):571–576

Mahant S, Jovcevska V, Wadhwa A (2012) The nature of excellent clinicians at an academic health science center: a qualitative study. Acad Med 87(12):1715–1721

McKneally MF, Singer PA (2001) Bioethics for clinicians: 25. Teaching bioethics in the clinical setting. Can Med Assoc J 164(8):1163–1167

Minter RM, Angelos P, Coimbra R et al (2011) Ethical management of conflict of interest: proposed standards for academic surgical societies. J Am Coll Surg 213(5):677–682

Miulli DE, Valcore JC (2010) Methods and implications of limiting resident duty hours. J Am Osteopath Assoc 110(7):385–395

Morris L, Taitsman JK (2009) The agenda for continuing medical education – limiting industry's influence. New Engl J Med 361(25):2478–2482

Neurosurgery residents oppose restrictions on work hours (2011). Available at: http://www. wolterskluwerhealth.com/News/Pages/Neurosurgery-Residents-Oppose-Restrictions-on-Work-Hours.aspx

Parmar MS (2002) What's a good doctor, and how can you make one? The ABC of being a good doctor. BMJ 325:711

Robertson JH (2008) Neurosurgery and industry. J Neurosurg 109(6):979–988

Royal College of Physicians and Surgeons of Canada maintenance of competence. Available at: http://www.royalcollege.ca/portal/page/portal/rc/members/moc

The AANS Professional Conduct Program (2001). Available at: http://www.aans.org/en/About%20 AANS/~/media/38D91B03C04540D999ED76D3B58784B9.ashx

The Accreditation Requirements of the Accreditation Council for Continuing Medical Education (2012). Available at: https://medschool.vanderbilt.edu/cme/files/cme/u8/ACCME%20Accreditation%20 Requirements%206-1-12.pdf

Troppmann KM, Palis BE, Goodnight JE et al (2009) Career and lifestyle satisfaction among surgeons: what really matters? The national lifestyles in surgery today survey. J Am Coll Surg 209(2):160–169

Warschkow R, Steffen T, Spillmann M et al (2010) A comparative cross-sectional study of personality traits in internists and surgeons. Surgery 148(5):901–907

White AP, Vaccaro AR, Zdeblick T (2007) Counterpoint: physician-industry relationship can be ethically established, and conflicts of interest can be ethically managed. Spine (Phila Pa 1976) 32(11 Supp):S53–S57

Wolpe PR (2002) What's a good doctor, and how can you make one? We are trying to make doctors too good. BMJ 325:711

Woodrow SI, Park J, Murray BJ et al (2008) Differences in the perceived impact of sleep deprivation among surgical and non-surgical residents. Med Educ 42(5):459–467

World Federation of Neurosurgical Societies and European Association of Neurosurgical Societies (1999) Good practice: a guide for neurosurgeons. Acta Neurochir (Wien) 141(8):793–799

Ethical Decision-Making

12

Mark Bernstein and Vijendra K. Jain

12.1 Introduction

Neurosurgeons are faced with many clinical decisions every day. Decision-making is a complex process and the subject of research in its own right (Croskerry et al. 2014). It is not formally taught but acquired by practicing physicians, and it is essential that the practice of value-based medicine guide the neurosurgeon's decisions. In everyday decision-making not only must our skill and knowledge be honed and nurtured, but so must our attention to the ethical dimensions of what we do (Groopman 2007). For many neurosurgical conditions, there are multiple options available to treat them (Bernstein and Khu 2009). This must be disconcerting to patients who seek multiple opinions about their condition only to receive a different recommendation from each surgeon they meet. Not only is it confusing, adding to their anxiety and fear, but it must make the patient feel a little insecure that the noble profession of neurosurgery has not evolved sufficiently to have answered some basic questions, like how best to treat their condition.

In neurosurgery, there are many treatment protocols that are the subject of intense personal, local, and international debate. Through residency training, and then continuing education in the form of conferences, seminars, and the medical literature, and personal experience, each neurosurgeon develops his/her own preferred option

M. Bernstein, MD, MHSc, FRCSC
Division of Neurosurgery, Toronto Western Hospital, University of Toronto,
399 Bathurst Street, Toronto, ON M5T 2S8, Canada
e-mail: mark.bernstein@uhn.ca

V.K. Jain, MCh (✉)
Department of Neurosurgery, Max Super Speciality Hospital,
New Delhi, India
e-mail: vkjneuro@gmail.com

A. Ammar, M. Bernstein (eds.), *Neurosurgical Ethics in Practice: Value-based Medicine*,
DOI 10.1007/978-3-642-54980-9_12, © Springer-Verlag Berlin Heidelberg 2014

to approach a particular situation. What ethical principles should guide a neurosurgeon in choosing a particular mode of treatment over another in a particular case? Decision-making is an important issue in every area of neurosurgery – from common "routine" conditions like lumbar disc disease to more "exotic" and rare conditions like large basilar tip aneurysms.

12.2 Illustrative Case (Which Treatment Option Is the Right One?)

A 37-year-old woman with melanoma has known lung lesions which are essentially stable on chemotherapy. She presents with a single seizure but no neurological deficit. MRI shows a sizable right anterior frontal hemorrhagic lesion with surrounding edema and a small second lesion superficially in the right posterior frontal lobe (Figs. 12.1 and 12.2). The presumption is made that they are metastatic tumors. The multidisciplinary brain metastasis team consisting of neurosurgery, radiation oncology, and medical oncology discusses her case at conference trying to decide on the best strategy for her. What should they recommend?

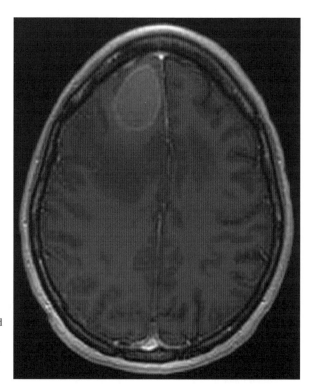

Fig. 12.1 Axial T1-enhanced MRI showing a hemorrhagic metastasis in the right frontal lobe of a 37-year-old woman with metastatic melanoma

Fig. 12.2 A smaller second
lesion is seen on another cut

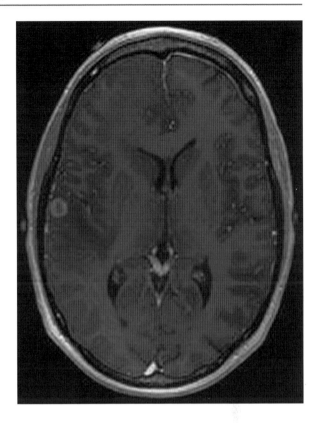

12.3   Approach to the Case

The team approached the case considering available evidence from the literature including as many as possible randomized studies, the patient's eligibility for ongoing clinical trials, their collected clinical experience, analysis of risks and benefits, and patient preference. The options they listed include:

1. Whole brain radiation alone (WBRT)
2. Resection of the larger lesion followed by WBRT
3. Resection of the larger lesion plus stereotactic radiosurgery (SRS) to the resection bed and the smaller tumor
4. Resection of the larger lesion plus stereotactic radiosurgery (SRS) to the smaller tumor
5. Resection of both tumors alone
6. Resection of both tumors followed by WBRT
7. Resection of both lesions followed by SRS to both resection beds
8. SRS for both lesions alone
9. SRS for both lesions followed by WBRT

While there is some validity for all of these options, the team decided on option 4 which the patient accepted, and the treatment plan proceeded without problem.

12.4 Discussion

12.4.1 General Ethical Approach

Rapid evolution and development in neurosurgery has resulted in several different approaches to treat the same neurosurgical problems, and this will increase in the future with the development of more and more sophisticated and complex technologies and treatments. The absence of national or international guidelines, and the lack of class I evidence supporting one method over another for most of the conditions we treat, has given the neurosurgeon the possibility to choose both what he/she feels is best and what is within his/her own capabilities and still offer the best treatment he/she is able to give the patient. Patients may get confused receiving different suggestions. The principle of autonomy dictates that the patient should know everything about the disease and should know the different methods of treatment. Although patients should make the final decision on treatment, it is wrong to presume that they can reach the decision with minimal input from the neurosurgeon. The neurosurgeon should explain all equally successful methods and then state his/her preferred method for treating the case. Ultimately the patient must decide if he/she is willing to undergo the treatment method preferred by the neurosurgeon.

> **Pearl**
> Arguably the most important single manifestation of the sacred trust between the patient and surgeon is the course of treatment the surgeon recommends. This trust is truly sacred and the surgeon must bring everything to bear to make the best decisions for his/her patients.

12.4.2 Disease-Specific and Modality-Specific Examples of Sources of Ambiguity in Decision-Making

12.4.2.1 Spine Surgery

In a patient with intractable S1 sciatica and a moderate-sized herniated lumbar disc, should the neurosurgeon try an epidural nerve root block prior to surgery? If it comes to surgery, should a standard microsurgical discectomy be done or a minimally invasive "tubular" discectomy (Dasenbrock et al. 2012)? Is an interbody fusion needed? Should the procedure be done as an outpatient procedure or should the patient be admitted (Purzner et al. 2011)? The same dilemmas exist regarding cervical disc disease. A retrospective database analysis was done to compare the perioperative patient characteristics, early postoperative outcomes, and costs between anterior cervical discectomy and fusion and a cervical total disc replacement surgery in one US center (Nandyala et al. 2014), and they found out that both cohorts demonstrated comparable incidences of early postoperative complications and costs. There were no significant differences in the risks for postoperative complications between the surgical cohorts. There are no fixed proven-beyond-doubt guidelines for spinal instrumentation. A lot depends on the experience of the neurosurgeon and the availability of instrumentation and affordability for patients; the last two factors are particularly relevant for neurosurgeons practicing in the developing world. Some people argue that spinal instrumentation may be being overused and is an industry-driven practice.

12.4.2.2 Gliomas

In a patient with a presumed low-grade glioma, should the patient be treated up front or observed in a "wait and see" protocol (Deekonda and Bernstein 2011; Hayhurst et al. 2011)? Should a biopsy be done either way? If open surgery is opted for, should a radical resection be attempted or as aggressive as the surgeon is comfortable doing? Should the surgery be done under general anesthesia or using awake craniotomy with functional mapping (Kirsch and Bernstein 2012)? Is surgical navigation based on archived imaging sufficient or is operating in an open MRI unit to provide real-time imaging the gold standard? Should the procedure be done as an outpatient procedure, or does the patient require admission to hospital (Purzner et al. 2011)?

Regarding lesions with the imaging features presumed to be high-grade glioma, the imaging findings do not predict the exact pathology in 100 % of these cases. Many times, particularly in the developing world, tuberculoma is also a differential diagnosis. Should all patients presumed to have a tuberculoma which can be treated pharmacologically first have an image-guided biopsy or resection to avoid treating a glioblastoma erroneously (Fath-Ordoubadi et al. 1997)? Should patients with glioblastoma receive, after best standard care (i.e., surgery, radiation, temozolomide), additional therapy with Gliadel wafers, Avastin, or other marginally effective treatments? The surgeon and his/her team can be challenged both when these therapies are used and when they are not used.

12.4.2.3 Aneurysms

In a patient with a subarachnoid hemorrhage, is CT angiography sufficient for surgical planning, or is a catheter angiogram needed? Should an endovascular procedure like coiling be done, or should open surgery be done? If surgery is done is a ventricular drain or lumbar drain needed routinely? Some evidence is available to help guide our approach. The effect of coiling versus clipping of ruptured and unruptured cerebral aneurysms on length of stay, hospital cost, hospital reimbursement, and surgeon reimbursement was studied in one US center and surgery, compared with endovascular treatment, was associated with longer hospitalization, but lower hospital costs, higher surgeon reimbursement, and similar hospital reimbursements (Hoh et al. 2009). It is easy for those who practice endovascular coiling to scare people about open surgery required for clipping. They may say that for clipping, the skull will be opened, the brain may get damaged, and therefore there are more chances of bad results, while endovascular treatment is safer as there is no open operation. The patient and family may not understand the importance of the experience of the surgeon or that sometimes something that sounds riskier is still the best for them. What they are told is that in coiling, the patient is being treated without a major brain operation. Is it ethical for those who practice coiling to focus mainly on the risks of clipping? On the other hand, how far is a surgeon who practices clipping justified in advocating clipping over coiling?

12.4.2.4 Radiosurgery Versus Surgery

The same ethical issues may apply regarding treatment by any radiosurgery modality, such as Gamma Knife, CyberKnife, etc. (Gottfried et al. 2004). The radiosurgery clinic neurosurgeon promises treatment without any immediate complications for a 1.3 cm vestibular schwannoma, while the operating neurosurgeon must always warn of the possibility of some complications of open surgery. Sometimes it can be very difficult to make patients and their relatives understand the balanced approach in any given situation.

12.4.2.5 Endoscopic Versus Conventional Microsurgery

Controversy exists over the benefits, efficacy, and safety of the endoscopic approach for complex skull base pathology over the microscopic approach, and endoscopy is becoming more widespread due to its obvious advantages (Mortini et al. 2003) and satisfaction for patients (Edem et al. 2013). In the absence of class I evidence to favor one method over the other, either method should be acceptable, and practitioners of one technique or the other must be mindful of not overemphasizing the negative aspects of the other method.

> **Pearl**
> Several factors affect how surgeons make decisions about treatment recommendations. They include surgeon comfort, surgeon bias, presence of class I evidence, existence of ongoing clinical trials, the impact of the surgeon's training, and conflicts of interest (financial and others).

12.4.3 Factors Affecting Surgeons' Decision-Making

12.4.3.1 Surgeon Comfort Level

There are many neurosurgeons who are not comfortable to operate on aneurysms, complex skull base tumors, complex spine surgery, and other conditions due to (1) their perceived level of expertise in various areas of neurosurgery, (2) the nature of their training, and (3) the nature of their hospital group in which subspecialization may be so developed that they focus on only one or maybe two areas of neurosurgery and there may be pressure to refer specialized cases to one's partners.

12.4.3.2 Surgeon Bias

Surgeons are definitely subject to bias about what is the best treatment, and they may openly or inadvertently convey this bias to patients (Deekonda and Bernstein 2011). If a nonaneurysm expert feels coiling is generally safer than open microsurgery for an anterior communicating aneurysm, or a non-skull base surgeon feels that radiosurgery is safer than microsurgery for a 1.3 cm vestibular schwannoma, he/she may refer these patients for coiling or radiosurgery, respectively, by enumerating the high risks of surgery to the patients and extolling the advantages of the recommended approach. There is great asymmetry of power between surgeon and patient in that the surgeon is in control and authority and the patient is vulnerable. This gap is decreasing as patients become more informed about their disease, partly due to the internet, and more involved in their care. But in any given interaction, it is relatively easy for a surgeon to "sell" his/her preferred treatment option by the way he/she presents the information.

12.4.3.3 Available Class I Evidence

Clearly, neurosurgeons have their patients' best interests at heart, and if definitive scientific evidence demonstrates the superiority of one treatment over another, that will color their decision-making in a powerful way. Unfortunately we do not have class I evidence to guide many of our clinical decisions in everyday practice. For example, no class I evidence exists to recommend radical resection of either low-grade or high-grade gliomas although there is some class II evidence (Lacroix et al. 2001), and substantial debate remains over this issue. However some randomized studies have helped significantly over the years. For example, over a decade ago two negative randomized trials essentially removed high-activity interstitial brachytherapy from the decision-making algorithm of neurosurgeons caring for patients with malignant glioma (Laperriere et al. 1998).

12.4.3.4 The Act of Seeking Class I Evidence

If clinical trials exist in a neurosurgeon's institution or larger research network (e.g., Radiation Therapy Oncology Group), a moral obligation to support such trials exists. Sometimes the presence of multiple clinical trials for which a patient is eligible can actually complicate the problem of decision-making for the surgeon because it is impossible to decide which trial might be most appropriate for the patient (Ibrahim et al. 2011). Neurosurgeons also have an obligation to be on the forefront of generating clinical studies especially if they are primarily surgical in nature.

12.4.3.5 The Impact of the Surgeons' Training

Obviously, neurosurgeons will be strongly influenced by the training they received from individual neurosurgeons and also institutional or even countrywide biases. For example, a German study showed that about 50 % of neurosurgery departments routinely exercise the "wait and see" approach for patients with presumed low-grade gliomas not requiring surgery for the usual indications such as focal deficit or increased intracranial pressure (Seiz et al. 2011). A neurosurgeon graduating from such a program will clearly look at low-grade gliomas differently than one who graduates from a program where every such case is operated early and aggressively. Similarly an institution with a champion of awake craniotomy will influence how graduates of their program conduct their glioma and metastasis surgery when they are consultants, and these biases must be recognized by teachers and attempts made at mitigating these biases. Some of these ethical dilemmas have been addressed and examined by some commentators (Kirsch and Bernstein 2012).

12.4.3.6 Conflicts of Interest

Neurosurgeons are committed hardworking people who have their patients' best interests at heart. However, they are human and are subject to personal conflicts of interest, both financial and nonfinancial. If the surgeon wants the patient to accept an operation because they feel in their heart it is really the best for the patient or because it will help him/her gain experience and numbers for research, this is a conflict of interest which must be recognized so the surgeon can deal with such situations as ethically as possible (Bernstein 2003). Conflicts may be very banal such as simple logistic issues such as a surgeon thinking: "I have an empty OR slot next Tuesday and that looks bad for me to my partners and residents and it's a sin to waste OR time – I think this patient needs her disc operated and I'll convince her to have it done next Tuesday."

Regarding financial conflicts of interest, if the surgeon works in a fee-for-service system and believes there is equipoise between two treatment options, one of which will reimburse better (e.g., microsurgery over radiosurgery for a 1.3 cm vestibular schwannoma), he/she may well pick the option which benefits him/her more. This is an uncomfortable reality that no one likes to discuss, but if these conflicts are recognized and approached head-on, they are more likely to become less common. The competition present in some systems is also conducive to these conflicts as demonstrated by a surgeon thinking: "If I don't operate on this equivocal case, the surgeons down the road will, so it might as well be me." The other important financial conflict is that incurred due to the participation of industry in neurosurgical care, without which all of medicine could not function (Robertson 2008). But, if a surgeon has developed an excellent working relationship with a supplier of spinal instrumentation, for example, and enjoys fringe benefits of that relationship, he/she may be more prone to recommend fusion in equivocal cases which represents a conflict of interest.

> **Pearl**
> Conflicts of interest are ever present for neurosurgeons when they are recommending treatments to patients. It is not unethical for neurosurgeons to be subject to human weaknesses, but these conflicts must be recognized and acknowledged to oneself in order to decrease their negative impact on patients.

12.4.4   Strategies to Ensure the Best Possible Decision-Making

12.4.4.1 Teamwork

What seems the right course of action to one surgeon may not seem right to another surgeon. One of the best ways to combat these differences of opinion and for a surgeon to ensure he/she has made a good and justifiable decision is to get help through teamwork. This can take the form of informal consultations with one's colleagues either locally or by internet or in a more organized way such as a tumor board or other multidisciplinary conferences. For example, if in a team there are surgeons and/or interventional radiologists who practice coiling and other surgeons who practice clipping, then they can both discuss the case and together decide the course that is best suited to that particular patient. Needless to say, the surgeons would have to enter the discussion with an open mind and be prepared to give way and even "lose the case" with its financial and other implications. This approach ensures that the patient is being offered the best possible treatment option and, just as importantly, reassures the patient of this. It may even mitigate medico-legal problems which may rarely arise, if a team has recommended a treatment instead of one person.

Along the same vein as teamwork, in case this team approach to decision-making is not possible in one's own institution, a surgeon should recommend his treatment plan to the patient, inform him/her of all alternatives, and be prepared to suggest to the patient that they might benefit from a second opinion elsewhere. Patients may be too shy or respectful to request a second opinion on their own, but if the neurosurgeon suggests it and offers to facilitate it, they will be receptive. The surgeon may complicate things by making the time line longer, and may even "lose the case," but he/she would be comfortable in the knowledge that the right thing has been done.

> **Pearl**
> One who desires to practice medicine ethically should not keep facts from patients and their relatives. The neurosurgeon should not claim or even try to be infallible but should try to do his/her best in every case. He/she should allow patients to make their own decisions and should not try to influence their decision-making beyond giving them the relevant medical information.

12.4.4.2 The Patient's and Family's Role in Decision-Making

It is not sufficient for a doctor to simply act in an ethical manner. It is also important that the patients and their families see him as ethical. It is a fact that many people believe that doctors are more interested in their own interests (including financial gain) than the patient's welfare. It therefore becomes important that not only should the doctor be ethical but should also appear to be so. The challenge here is that the patients are of different types and have to be dealt with differently; they fall broadly into four groups:

1. The patient and the family communicate well and clarify their doubts during the course of the treatment. They take their own decisions and feel responsible for them. This is the best group for a doctor who is sincerely doing his/her best.

2. The patient and family are not interested in discussions and do not want to understand the gravity of the disease. They believe it is the clinician's duty to do his/her best and "fix the problem." In the eyes of this group, if the result of the treatment is good, the doctor is good and has done everything right. However, if the result is not as good as expected, the doctor has either committed some mistake or neglected to perform his/her duty.

3. The patient and family want to repeatedly discuss not only what you have already explained but also their own experiences, citing examples of what happened to someone they know who was suffering from the same disease (which often ends up being something different) and was treated somewhere else. If the result was bad, they do not want the same to happen in your hands, and if the result was good, they want the same result in your hands. They complain about minor issues and frequently a new relative or friend wants to discuss everything all over again. This group is difficult to deal with and hard to satisfy.

4. Some families do not want to reveal the seriousness of the operation to the patient. They ask the doctor not to reveal the disease and the possibility of an unfavorable outcome to the patient. This creates a problem when it comes to taking informed written consent from the patient instead of the relative.

It is clear that with all groups but the first it is not easy for the doctor to prove that he/she is doing his/her best and is following best practices. Decision-making on behalf of the patient is challenging for the surgeon in these scenarios. A psychological game begins between the relatives and doctor who has to weigh the pros and cons of accepting the responsibility of treatment of a particular patient. What is the best course for a doctor to follow in situations like these? The doctor should sincerely explain and discuss the disease of the patient, the natural course of the disease, various options of treatment, his/her own experience and capabilities, and his/her recommendation and then let the patient and family decide. This should be done honestly and without bias. Some doctors explain the various aspects of treatment in such a way that at the end of their explanations, the patient and family are left with only one choice, the one that the doctor wishes them to accept. This is not ethical. At the same time one should not confuse the patient and the family by teaching them a lot of medical literature which they cannot be expected to understand. In the worst scenario if an irreconcilable personality conflict arises, the surgeon may have to recuse him/herself from the case and find the patient another neurosurgeon, fortunately an extremely rare occurrence (Bernstein and Upshur 2008).

12.4.4.3 Living Within Financial/Resource Constraints

It is not difficult to understand that the finances available to a doctor and his/her patient play a huge role in decision-making in neurosurgery. The financial angle becomes especially important in developing world countries where money is scarce (Howe et al. 2013). In such places, the doctor is faced with difficult choices and often has to agonize over them. Difficult decisions have to be taken in situations in which the outcome is doubtful and the financial implications are substantial. For example, children with blindness due to hydrocephalus from a complex suprasellar tumor may often be treated with a shunt only because of the technical comfort level of the surgeon, lack of proper equipment, and financial limitations for the patient's family. If the tumor is approached, a very subtotal resection may be performed and the wait for radiotherapy may be very long. Neurosurgeons may have to recommend treatments they know are "second best" given various constraints. These issues also exist to a lesser degree in more resource-rich settings in which private health-care systems dictate that the patient must pay to receive a costly treatment.

Conclusion

To conclude, best ethical standards are followed if one treats a patient in the same way one would like to be treated oneself. At all times, the surgeon must make as certain as possible that he/she is making good decisions with the patient's best interests at heart and if anything gets in the way of this, the surgeon must recognize and acknowledge the problem and deal with it head-on.

The doctor should sincerely explain and discuss the disease of the patient, the natural course of the disease, various options of treatment, his/her own experience and capabilities, and his/her recommendation and then let the patient and family learn through their own resources about all these aspects to decide the final course of action. Such a process, if followed, helps the patient have faith in the treatment that the surgeon offers. There is a general feeling among doctors that the result of treatment is best when one has faith in the treating doctor and the doctor feels at ease in treating the patient. Teamwork, open discussions with colleagues, and most of all an open mind will help the doctor to make balanced ethically and medically sound decisions in the best interest of the patient.

References

Bernstein M (2003) Conflict of interest: it is ethical for an investigator to also be the care-giver in a clinical trial. J Neurooncol 63:107–108

Bernstein M, Khu LJ (2009) Is there too much variability in technical neurosurgery decision-making: virtual tumour board of a challenging case. Acta Neurochir 151:411–413

Bernstein M, Upshur REG (2008) The challenge of difficult patients. Parkhurst Exchange 16:74–75

Croskerry P, Petrie DA, Reilly JB et al (2014) Deciding about fast and slow decisions. Acad Med 89(2):197–200

Dasenbrock HH, Juraschek SP, Schultz LB et al (2012) The efficacy of minimally invasive discectomy compared with open discectomy: a meta-analysis of prospective randomized controlled trials. J Neurosurg Spine 16:452–462

Deekonda P, Bernstein M (2011) Decision making, bias, and low grade glioma. Can J Neurol Sci 38:193–194

Edem IJ, Banton B, Bernstein M et al (2013) A prospective qualitative study on patients' perceptions of endoscopic endonasal transsphenoidal surgery. Br J Neurosurg 27:50–55

Fath-Ordoubadi F, Lane RJ, Richards PG (1997) Histological surprise: callosal tuberculoma presenting as malignant glioma. J Neurol Neurosurg Psychiatry 163:98–99

Gottfried ON, Liu JK, Couldwell WT (2004) Comparison of radiosurgery and conventional surgery for the treatment of glomus jugulare tumors. Neurosurg Focus 17(2):E4

Groopman J (2007) How doctors think. Houghton Miflin Company, Boston

Hayhurst C, Mendelsohn D, Bernstein M (2011) Low grade glioma: a qualitative study of patients' perspectives on the wait and see approach. Can J Neurol Sci 38:256–261

Hoh BL, Chi YY, Dermott MA et al (2009) The effect of coiling versus clipping of ruptured and unruptured cerebral aneurysms on length of stay, hospital cost, hospital reimbursement, and surgeon reimbursement at the University of Florida. Neurosurgery 64(4):614–619

Howe KL, Malomo AO, Bernstein M (2013) Ethical challenges in international surgical education, for visitors and hosts. World Neurosurg 80:751–758

Ibrahim GM, Chung C, Bernstein M (2011) Competing for patients: an ethical framework for recruiting patient with brain tumors into clinical trials. J Neurooncol 104:623–627

Kirsch BM, Bernstein M (2012) Ethical challenges with awake craniotomy for tumor. Can J Neurol Sci 39:78–82

Lacroix M, Abi-Said D, Fourney DR et al (2001) A multivariate analysis of 416 patients with glioblastoma multiforme: prognosis, extent of resection, and survival. J Neurosurg 95:190–198

Laperriere NJ, Leung PMK, McKenzie S et al (1998) Randomized study of brachytherapy in the initial management of patients with malignant astrocytoma. Int J Radiat Oncol Biol Phys 41:1005–1011

Mortini P, Roberti F, Kalavakonda C et al (2003) Endoscopic and microscopic extended subfrontal approach to the clivus: a comparative anatomical study. Skull Base 13:139–147

Nandyala SV, Marquez-Lara A, Fineberg SJ et al (2014) Comparison between cervical total disc replacement and anterior cervical discectomy and fusion of 1–2 levels from 2002–2009. Spine (Phila Pa 1976) 39(1):53–57

Purzner T, Purzner J, Massicotte EM et al (2011) Outpatient brain tumor surgery and spinal decompression: a prospective study of 1003 Patients. Neurosurgery 69:119–127

Robertson JH (2008) Neurosurgery and industry. J Neurosurg 109:979–988

Seiz M, Freyschlag CF, Schenkel S et al (2011) Management of patients with low-grade gliomas – a survey among German neurosurgical departments. Cen Eur Neurosurg 72:186–191

Errors

13

Daniel Mendelsohn and Mark Bernstein

13.1 Introduction

Patient safety in medicine is the reduction of harm to patients caused by health-care interventions administered to them (Kohn et al. 2000). This should be at the core of value-based medicine. In the past two decades, errors in medicine have been increasingly publicized in the media and increasingly scrutinized within the health-care profession. The 1999 Institute of Medicine's report titled "to Err is Human" found errors in health care accounted for 100,000 deaths in the United States annually (Kohn et al. 2000).

Errors can be categorized into errors of execution (Fig. 13.1) or errors of planning, the former being the failure of a planned action to completed as intended and the latter meaning the implementation of the incorrect plan to achieve a goal (Reason 1990). Errors are assumed to be avoidable and patient safety measures are dedicated toward reducing the chance of errors bringing harm to a patient.

Adverse events are unintended outcomes of medical treatment that cause patient morbidity, mortality, or prolonged hospital stay (Kohn et al. 2000). Adverse events are either preventable, that is, caused by errors, or non-preventable. Not all errors lead to adverse events; an error which does not cause harm to the patient is referred to as a "near miss" (Reason 1990). Approximately half of all surgical adverse events are preventable (Gawande et al. 1999). In the surgical literature, no universally accepted definition of complications exists. One attempt defines surgical

D. Mendelsohn, MD, MSc
Division of Neurosurgery, University of British Columbia, Vancouver, BC, Canada
e-mail: danny.mendelsohn@gmail.com

M. Bernstein, MD, MHSc, FRCSC (✉)
Division of Neurosurgery, Toronto Western Hospital, University of Toronto,
399 Bathurst Street, M5T 2S8 Toronto, ON, Canada
e-mail: mark.bernstein@uhn.ca

A. Ammar, M. Bernstein (eds.), *Neurosurgical Ethics in Practice: Value-based Medicine*, 147
DOI 10.1007/978-3-642-54980-9_13, © Springer-Verlag Berlin Heidelberg 2014

Fig. 13.1 Planning CT (for fusion with MRI) after frame placement of a patient about to receive Gamma Knife radiosurgery for a small metastasis – a large right frontal one has been previously resected. In spite of the neurosurgeon taking care, the right frontal pin has been placed into the bone flap and has depressed it. Fortunately there were no negative sequelae

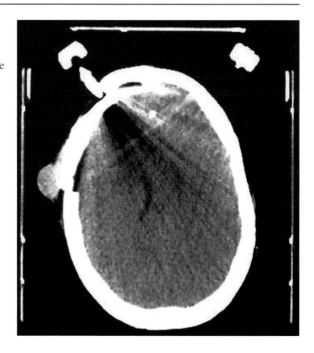

complications as "any undesirable, unintended and direct results of an operation affecting the patient which would not have occurred had the operation gone as well as could reasonably be hoped" (Sokol and Wilson 2008). "Complications occur, whereas errors are committed" according to one commentator (Angelos 2009). Under this definition, if an action or omission during surgery leads to an adverse event, it is considered an error and the adverse event was preventable. In contrast if despite best practices the adverse event occurred anyway, a complication occurred and the adverse event was non-preventable. In reality, most surgeons use the word complications in reference to adverse events that occurred as a result of surgery whether they were preventable or not.

> **Pearl**
> Adverse events are unintended outcomes of medical treatment that cause patient morbidity, mortality, or prolonged hospital stay. Preventable adverse events are caused by errors. Non-preventable adverse events are complications of care and treatment.

Errors and complications in neurosurgery have the potential for devastating outcomes and tragic patient harm. The eloquence and frailty of the nervous system structures and their critical role in human function make errors and complications in neurosurgery all the more harmful and regrettable. It is the neurosurgeon's obligation to take every precaution possible to prevent errors.

13.2   Illustrative Cases

Case 1 (An Error of Execution Occurs and the Patient Is Not Harmed)

A 60-year-old male with a right frontal glioma undergoes craniotomy for resection of tumor. While the nurse is draping the microscope, the surgeon makes use of the time to prepare the bone flap with titanium plates and screws and returns it to a basin on edge of the back table without informing the scrub nurse. A few minutes later the scrub nurse knocks the bone flap basin to the floor. The bone flap is discarded and a cranioplasty fashioned from a titanium mesh. The patient awakens without neurologic deficits and an infection never occurs.

Case 2 (An Error of Planning Occurs and the Patient Is Harmed)

A 45-year-old female presents with aneurysmal subarachnoid hemorrhage on Saturday afternoon. Vascular imaging reveals a 1.2 cm left supraclinoid internal carotid artery. The next best available opportunity for clipping the aneurysm is at 9:00 a.m. Sunday morning. The neurosurgeon specializes in functional neurosurgery and the two aneurysm surgeons are both away until Monday, but she decides to proceed. During the dissection around the aneurysm, an intraoperative rupture occurs and the surgeon struggles for 20 min to obtain proximal control leading to intraoperative hypotension from blood loss and prolonged cerebral ischemia from temporary clipping. Following the surgery, the patient awakens with complete hemiplegia and global aphasia.

Case 3 (No Error Occurs but the Patient Experiences a Complication)

A 70-year-old patient with normal pressure hydrocephalus is admitted to undergo an elective ventriculoperitoneal shunt insertion. The surgeon had recently reviewed the guidelines for prevention of shunt infections and adhered to current best practices including double-gloving and perioperative antibiotics. The surgery goes as planned and sterile technique is maintained throughout the procedure. The patient's initial postoperative course is uncomplicated and he is discharged on the second postoperative day. Two months later the patient returns with a shunt infection requiring a hospital admission, shunt removal, antibiotics, and eventual reinsertion.

13.3   Detection and Surveillance of Errors

Harvey Cushing, the "father" of modern neurosurgery recognized the importance of learning from errors and sharing them with peers. In a classic paper on the use of bony decompression for treating cerebral herniation, Cushing stated: "Surgical knowledge of value is built up more on the mistakes than on the successes of past experience" (Cushing 1905). Cushing also recognized the importance of strict prospective recording of errors.

There are several methods for detecting errors and adverse events. The most sensitive methods involve direct prospective observation and documentation of clinical care, frequent review of charts, and interviewing caregivers (Stone and Bernstein 2007). An increasing number of surgical practices are incorporating prospective error recording – one general surgery group demonstrated that continuous monitoring of adverse events reduced the number of errors during the study period by more than half (Rebasa et al. 2009). In comparison to prospective error recording, retrospective chart review detects far fewer errors and adverse events. Ten times as many postoperative adverse events following major spinal surgery were discovered when they were recorded prospectively compared to retrospective chart abstraction (Street et al. 2012).

> **Pearl**
> The most effective method of error recording is prospective observation and documentation of errors.

Prior to the increased focus on patient safety of the past decade, voluntary reporting was the major method for detecting adverse events. The Joint Commission, an oversight body that accredits hospitals in the United States, recommends voluntary reporting of sentinel events and "never events" such as wrong-site surgery and gossypiboma (retained foreign object), by accredited hospitals (Joint Commission 2012). Voluntary reporting of errors alone has a low detection rate for adverse events, but one advantage of voluntary reporting systems is that they enable systematic reviews of specific events and the development of systems for prevention. The Joint Commission performs root cause analysis on reported sentinel events, a system developed in psychology to identify factors that underlie variations in performance (Wu et al. 2008). Morbidity and mortality rounds are a form voluntary reporting commonly practiced in surgery. Although these rounds only detect a small proportion of adverse events, they are capable of teaching surgical residents to reflect on adverse events and can encourage openness in error reporting among colleagues.

The gold standard for error and adverse event detection and recording is prospective collection and documentation with frequent event review. However, voluntary reporting systems can raise awareness of the most significant errors and adverse events and can allow for analysis and development of systems for prevention.

13.4   Causes of Errors and Adverse Events

All errors can be ultimately attributed to human error in some way. The goal of patient safety initiatives is to minimize the chance of an error becoming an adverse event that harms a patient in some way; this is the error that is blocked from hurting the patient by systems put in place. A useful visible model for errors and adverse events is the Swiss cheese model or cumulative act effect. Many slices of Swiss cheese line up each representing a barrier. When the holes in all the slices line up, an error passes through them causing the error to become an adverse event (Reason 2000). The systems approach to patient safety views errors as inevitable and attempts to reduce the likelihood of systemic factors from contributing to errors and creates barriers for error prevention. The causes of errors and the reasons errors evade prevention can be classified as organization, situational, team, individual, task, and patient factors (Vincent et al. 2000).

> **Pearl**
> The systems approach to patient safety views errors as inevitable and attempts to promote the development of systems to create barriers to errors causing harm to patients. The most important step in error prevention is endorsing and embracing a culture of safety.

13.4.1 Organizational Factors

Organizational factors are underlying system conditions that predispose to errors (Vincent et al. 2000). Examples of organizational factors include adequacy of personnel and quality and availability of equipment, scheduling and timing of procedures, and substitution of usual team members with new team members. For instance, in Case A, an organizational policy mandating that the surgeon should inform the nurse when he/she returns the bone flap to the back table could have prevented the bone flap from being knocked to the floor. In neurosurgery, having specialized scrub nurses with experience in neurosurgery is critical for providing safe surgery. Hospitals are obliged to ensure adequate scrub nurse coverage for the types of elective operations that occur during regular working hours and the types of emergencies occurring afterhours.

13.4.2 Situational Factors

Situational factors are work environment conditions such as distractions and interruptions and equipment design elements such as monitors and displays (Bernstein et al. 2003). One study examining the type and timing of pages received by the on-call junior neurosurgery resident found that two-thirds of pages were classified as nonurgent and two-thirds occurred during and potentially interrupted patient care activities (Fargen and Friedman 2012). Several organizational approaches can minimize nonessential interruptions by establishing policies for managing nonurgent ward issues such as doctor's notes on patient's charts or specific times during the day for handling nonurgent concerns. Regarding equipment, if surgical equipment fails causing an error or adverse event, the equipment may require redesign. Furthermore, in this situation is the surgeon, hospital, or manufacturer culpable for the adverse event, or all three?

13.4.3 Team Factors

Team factors encompass verbal and written communication among team members, team structure such as leadership and supervision, confidence among team members, and the ability of teams to manage unexpected events (Vincent et al. 2000). In a review of 35 cases of wrong-site neurosurgery, communication breakdown among team members and between hospital departments was determined to be the most prevalent contributing factor to wrong-site neurosurgery (Cohen et al. 2010). In Case A, had the surgeon communicated to the scrub nurse he/she was returning the bone flap, the nurse may have positioned it away from the edge of the table and error could have been prevented.

13.4.4 Individual Factors

Individual factors include mental readiness, technical performance, and fatigue. Individual factors contribute to human errors that may become adverse events if barriers are not in place or are ineffective. Sleep deprivation impairs surgeon concentration and worsens performance (Taffinder et al. 1998). A significant number of wrong-site craniotomies occur during late hours and emergency situations (Cohen et al. 2010). Each surgeon is responsible for recognizing the individual factors that may affect their performance and for developing strategies to cope with fatigue and emergent situations.

13.4.5 Task Factors

Task factors relate to the task at hand including clear protocols and accurate available information. The omission of necessary task steps may be the most common type of human error. In Case B, the surgeon decided to proceed with a difficult aneurysm without proper backup from more experienced colleagues on a weekend (an example of task factors and individual factors). Surgery involves executing many different complex tasks in a coordinated fashion. In order to reduce the likelihood of omitted steps becoming adverse events, one may first determine whether the omission of a step in surgery could harm the patient. Second, decide if a particular step is predisposed to omission in particular. Lastly, develop a method for ensuring that a particular step is performed when necessary. For instance, in spine surgery, to prevent a wrong-level surgery, one should always obtain an intraoperative x-ray (or several as needed) verifying the correct level (Bernstein et al. 2003).

13.4.6 Patient Factors

Patient factors that may contribute to errors in surgery include obesity, anatomical variations, disease severity, and comorbidities. A large body habitus increases the task difficulty of lumbar puncture, increasing the likelihood of inadvertent injury to local structures. The location of certain tumors to eloquent neurologic structures increases the risk of postoperative deficits. Elderly patients experience more preventable adverse events because their comorbidities necessitate more complex care.

13.5 Error Prevention

13.5.1 Endorse a Culture of Safety

Reducing errors and adverse events in health care requires a multifaceted approach. The most important component to patient safety initiative is endorsing a culture of safety. Rather than a shame and blame approach that targets the individual for error culpability, the systems approach encourages learning from errors and ensuring they do not recur through systems-based initiatives. When a health-care professional mentions concerns about danger in the workplace or alerts leadership about an error that took place, their efforts should be commended. Today's generation of residents needs to experience and support a culture of safety in order to overcome the counterproductive traditional approach of shame and blame.

13.5.2 Improve Error Detection, Measurement and Reporting

In order to identify systemic factors contributing to errors, errors must be detected, measured, reported, and analyzed. The major barrier to error reporting is the existing culture of shame and blame and the public's view that physicians, especially surgeons, should be flawless. Near misses provide opportunities for analyzing situations where a patient was not harmed but still expose the factors that predispose to potentially devastating errors so the surgeon and the team can learn. For example, suppose a surgeon nearly performed a wrong-site craniotomy but realized at the last minute and no error occurred. The system failures that nearly enabled the error to take place can be scrutinized and future related adverse events can be prevented without casting shame or blame on an individual. The most effective method of detecting and measuring errors is the prospective recording of errors. Although at present, few oversight bodies require mandatory reporting of certain errors, reporting errors and adverse events allows for root cause analysis and future error prevention.

13.5.3 Embrace a Systems Approach

There are three principles underlying the systems approach:
1. Human error is unavoidable.
2. Faulty systems allow human errors to harm the patient.
3. Systems can be designed that prevent human error from causing patient harm.

These principles have been applied in other industries and have led to dramatic error reduction. In aviation, pilot error decreased 40 % over two decades, in part due to mandatory reporting of accidents, rigorous error analyses, and the development of meticulous error-prevention systems. An important component of the systems approach is the emphasis on "human factors." Understanding human abilities and limitations and applying this knowledge to equipment, machines, systems, and work environments can improve the safety and the effectiveness of task performance.

Surgeons tend to ignore human limitations. Compared to nonsurgical residents, residents in surgical training programs tend to perceive a lesser impact of sleep deprivation on their performance (Woodrow et al. 2008). In the aviation industry, strict limitations on works hours are enforced. In response to growing concerns by the public regarding the impact of sleep deprivation among residents on patient safety, the Accreditation Council for Graduate Medical Education has mandated an 80-h work week restriction for all American residency training programs. Whether these work hour limitations have improved patient safety remains unclear. The impact of fatigue on performance in surgery is a complex issue, and for now, it is the individual surgeon's responsibility to recognize their fatigue level and the potential impact on patient care and to do their best to modify work demands as much as possible to ensure patient safety is prioritized.

13.5.4　Know What to Fix

In order to develop safety solutions, a thorough understanding of the problem is crucial; a systematic evaluation of the factors that led to an error is a necessary first step. The Veterans Affairs National Center for Patient Safety has developed a root cause analysis tool that investigates the human factors that may have precipitated a near miss or error. Suggestions are then formed to prevent recurrences (Bagian et al. 2002). Anesthesiology has excelled at identifying systemic problems and designing solutions to address these problems. Since the 1970s, anesthesiologists have scrutinized adverse events, embraced human factors analyses, applied technological solutions, created standards and guidelines, and incorporated patient simulation in residency training. As a result, anesthesia is now safer than ever (Gaba 2000).

13.5.5　Be Suspicious and Proactive

New ways of doing things create ample opportunity for doing things incorrectly (McKneally 1999). In particular, the use of new technologies introduces the possibility for new types of errors to occur. A dry run can ensure mistakes are intercepted or mitigated before harm occurs. For instance, new technologies can often be tested in a simulated operating room environment before they are used on patients. Surgeon input during innovation is a proactive method for ensuring new technologies are user-friendly and less error prone (Bernstein et al. 2003).

13.5.6   Adopt Forcing and Constraining Functions

Forcing functions essentially make it impossible for errors to happen, such as in the OR oxygen tubing cannot mistakenly be connected to nitrogen tanks because the connections are incompatible. Constraining functions diminish but do not completely prohibit the chance of an error such as a preoperative surgical site marking policy. One example of a dramatic error that should always be preventable is wrong-sided surgery. The World Health Organization has devised a safe surgery checklist; in the initial multicenter study, this checklist reduced mortality and complications associated with surgery (Haynes et al. 2009). The routine use of surgical navigation systems would also make a wrong-sided craniotomy almost impossible to occur.

> **Pearl**
> Adherence to checklists and guidelines can minimize the chance of major errors occurring in surgery and must be incorporated into the standard of care.

13.5.7   Communicate Against Authority Gradients

The operating room has traditionally been a hierarchical environment with the surgeon serving as the captain. In the past, questioning the leading surgeon has been frowned upon and avoided by operating team members. Effective error prevention requires an open environment where team members can communicate concerns freely. A reluctance to voice concerns contributed to at least one wrong-sided craniotomy in the past (Cohen et al. 2010). In aviation training, crews use a two-check override system to voice concerns to a senior member. If a satisfactory explanation is not given after two challenges, a junior member can override a senior member's decision. This system allows for lines of authority to be challenged for the purposes of safety.

13.5.8   Prevent the "Unpreventable"

Not all adverse events are preventable. This is illustrated in Case C; the surgeon employed all the best sterility practices and despite their best efforts, the patient suffered a shunt infection. Surgeons must strive to make adverse events previously considered unpreventable preventable by developing and researching new practices. The Hydrocephalus Clinical Research Network is an exemplary initiative illustrating this point. Twenty-one pediatric neurosurgeons at four centers developed a protocol designed to reduce shunt infections and its implementation reduced the number of shunt infections by 36 %. Simple measures such as restricting OR traffic, positioning the head away from the OR entrance, and double-gloving were included in the protocol (Kestle et al. 2011). Preventing the "unpreventable" adverse events in the future will require similar innovative and collaborative efforts among neurosurgeons in multiple centers.

13.6   Disclosure of Errors and Complications

Once an error has occurred, when is the surgeon and institution obligated to disclose the error to the patient and/or family? Disclosure of errors has practical, legal, and ethical dimensions.

13.6.1   The Ethics of Disclosure

Patients (or their substitute decision-makers if the patient is considered incapable) have a right to know information affecting their medical care. Out of respect for patients as autonomous human beings, physicians are required to keep patients informed about major events, like errors. Several studies have demonstrated that patients want to be informed about all harmful medical errors (Gallagher et al. 2003; Hobgood et al. 2002). Failure to disclose significant errors constitutes deceptions and suggests the prioritization of professional self-interests over the best interests of the patient. The practical challenge is determining what to disclose.

The ethical principle of underlying the necessity for disclosure is that the greater the harm, or risk of harm, the greater the requirement of disclosure (Bernstein et al. 2003). If an error occurs and there is no harm or potential of future harm to the patient, this error does not need to be disclosed. For instance, if during a tumor resection, the image guidance system fails and troubleshooting leads to a 5 min delay, such an error does not necessitate disclosure because the error did not cause any foreseeable harm to the patient. However, if an error has the potential for future harm, such an error necessitates disclosure. For example, if during a craniotomy the bone flap falls to the floor and is discarded and synthetic cranioplasty fashioned, the patient must be informed of such an error. This type of error would increase the patient's risk of an infection in the future. Given that the error carries the potential for future harm, disclosure is necessary. Furthermore, any reasonable patient would want to know that "there is a plate in their head." Surgeons must exercise judgment in determining what to disclose. Near misses or trivial events that are inconsequential to a patient's care do not require disclosure. In contrast, errors that have any potential for immediate or future harm necessitate disclosure.

> **Pearl**
> Surgeons are obliged to disclose errors that harmed or have the potential to cause harm to the patient and those that any reasonable person would want to know. An apology does not constitute an admission of guilt or liability.

13.6.2   The Legal Aspects of Disclosure

Physicians are legally obliged to disclose an error "if it is something a reasonable person in the patient's position would want to know" (LeBlang 1981). Physicians face a number of barriers to disclosure including uncertainty about reporting

Table 13.1 Guidelines for disclosing adverse events (adapted from Bernstein et al. 2003)

1. Prepare patients and families in advance for the possibility of poor outcomes by comprehensively explaining the risks of a procedure and the potential for complications
2. If a complication or adverse event occurs, do not act defensively
3. If uncertain about how to disclose an error, seek counsel from others if time permits
4. Take the lead in error disclosure; do not wait for patients to ask
5. Explain in an objective manner the events that occurred and their implications for the patient. Do not attribute responsibility for the error
6. If events are not entirely clear or not all information is available at the time of error disclosure, only disclose what you know. Do not feel compelled to answer every question in the first meeting. Promise to get back to the patient/family in a timely manner
7. Document all events including discussions with the family
8. Do not attribute blame to individuals – to either yourself or coworkers. Never use the term negligence. Not all mistakes are culpable errors
9. Do not actively distance yourself from the patient/family. Open communication with the patient/family is an important legal defense
10. If the patient requires further medical attention, focus on the next steps in care. Offer the opportunity to seek a second opinion and/or have another surgeon assigned
11. Always be prepared to apologize. An apology is an empathetic statement and not an admission of guilt or liability

requirements, the desire to avoid upsetting patients, and concerns for the consequences of disclosure. One survey-based study from the 1980s found a third of physicians would offer incomplete misleading information to a patient's family about an error that led to the patient's death (Novack et al. 1989). This innate fear of retaliation is misguided. In the United States, only 2 % of negligent adverse events led to litigation in the form of malpractice claims and a policy of active disclosure of adverse events in one American hospital led to reduction in malpractice claims (Kraman and Hamm 1999). A survey-based study of primary care patients revealed patients were more likely to sue the physician if they were not informed of an error in their care (Witman et al. 1996). A qualitative study on errors in patients with brain tumors found that trust in the surgeon was of critical importance (Bernstein et al. 2004). Failure to disclose errors can compromise a patient's trust in their surgeon.

Pearl
Patients/families are less likely to seek legal action if they are promptly informed of errors that occurred in the course of their care.

Physicians may fail to disclose errors because of a lack of clear policies and guidelines for error disclosure at their institution. The Joint Commission now requires hospitals to have mechanisms in place for informing patients about untoward incidents (Wojcieszak et al. 2006). Individual hospitals are responsible for ensuring policies are in place for disclosing errors to patients (Table 13.1) and that support mechanisms are available to help clinicians, patients, and families cope with errors and adverse events.

Conclusion

Surgery and medical care are complex human tasks that will inevitably be affected by errors. Surgeons and health-care providers must embrace a culture of openness toward errors and adverse events and must prioritize patient safety. The active prevention of errors and adverse events requires systems for error detection, reporting, and rigorous analyses of root causes. Systems for prevention depend on checklists, guidelines, open communication, and teamwork among health-care providers. Research initiatives and collaboration among clinicians can improve adverse event prevention. Surgeons are obligated to educate themselves on their individual institution's policies and guidelines for error disclosure. If an error occurs that harms a patient or has the potential for future harm, surgeons must actively disclose errors in a practical and socially responsible manner.

References

Angelos P (2009) Complications, errors, and surgical ethics. World J Surg 33(4):609–611

Bagian JP, Gosbee J, Lee CZ et al (2002) The Veterans Affairs root cause analysis system in action. Jt Comm J Qual Improv 28(10):531–545

Bernstein M, Hebert PC, Etchells E (2003) Patient safety in neurosurgery: detection of errors, prevention of errors, and disclosure of errors. Neurosurg Q 13(2):125–137

Bernstein M, Potvin D, Martin DK (2004) A qualitative study of attitudes toward error in patients facing brain tumour surgery. Can J Neurol Sci 31(2):208–212

Cohen FL, Mendelsohn D, Bernstein M (2010) Wrong-site craniotomy: analysis of 35 cases and systems for prevention. J Neurosurg 113(3):461–473

Cushing H (1905) The establishment of cerebral hernia as a decompressive measure for inaccessible brain tumors: with the description of intermuscular methods of making the bone defect in temporal and occipital regions. Surg Gynecol Obstet 1:297–314

Fargen KM, Friedman WA (2012) An observational study of junior neurosurgery resident call at a large teaching hospital. J Grad Med Educ 4(1):119

Gaba DM (2000) Anaesthesiology as a model for patient safety in health care. BMJ 320(7237):785–788

Gallagher TH, Waterman AD, Ebers AG, Fraser VJ, Levinson W (2003) Patients' and physicians' attitudes regarding the disclosure of medical errors. JAMA 289(8):1001–1007

Gawande AA, Thomas EJ, Zinner MJ et al (1999) The incidence and nature of surgical adverse events in Colorado and Utah in 1992. Surgery 126(1):66–75

Haynes AB, Weiser TG, Berry WR et al (2009) A surgical safety checklist to reduce morbidity and mortality in a global population. N Engl J Med 360(5):491–499

Hobgood C, Peck CR, Gilbert B et al (2002) Medical errors-what and when: what do patients want to know? Acad Emerg Med 9(11):1156–1161

Joint Commission (2012) Sentinel event policy expanded beyond patients. Jt Comm Perspect 32(12):1–3

Kestle JR, Riva-Cambrin J, Wellons JC et al (2011) A standardized protocol to reduce cerebrospinal fluid shunt infection: the Hydrocephalus Clinical Research Network Quality Improvement Initiative. J Neurosurg Pediatr 8(1):22–29

Kohn LT, Corrigan J, Donaldson MS (2000) To err is human : building a safer health system. National Academy Press, Washington, DC

Kraman SS, Hamm G (1999) Risk management: extreme honesty may be the best policy. Ann Intern Med 131(12):963–967

LeBlang TR (1981) Disclosure of injury and illness: responsibilities in the physician-patients relationship. Law Med Health Care 9(4):4–7

McKneally MF (1999) Ethical problems in surgery: innovation leading to unforeseen complications. World J Surg 23(8):786–788

Novack DH, Detering BJ, Arnold R et al (1989) Physicians' attitudes toward using deception to resolve difficult ethical problems. JAMA 261(20):2980–2985

Reason JT (1990) Human error. Cambridge University Press, Cambridge England

Reason J (2000) Human error: models and management. BMJ 320(7237):768–770

Rebasa P, Mora L, Luna A et al (2009) Continuous monitoring of adverse events: influence on the quality of care and the incidence of errors in general surgery. World J Surg 33(2):191–198

Sokol DK, Wilson J (2008) What is a surgical complication? World J Surg 32(6):942–944

Stone S, Bernstein M (2007) Prospective error recording in surgery: an analysis of 1108 elective neurosurgical cases. Neurosurgery 60(6):1075–1080

Street JT, Lenehan BJ, DiPaola CP et al (2012) Morbidity and mortality of major adult spinal surgery. A prospective cohort analysis of 942 consecutive patients. Spine J 12(1):22–34

Taffinder NJ, McManus IC, Gul Y et al (1998) Effect of sleep deprivation on surgeons' dexterity on laparoscopy simulator. Lancet 352(9135):1191

Vincent C, Taylor-Adams S et al (2000) How to investigate and analyse clinical incidents: clinical risk unit and association of litigation and risk management protocol. BMJ 320(7237): 777–781

Witman AB, Park DM, Hardin SB (1996) How do patients want physicians to handle mistakes? A survey of internal medicine patients in an academic setting. Arch Intern Med 156(22): 2565–2569

Wojcieszak D, Banja J, Houk C (2006) The sorry works! coalition: making the case for full disclosure. Jt Comm J Qual Patient Saf 32(6):344–350

Woodrow SI, Park J, Murray BJ et al (2008) Differences in the perceived impact of sleep deprivation among surgical and non-surgical residents. Med Educ 42(5):459–467

Wu AW, Lipshutz AK, Pronovost PJ (2008) Effectiveness and efficiency of root cause analysis in medicine. JAMA 299(6):685–687

Workplace Ethics and Professionalism

14

Ross Upshur and Mark Bernstein

14.1 Introduction

There was a time when the words and actions of the surgeon were paramount – life in the hospital was nondemocratic but simple. But the delivery of health care has undergone significant transformation in the past few decades. Health care has become more complex, delivered in multiple contexts by a growing number of recognized health professionals (Breitbach et al. 2013; Clark 2014). In the past health-care institutions were dominated by physicians and nurses, who, in addition to service delivery, also played most of the key administrative roles. Concerns for quality of care and patient safety have motivated initiatives to foster team-based care. This requires consideration of both interdisciplinary and interprofessional aspects of ethics, essential to the practice of value-based medicine. In addition, health-care institutions and their functions have become more complex. Health sciences centers often combine missions of service delivery, research, and education which brings additional human resources into the mix. Neurosurgeons are increasingly recognizing the importance of professionalism and teamwork (Apuzzo 2013; Bernstein 2005; Dacey 2013; Harnof et al. 2013; Kanat and Epstein 2010; McLaughlin et al. 2013; Sekhar and Mantovani 2013). There is also a recognition that the ethic of an institution percolates down to the workers and can positively influence workplace professionalism (Silva et al. 2008).

R. Upshur, MD, MSc (✉)
Division of Clinical Public Health, Department of Family and Community Medicine,
Clinical Research, Dalla Lana School of Public Health, Bridgepoint Health,
University of Toronto, Toronto, ON, Canada
e-mail: ross.upshur@gmail.com

M. Bernstein, MD, MHSc, FRCSC
Division of Neurosurgery, Toronto Western Hospital, University of Toronto,
399 Bathurst Street, Toronto, ON M5T 2S8, Canada
e-mail: mark.bernstein@uhn.ca

A. Ammar, M. Bernstein (eds.), *Neurosurgical Ethics in Practice: Value-based Medicine*,
DOI 10.1007/978-3-642-54980-9_14, © Springer-Verlag Berlin Heidelberg 2014

The reality of health care is that there are multiple health professions, administrators, and others involved in a complex web of relationships. The playing field has been leveled such that all members of the health-care team have voices that count, which is a good thing for patients. The advent of team-based care has forced health-care providers, educators, and administrators to rethink the roles and responsibilities of health-care providers in the context of teams. However, the bulk of the literature in bioethics focuses on specific and easily identifiable issues related to the extremities of life such as end of life decisions, intensive care unit experience, and neonatology. Much of workplace ethics will be of the everyday nature and deal with the interactions of the varied and heterogeneous providers. Each of these has their own codes of ethics and organizations which also instill particular cultures which influence ethical considerations.

Ethical issues are common in health care. The last two decades have witnessed increased attention to ethics training in the health-care professions. Many academic programs need to demonstrate proof of ethics training as a condition for accreditation. Similarly, many health-care institutions have devoted more resources to ethics services in terms of full time ethicists and support for ethics committees.

It is commonly thought that health professionals work from a well-established common ground of shared values. This, however, has been shown in numerous studies to be untrue (Bleakely 2006; Stiggelbout et al. 2006). Empirical studies have demonstrated that there are considerable intra- and interprofessional differences in how various ethical issues are understood and weighed (Miyashita et al. 2007). Personal and professional morality may also come into conflict in the conduct of daily work and may be particularly evident in interprofessional contexts (Upshur and Bernstein 2008). Formal effort is increasingly being directed at teaching professionalism (Hochberg et al. 2010; Parran at al 2013).

However, ethics training focuses largely on the roles and responsibilities of health-care providers with respect to the provision of care to individual patients. Ethics consultations also focus largely on issues related to the care of individual patients. This leaves a gap in terms of how to manage ethical issues that arise in the context of the workplace. This is particularly important in terms of addressing the ethics of interprofessional and team-based care. There is comparatively little literature and scholarship on this topic in the literature (Clark et al. 2007).

Despite the rapid move towards team-based care, the literature has not kept pace. It is clear that competency in workplace ethics is desirable as it is highly unlikely that health-care institutions will become simpler in the near future. As well, the days of physicians being the unquestioned leader and decision maker are likely in the past.

The well-known principles of autonomy beneficence, non-maleficence, and justice do not adapt easily to workplace ethics as they were specifically formulated to address issues related to care of patients by health-care providers. It may be necessary to draw from other ethical frameworks and theories (Bernstein and Fundner 2003) to assist in workplace ethics as it requires the framing and analysis of ethical issues in a manner that is not explicitly focused on the patient, but rather on the team or the organization.

> **Pearl**
> High-profile ethical issues like end of life conflicts and treatment of other vulnerables like neonates are actually relatively uncommon but get a lot of attention. Workplace ethics and breaches of professionalism are everyday occurrences, and continual vigilance is required by all members of the health-care team, mainly not only about their own behavior but also that of others.

14.2 Illustrative Case (Numerous Breaches of Professionalism)

A neurosurgeon is editing a multiauthored book and three of his chapter authors are late weeks after the deadline. When he e-mails them to find out what's going on, two respond that they have been very busy and will get to it when they can, and the third does not respond at all. That night the neurosurgeon is on call and is paged in the middle of the night by an emergency physician at another hospital an hour away without neurosurgical services. The ER doctor has an 87 year-old woman, with a very small traumatic brain contusion following a fall at home; her GCS is 15. The neurosurgeon yells at the emergency doctor stating, "This is not an emergency – why are you bothering me? You could have called me later in the morning for some advice." A few hours later at morning rounds, he tells his residents about the "stupid idiot" who woke him up in the middle of the night. An hour later he is performing an awake craniotomy in the OR and while doing so he chats with his residents about his other patients who are in hospital. Later that day on the ward, he shakes his head in desperation at a physiotherapist who is blocking his order to discharge one of his postoperative patients to her home. On the way home in the evening, he rides down in a full elevator in which two medical residents are animatedly discussing a complex patient, but says nothing to them.

14.3 Approach to the Case

As the vignette illustrates, lapses of professionalism and tensions often occur between health-care professionals in the conduct of everyday work. Examples of some which occur commonly and appear in our case include failure to respond to e-mails in a timely way (Bernstein 2006), violating patients' privacy by speaking about other patients within earshot of patients or loved ones (Zener and Bernstein 2011; Howe and Bernstein 2014), and speaking disrespectfully to colleagues (Upshur and Bernstein 2008). While much of this may relate to the quite heterogeneous personalities, perfectionist temperaments, and multitasking skills of health-care providers, it would be a mistake to simply relinquish many of these issues to personality conflicts and/or personality flaws. The ability to be a good collaborator is often included in discussions of professionalism. Exemplary professional behavior would entail acting in a collegial manner, the manner in which one would want to be treated by others.

Personality conflicts may raise ethical issues particularly when they threaten patient safety. Some of these conflicts may legitimately arise from competing values between clinicians. It is seldom required of a physician that they be familiar and conversant with the codes of professional ethics of their colleagues. But ethics entails more than just considerations of etiquette and manners. Ethics drills deeper into the underlying value structure and addresses arguments to support or rebuff preferred courses of action.

Workplace ethics makes us reflect on the fact that our work is not carried out in isolation and that our behavior may have significant impact on those around us. The neurosurgeon in the case may be rightly frustrated by the actions of his professional colleagues, but this does not justify his actions to others and the implications of the behavior on team function.

It is easy to pass summary judgment on the surgeon. Yelling at colleagues is clearly not an acceptable behavior. Is it unethical though? To make this case we need an analytical framework that will help us determine where the ethical problems exist and how they can be interpreted.

Pearl
Surgeons will always have bad days, but a systemic culture of collegiality and tolerance must exist in the workplace so that occasional breakdowns do not have pervasive negative effects. This is not dissimilar to the patient safety culture in which systemic safeguards are in place to help prevent human errors from hurting patients.

14.4   A Framework for Interprofessional Teamwork Ethics

Ethical frameworks are commonly employed as a means of aiding in the explicit recognition of value issues in health care. The idea of a framework is a metaphor that directs attention to how we organize our thinking about a topic. Frameworks can take many formats and include substantive and procedural dimensions. It has been argued that the primary role of ethical frameworks is to aid in the process of deliberation about what ought to be done in a particular situation (Dawson 2009). Frameworks are not the same as overarching ethical theories in that they do not seek to justify actions on the basis of consistent theoretical considerations. It is argued: "…there is nothing wrong with a framework taking certain theoretical considerations for granted and concentrating upon aiding busy decision makers through the provision of a checklist of relevant considerations, principles and issues to keep in mind" (Dawson 2009). As such ethical frameworks are pragmatic and action oriented.

A conceptual framework has been created to aid in the understanding of ethical issues involved in teamwork (Clarke et al. 2007). This group conducted a systematic review of the literature and identified significant gaps in the understanding of inter-professional ethics. While policy documents and regulatory bodies have advocated for greater collaboration and teamwork, there was a paucity of scholarship in this domain. As they note:

> Despite the recognition by professional bodies of the moral responsibilities of health care professionals to act collaboratively, there is little discussion in the literature of the unique ethical issues encountered when a group of health care providers interact with each other. To practice teamwork, health care professionals need to have an understanding both of their own discipline and of how other disciplines function, their views of the patient, and their strengths and limitations. However, even this knowledge is not sufficient, as there will be disagreements between providers and disciplines. The efficiency of teamwork has to do with establishing ongoing methods to capture the strength of these disagreements, and to use this strength to increase the effectiveness of care. Further, the goals and rules of the organization need to support the efforts of the team at achieving this efficiency and effectiveness. (Clark et al. 2007)

To address these shortcomings the authors propose a comprehensive framework for understanding and addressing ethical issues in teamwork. Their framework is oriented as a matrix that shows the linkage between principles to guide behavior, structures within organization that facilitate or impair teamwork and collaboration, and processes that enable professional activity. They argue that each of these three elements can be approached from the individual level (micro), the team level (meso), and the organizational level (macro).

Many other chapters in this book focus on individual level analysis of ethical issues. Teamwork and team-based ethics competency should be integrated into everyday practice. Many approaches to ethics foster self-reflection and concern for the justification of personally held beliefs; team-based ethics requires that we all use that self-knowledge explicitly as a basis for engaging others. Not only is it required that we are cognizant of the standards and expectations of our own particular profession, it is also required that we understand other professions as well. Structures may need to be put in place to facilitate this so that all team members have basic competencies. The framework described above further integrates reflection at several levels of application and focuses beyond the individual to the team and organizational level.

Pearl
Bioethical frameworks provide a way to approach ethical dilemmas and organize thinking about a problem. The one presented herein helps focus on teamwork and professionalism.

14.4.1 Team Level Approaches

At the team level, four principles are recommended as general guidelines of behavior (Clark et al. 2007):

1. Promote respect, truth telling, beneficence, and justice in relationships with other team members.
2. Address communication and conflict problems.
3. Develop understanding of differences in values, methods, and contributions of other team members.
4. Share responsibility for promoting team and accountability for its decisions and outcomes.

Three structures are identified to analyze forms of knowledge and patterns of behavior:

1. Integrate professional knowledge with other team members.
2. Develop integrated patient problem definitions and a structure for assessment and care planning.
3. Promote and protect the team as a distinct structure.

Finally, three processes are identified on how interprofessional ethics can be done:

1. Develop an ethic of open communication and dialogue.
2. Arrive on time for meetings.
3. Develop and implement integrated patient care plans.

14.4.2 Organizational Level Approaches

Three principles guide organizational behavior:

1. Respect unique relationships between the team and the patient.
2. Understand basic principles of teamwork.
3. Provide sufficient resources for the team to accomplish its work and fulfill its mission.

Two enabling structures:

1. Provide sufficient resource foundation for the team.
2. Establish evaluative structures for assessment of the team's work.

Two processes:

1. Support team development and function.
2. Appoint a facilitator to address communication and ethical issues and mediate team conflicts.

14.5 Applying the Framework to the Case

Clearly the neurosurgeon in the case example is having a bad day. Academic colleagues have failed to uphold their responsibilities as collaborators, a clinical case referred to him by a clinical colleague was considered inappropriate, and an allied health professional thwarted his discharge plans. To top it all off, he was witness to questionable professional behavior by trainees.

A straightforward analysis of this may suggest that the neurosurgeon failed to meet professional standards by acting out and verbally abusing his clinical colleagues, mocking one to his residents, and failing to correct the behavior of the trainees. At the same time he was disrespected by his colleagues who had promised him a chapter and/or did not respond to his e-mails. An analysis of the ethics of such behavior would be well covered in terms of theories that provide principles to adjudicate such behavior. A consequentialist, or utilitarian, would point out the net disutility associated with the negative atmosphere created by such behavior. A deontologist would point out that this type of action is wrong on its own merits and could not be willed to be made universal. A virtue theorist would point out that the qualities and characteristics manifest in such behavior fail to exemplify positive professional virtues and are not worthy of emulation. It is interesting that all three major universalist theories would converge on similar analysis. The corrective action to this case in each of these accounts would focus on remediation of the agent, as if the neurosurgeon himself or the other individuals were entirely to blame.

However, there is good reason to examine this case in light of interprofessional ethics. Modern health-care institutions frequently use the language of teams when describing the range of health-care providers that will be associated with any patient's care. Could some of the issues in this case be related to organizational failures in terms of supporting and facilitating team-based care?

In two instances in the case a more robust team-based approach to care would have provided ground rules for mutual respect and communication. The organization would have invested time and resources into building respect and appropriate communication in the team. If team-based care existed, the neurosurgeon would have had a better understanding of the referral patterns of the outside hospital emergency department, and so might the referring doctor, and may have the language to better understand and engage with the physiotherapist's concerns. In both cases, teamwork would have entailed the creation of integrated care plans where each member of the health-care team would be aware of their roles and responsibilities, thus diminishing interpersonal and interprofessional conflict.

The case may also represent an organizational failure. There may be a pervasive institutional culture that tolerates and perhaps rewards intemperate, non-collegial, and unprofessional behavior. The framework described above (Clark et al. 2007) directs attention to the organizational dimension of ethical concerns in ways that escape some of the more commonly used approaches in medical ethics.

At the organizational level, elements of basic principles, structures, and processes are not evident. It is clear that there is insufficient understanding of the basics of teamwork. This may be due to the organization failing to provide or commit to ensuring the required resources to build, nurture, and support teams. It is also evident that no facilitator is in place for mediation and resolution of conflict among the clinical team. Leaders in health-care organizations should take steps to support the function of teams.

Pearl

Neurosurgeons should try to always treat others as we would wish to be treated and take every opportunity to reflect on our own behavior and make sure it satisfies the level of quality we would expect of others.

Conclusion

The strengths of the framework are that it moves consideration of ethical issues in health care beyond simply the individual and begins the process of outlining the ethical responsibilities of team members. Furthermore, it directs attention to the organizational context of care and therefore explains the duties and responsibilities of organizations to foster optimal team performance.

Addressing ethical issues in health care from the team and organizational level in addition to the individual level adds nuance and sophistication to ethical analysis. It also creates insights that may prevent hasty conclusions regarding alleged unethical or unprofessional behavior of individuals by looking at how organizations can create the context for better standards of behavior. Below is presented a simplistic list of goals and tips to improve the ethics and culture of the workplace.

Long-term broader goals:

1. Learn about the codes of ethics of your fellow health professionals.
2. Reflect upon your own core values and how they may influence your work with others.
3. Educate referring doctors and others about the most effective way to interact with you.
4. Develop a relationship with your ethics service.
5. Include workplace ethics topics in your academic rounds.
6. Advocate for your institution to support interprofessional ethics initiatives.
7. Be a positive role model to your residents and students so that they will be acculturated to professional workplace behavior.
   Practical personal everyday tips:
1. Respond to communications from colleagues (e.g., e-mails, telephone calls) in a timely manner.
2. Attend meetings or other commitments on time.
3. Keep promises and commitments to colleagues.
4. Do not enter into acrimonious exchanges with colleagues, and if you absolutely feel you must provide some "constructive criticism" in this way, do it in private.
5. Do not speak badly about colleagues to other colleagues, especially those junior to you.
6. Do not discuss clinical cases within earshot of any member of the lay public.
7. Try to treat others as you would wish to be treated.
8. If you perpetrate a breach of professionalism and/or poor teamwork, apologize to the affected parties. If you witness such behavior in others, address it to them, and if they are unreceptive, be prepared to speak to their manager.

References

Apuzzo ML (2013) Facets of professionalism. World Neurosurg 79(1):1

Bernstein M (2005) Professionalism. We know it when we see it. Parkhurst Exchange 13

Bernstein M (2006) E-mail etiquette. Parkhurst Exchange 14:210

Bernstein M, Fundner R (2003) House of healing, house of disrespect: a Kantian perspective on disrespectful behaviour among hospital workers. Hosp Q 6:62–66

Bleakely A (2006) A common body of care: the ethics and politics in the operating theatre are inseparable. J Med Philos 31:305–327

Breitbach AP, Sargeant DM, Getlemeier PR et al (2013) From buy-in to integration: melding an interprofessional initiative into academic programs in the health professions. J Allied Health 42(3):e67–e73

Clark PG (2014) Narrative in interprofessional education and practice: implications for professional identity, provider-patient communication and teamwork. J Interprof Care 28(1):34–39

Clark P, Cott C, Drinka T (2007) Theory and practice in interprofessional ethics: a framework for understanding ethical issues in health care teams. J Interprof Care 21:591–603

Dacey RG (2013) Challenges to neurosurgical professionalism: 2012. Neurosurgery 2013(60 Suppl 1):30–33

Dawson A (2009) Theory and practice in public health ethics: a complex relationship. In: Peckham S, Hann A (eds) Public health ethics and practice. Policy Press, London, pp 191–209

Harnof S, Hadani M, Ziv A et al (2013) Simulation-based interpersonal communication skills training for neurosurgical residents. Isr Med Assoc J 15(9):489–492

Hochberg MS, Kalet A, Zabar S et al (2010) Can professionalism be taught? Encouraging evidence. Am J Surg 199(1):86–93

Howe K, Bernstein (2014) Privacy concerns in the surgical environment. J Clin Res Bioeth 4:3

Kanat A, Epstein CR (2010) Challenges to neurosurgical professionalism. Clin Neurol Neurosurg 112(10):839–843

McLaughlin N, Carrau RL, Kelly DF et al (2013) Teamwork in skull base surgery: an avenue for improvement in patient care. Surg Neurol Int 25:4–36

Miyashita M, Morita T, Shima Y et al (2007) Nurse views of the adequacy of decision making and nurse distress regarding artificial hydration for terminally ill cancer patients: a nationwide survey. Am J Hosp Palliat Care 24:463–469

Parran TV, Pisman AR, Youngner SJ et al (2013) Evolution of a remedial CME course in professionalism: addressing learner needs, developing content, and evaluating outcomes. J Contin Educ Health Prof 33:174–179

Sekhar LN, Mantovani A (2013) Teamwork mentality in neurosurgical teams to improve patient safety. World Neurosurg. [2013 Sept 6 Epub ahead of print]

Silva DS, Gibson JL, Sibbald R et al (2008) Clinical ethicists' perspectives on organisational ethics in healthcare organisations. J Med Ethics 34(5):320–323

Stiggelbout AM, Elstein AS, Molewijk B et al (2006) Clinical ethical dilemmas: convergent and divergent views of two scholarly communities. J Med Ethics 32:381–388

Upshur R, Bernstein M (2008) Conflicts with colleagues. We're just human, after all. Parkhurst Exchange 16:62–64

Zener R, Bernstein M (2011) Gender, patient comfort, and the neurosurgical operating room. Can J Neurol Sci 38:65–71

Neurosurgical Innovation

15

Karen M. Devon and Mark Bernstein

15.1 Introduction

The history of surgical progress cannot be told without reference to the creativity of surgeons. In neurosurgery, examples include the development of surgical navigation from stereotactic frames to frameless stereotaxy to intraoperative MRI, the invention of stereotactic radiosurgery and specifically the Gamma Knife, the introduction of the operating microscope and then its application to routine procedures such as lumbar discectomy, and the development of spinal instrumentation. These surgeon-driven innovations revolutionized the specialty, and the practice of modern neurosurgery would be unthinkable without these and many other innovations. However, some innovations fail, despite initial hopes that they might be better, and thus unbridled enthusiasm toward interventions that are new can be harmful. Unlike new drugs, when a surgeon thinks that he/she can do something differently to make it better, there is no regulatory oversight he/she must obtain prior to trying it, thus the importance of value-based medicine to guide them.

Surgeons also know that they are constantly making choices in an individual's operation since no two are exactly alike (Riskin et al. 2006) and thus even defining what is actually "new" may be difficult (Reistma and Moreno 2002). Furthermore, in some cases where overall complications are low, in order to determine whether an approach is better than a preexisting one, thousands of patients would need to be enrolled in a randomized trial (Morreim et al. 2006).

K.M. Devon MD, MSc, FRCSC (✉)
Division of General Surgery, Women's College Hospital, University Health Network,
University of Toronto, 76 Grenville Street, Toronto, ON, Canada
e-mail: karen.devon@wchospital.ca

M. Bernstein, MD, MHSc, FRCSC
Division of Neurosurgery, Toronto Western Hospital, University of Toronto,
399 Bathurst Street, Toronto, ON M5T 2S8, Canada
e-mail: mark.bernstein@uhn.ca

A. Ammar, M. Bernstein (eds.), *Neurosurgical Ethics in Practice: Value-based Medicine*,   171
DOI 10.1007/978-3-642-54980-9_15, © Springer-Verlag Berlin Heidelberg 2014

Thus, traditional methods of research prior to implementation are not possible and most surgical innovation does not occur in this manner (Lotz 2013; Morreim et al. 2006). Furthermore, the innovators often lack equipoise since they have developed the new procedure in order to improve care (Angelos 2010; Johnson and Rogers 2012; Taylor 2010). All of this brings out several ethical issues which are addressed in this chapter.

15.2 Illustrative Case (Surgeon Innovates Without Oversight)

A neurosurgeon observes that his patients' lengths of stay for intra-axial brain tumor surgery have progressively decreased over his career. This is partly due to adjunctive care such as awake craniotomy and surgical navigation. He eventually feels that day surgery craniotomy, in which the patient does not spend a single overnight in hospital, is feasible, safe, cost-effective, and desirable in order to avoid in-hospital complications. To his knowledge this has never been done before anywhere in the world. He starts to perform day surgery craniotomy with his patients' full consent, but without any other oversight from the inception to the time he publishes the results in a peer-reviewed journal 5 years after starting this innovation.

15.3 Approach to the Case

The above example could be considered innovation, or it might be seen simply as a natural evolution of the art and science of clinical neurosurgical practice (Bernstein 2001; Bernstein and Bampoe 2004; Boulton and Bernstein 2008; Purzner et al. 2011). This highlights the difficult challenge of defining, analyzing the ethics of, and introducing surgical innovation.

Currently no widely accepted ethical framework by which to assess the ethicality of a surgical innovation exists. Both institutions and individual surgeons have two obligations with respect to new innovation. First, innovation must be supported in circumstances which merit it. That is, if the oversight required for any creative alteration of procedures is so extensive that it hinders progress, then it may also hinder potential benefits to society. Second, they must also ensure that when innovation does occur, it proceeds in an ethical manner. Surgeons must honestly explain the known risks, benefits, and alternatives of a new procedure. They must also express that which is currently unknown about the innovation and include their own experience. When appropriate, consultation from an ethics board or peer review (such as the surgeon-in-chief at one's hospital or a committee of surgeons in the same specialty) should be sought. In the case where a new procedure which has been done elsewhere is being introduced at a new institution, both parties must insure that there has been adequate patient selection, training and mentoring of health-care professionals, and the ability to collect process and outcome data.

> **Pearl**
> The appropriate treatment of surgical innovation is a balance of obligations – one's fiduciary responsibility to individual patients against potential benefits to future patients and to society at large.

15.4 Discussion

15.4.1 Definition of Innovation

The distinction between innovation and clinical care or research first appeared in the Belmont Report (National Commission 1978) as is described as "practice that departs significantly from the standard or accepted." However, this gives rise to further questions about what is considered standard or accepted and who defines these standards. The intent of "research," as opposed to that of some innovations, is not to directly improve the care of patients involved, but rather to test a hypothesis. Research allows one to draw conclusions that may contribute to generalizable knowledge (Bernstein and Bampoe 2004). With innovation, there is often no intent to publish the surgical series at a later time (Morreim et al. 2006). On the other hand, clinical practice refers to interventions designed solely to enhance the well-being of an individual (National Commission 1978). The precise definition of innovation is still one of considerable debate (Reitsma and Moreno 2005).

Several different categories of innovation have been articulated (Reitsma and Moreno 2005):
1. A novel procedure
2. A significant modification of a standard technique
3. A new application of or new indication for an established technique
4. A combination of an established technique with a new therapeutic modality
5. A procedure being used for the first time by a surgeon

While it is useful to distinguish between these categories, doing so is not always straightforward. In particular in the second case, determining what modifications are significant versus not can be challenging. In 2008, the Society of University Surgeons tried to clarify the difference between variations, innovations, and research (Biffl et al. 2008). Variation was defined as "the minor modification of a surgical procedure that does not have the reasonable expectation of increasing the risk to the patient. Variations should not extend the time of anesthesia." Furthermore, they state that these need not be routinely discussed during the consent process (Biffl et al. 2008). An innovation was described as "a new or modified surgical procedure that differs from currently accepted local practice, the outcomes of which have not been described, and which may entail risk to the patient" (Biffl et al. 2008). Our case example may fall into this category. Many of these are dictated, on an ad hoc basis by a clinical situation, and at the time they are performed and do not meet criteria for human subjects research (Biffl et al. 2008).

Finally, research is defined as it is above, as a systematic investigation designed to develop or contribute to generalizable knowledge. Arguably the most meaningful way to assess what is innovation and what is not is by using qualitative research to access the views of key stakeholders (Danjoux et al. 2007; Ehrlich et al. 2013; Rogers et al. 2014).

15.4.2 Conflict of Interest

Surgeons generally act in pursuit of the patient's best interests; however, several nonfinancial conflicts of interest inherently exist when surgeons become innovators: (1) there is the emotional excitement associated with the satisfaction of contributing to advances in medicine and (2) reputation and academic advancement can both be greatly enhanced by developing a new procedure. These can be mitigated by third-party review of outcomes (Awad 1996) as well as rigorous peer review at the developmental stage (Grimmett and Sulmasy 1998). While some recommend that all innovation ultimately be tested in a formal research study, there are difficulties with this as well. For instance, when rare diseases are involved, small numbers may preclude determining a statistically significant difference in outcome.

Next, there may be direct or indirect financial rewards provided as a result of new innovation. Direct rewards would be proceeds of a new patented device. Indirectly, a surgeon known to have invented a new technique might receive more patient referrals. Finally even when the study of a new innovation is feasible and desirable, the principle of equipoise, which is important in the conduct of clinical research, often does not exist since the person willing to learn or proceed with a new surgical technique should inherently believe that it will benefit his/her patient.

15.4.2.1 Inventor's Dilemma
A special type of conflict of interest related to innovation arises when a neurosurgeon invents a new piece of equipment (Ammar 1995) and promotes it to the exclusion of all others. For example, if the Head of Neurosurgery at a hospital invents a new image guidance system (i.e., frameless stereotaxy) and uses it for every case, insists that no other make of navigation system be bought by his/her hospital, insists that his/her residents are exposed to only it, and lectures about it passionately at national meetings, a conflict of interest is present as the surgeon is presumably receiving financial or reputational rewards each time it is used or sold. If the system is truly superior to others on the market, and proven to be so, then the surgeon is obliged to use it and there is no ethical breach. But if the system is equivalent to the others and of similar cost (or more expensive), then an ethically dubious situation clearly exists. The same obtains if it is a new operation which the surgeon champions – herein he/she may gain more patients and thus financial benefits or certainly at minimum reputational advancement. These are not common problems but ones which must be faced head-on by any neurosurgeon innovative enough to create a new device or operation.

15.4.3 Informed Consent

In modern society what is "new" is also often considered "improved." Even the term innovation has the connotation of added value and it has been suggested it be replaced by the term "nonvalidated procedure" (Levine 1988; McKneally 1999). Therefore, even when patients are objectively given information about a new procedure, they may not maintain such objectivity (Angelos 2010). Furthermore, framing has long been known to influence patient decisions, and thus, often the person obtaining consent is also the innovator who at the very least believes the innovation was worth spending time and effort on. Thus, the principles of informed consent which include disclosure, capacity, understanding, and voluntariness ought to be pursued even more stringently with new innovation than in our daily consent to "standard" operations (McKneally and Daar 2003). The patient should also know that while they may not be enrolled in a clinical trial, surgeons will study their outcomes in order to better understand the procedure. The consent form could be reviewed by a research ethics board (McKneally and Daar 2003).

> **Pearl**
> Informed consent is the primary method of exercising the ethical principle of respect for patient autonomy.

15.4.4 Teaching and the Learning Curve

The problem of the learning curve and its influence on the risk-benefit ratio (Jones et al. 2004) exists throughout surgical training and becomes even more acute when an experienced surgeon uses a new technique (Angelos 2010). We must somehow ensure that patient safety is being protected. The learning curve is also a very positive thing with respect to innovation, as it ensures progressive improvement in results with experience (Morreim et al. 2006). Deciding the appropriate timing at which to study an intervention is imperative.

One desirable method to mitigate the learning curve is the use of animal models, cadavers, or simulation techniques when possible (Angelos 2010). Another way to ensure patient safety is to ensure that an experienced preceptor is present during initial cases using a new technique (Angelos 2010; Biffl et al. 2008). While regulatory bodies may license a neurosurgeon to practice, individual surgeons may not be qualified to undertake all procedures (Bernstein and Bampoe 2004). For example, most neurosurgeons trained in an accredited program are still not safe to clip a complex giant basilar artery aneurysm on their own. Furthermore, the introduction of new equipment, procedures, or treatment disequilibrates the system for certifying continuing competence (McKneally 1999), and thus, self-regulation becomes a key element of professionalism and safe practice.

15.4.5 Cost

In most countries in the world, health-care costs are significant to the individual and/or to society. New technologies often increase these costs and therefore financial implications of innovation must be considered when implementing something new (Angelos 2010). On the other hand, considering only cost as the determining factor in supporting new innovation may undermine potential unseen future benefits of a technology. For example, surgical navigation systems require an initial outlay of significant amounts of money, but the resultant increased safety profile and shorter lengths of stay ultimately render these innovations cost-savers.

> **Pearl**
> The principle of justice is exercised when societal and personal costs are considered while evaluating new innovations.

15.4.6 Oversight of Innovation

While it is clear that the protection of all human subjects in research requires an institutional review, it is not quite as clear which surgical procedures require some form of regulation. The subject is one of considerable controversy about whether innovation ought to be regulated, can be regulated, and if so by whom? There are currently no formal regulations on surgical innovation; however, clearly surgical innovation cannot go completely unbridled (McKneally 1999). Some fear that introducing formal regulation will stifle innovation (Morreim et al. 2006). Many innovations today might not be acceptable to IRB's as innovations, and throughout history most certainly have had the possibility and the actuality of some patient risk (Bernstein and Bampoe 2004; Biffl et al. 2008). While we may not be able to avoid patient risks, we can certainly aim to reduce these (Morreim et al. 2006). Even if regulation is recommended, the stage at which an innovator ought to do so may vary. If peer review occurs too early, it may give a distorted sense of the utility or facility of the technique (Awad 1996). Some recommend that peer review ought to be the recommended course for new innovations of all types. It has been suggested than an idea that won't withstand collegial scrutiny may not be a good idea at all; even more importantly, getting perspectives from peers may introduce considerable improvement to a planned innovation (McKneally and Daar 2003). Requiring some evaluation by peers also necessitates a review of the literature and facilitates the surgeon's goal of providing good care (Jones et al. 2004).

A literature review may still reveal more positive results than failed attempts at innovation; thus, another suggestion is maintenance of international registries for reporting of innovations. A possible flaw of peer review in the institutional context is that it may be inappropriately influenced by peer relationships, such as when an individual in a position of power is submitting the new innovation for review. Several authors have suggested that the group evaluation of innovations could consist of peers on the same service as well as the surgeon-in-chief (Bernstein and Bampoe 2004; Jones et al. 2004; McKneally and Daar 2003). Alternatively, some cases of innovation which have clear benefits and are unlikely to portend any risks may not require regulation. One example of such innovation is changing postoperative orders to a standardized form so that essential medications are not forgotten. It has been suggested that journals ought to insist upon peer evaluation prior to publication of novel techniques (Morreim et al. 2006). Clearly a balance between innovation and regulation must be found. If any doubt exists in a surgeon's mind about a new innovation, they should obtain additional opinions either from peers or through formal review.

One framework has been proposed to rate surgical procedures according to their need for regulation and whether this is done by existing IRB or other methods such as peers, surgeons-in chief, or advisory committees (Bernstein and Bampoe 2004). This includes if the procedure was novel, amended, or novel to the particular surgeon. The urgency of the innovation and a surgeon's prior experience are important considerations. Some innovations are unplanned responses to intraoperative scenarios or new clinical problems, while others may be able to benefit from advance planning and training. The range of surgical innovation in the neurosurgical setting is represented in Table 15.1.

Table 15.1 Neurosurgery innovations requiring oversight/regulation, in descending acuity

Description of procedure	Example	Recommendation
New OR procedure not in RCT		
Elective	Spinal cord stem cell transplant	IRB/surgeon-in-chief
Urgent	Pattie to plug aneurysm	Post hoc discussion with peers
New procedure as part of RCT	Cervical interbody cage fusion	IRB
New application of established OR	DBS for Alzheimer's	IRB/surgeon-in-chief
New way of doing established OR	Outpatient aneurysm repair	Surgeon-in-chief/peer committee
New OR for an individual surgeon	First temporal lobectomy	Peer mentor

OR surgery, *RCT* randomized controlled trial, *IRB* institutional review board, *DBS* deep brain stimulation

Pearl
Peer review has traditionally been one of the key methods to ensure the principle of nonmaleficence.

15.5   Recommendations

1. Innovation in surgery should be driven by need for alternate approaches and improved outcomes, rather than cost and personal or institutional interests (Strasberg and Ludbrook 2003).
2. Institutions should guide/support a systematic approach to new innovations in surgery in order to maximize chances of success. This may be accomplished by a task force (McKneally and Daar 2003), guidelines, surgeon-in-chief, or ad hoc committee of peers.
3. An international registry should be maintained so that surgeons can learn about innovative advance and not repeat unsuccessful innovations.
4. The process of informed consent must be even more vigilant than usual, when a new technology or procedure is introduced.
5. Neurosurgeons should continue to teach and encourage ethical behavior in order to encourage thoughtful decision making around new innovations (Angelos 2010).

Conclusion

Our illustrative case demonstrates that a combination of new technologies and human creativity led to a neurosurgical innovation. This was not the sort of innovation that could be tested in a laboratory. It was critical to success that this surgeon believed his innovation would create improved results for his patients as well as result in decreased costs to society if successful, even though this creates some conflict of interest by way of indirect rewards. Some method of peer review and/or oversight might have aided the surgeon to ensure that the planned change in course of surgery would carry as little risk as possible. However, concerns over such a drastic change in practice by a committee of non-neurosurgeons may have hindered progress. Importantly, the surgeon acted as ethically as possible by truly informing his patients of his proposed new approach. Furthermore, now that this innovation has worked (or failed), he is ethically obligated to share this information with his professional community.

The conservative and careful tradition of surgery and commitment to patients engenders profound trust that must be respected (McKneally 1999). An ethical and systematic approach to new innovations may be the key to maintaining such trust, keeping in mind the balance of obligations, costs, honest communication, and open collaboration.

References

Ammar A (1995) Ammar shunt: an option to overcome shunt complications in premature and term neonates. Childs Nerv Syst 11(7):421–423

Angelos P (2010) The art of medicine: the ethical challenges of surgical innovation for patient care. Lancet 376:1046–1047

Awad IA (1996) Innovation through minimalism: assessing emerging technology in neurosurgery. Clin Neurosurg 43:303–316

Bernstein M (2001) Outpatient craniotomy for brain tumor: a pilot feasibility study in 46 patients. Can J Neurol Sci 28:120–124

Bernstein M, Bampoe J (2004) Surgical innovation or surgical evolution: an ethical and practical guide to handling novel neurosurgical procedures. J Neurosurg 100:2–7

Biffl WL, Spain DA, Reistma AM et al (2008) Responsible development and application of surgical innovations: a position statement of the Society of University Surgeons. J Am Coll Surg 206:1204–1209

Boulton M, Bernstein M (2008) Outpatient brain tumor surgery: innovation in surgical neurooncology. J Neurosurg 108:649–654

Danjoux NM, Martin DK, Lehoux PN et al (2007) Adoption of an innovation to repair aortic aneurysms at a Canadian hospital: a qualitative case study and evaluation. BMC Health Serv Res 7:182

Ehrich K, Cowie L, Sandall J (2013) Expect the unexpected: patients' and families' expectations and experiences of new clinical procedures. Health Expect [Epub ahead of print]

Grimmett MR, Sulmasy DP (1998) The call of the sirens: ethically navigating the sea of nonvalidated therapies. J Refract Surg 14:559–566

Johnson J, Rogers W (2012) Innovative surgery: the ethical challenges. J Med Ethics 38(1):9–12

Jones JW, McCullough LB, Richman BW (2004) Ethics of surgical innovation to treat rare diseases. J Vasc Surg 39:918–919

Levine RJ (1988) Ethics and regulation of clinical research, 2nd edn. Yale University Press, New Haven, pp 127–131

Lotz M (2013) Surgical innovation as sui generis surgical research. Theor Med Bioeth 34(6):447–459

McKneally MF (1999) Ethical problems in surgery: innovation leading to unforeseen complications. World J Surg 23:786–788

McKneally MF, Daar AS (2003) Introducing new technologies: protecting subjects of surgical innovation and research. World J Surg 27:930–934

Morreim H, Mack MJ, Sade RM (2006) Surgical innovation: too risky to remain unregulated? Ann Thorac Surg 82:1957–1965

National Commission for the Protection of Human Subjects of Biomedical and Behavioral Research (1978) The Belmont Report: ethical principle and guidelines for the protection of human subjects of research. US Government Printing Office, Washington, DC

Purzner T, Purzner J, Massicotte EM et al (2011) Outpatient brain tumor surgery and spinal decompression: a prospective study of 1003 patients. Neurosurgery 69:119–127

Reitsma AM, Moreno JD (2002) Ethical regulations for innovative surgery: the last frontier? J Am Coll Surg 194:792–801

Reitsma AM, Moreno J (2005) Ethics of innovative surgery: US surgeons' definitions, knowledge and research. J Am Coll Surg 200:103–110

Riskin DJ, Longaker MT, Gertner M et al (2006) Innovation in surgery: a historical perspective. Ann Surg 244:686–693

Rogers WA, Lotz M, Hutchison K et al (2014) Identifying surgical innovation: a qualitative study of surgeons' views. Ann Surg 259(2):273–278

Strasberg SM, Ludbrook PA (2003) Who oversees innovative practice? Is there a structure that meets the monitoring needs of new techniques? J Am Coll Surg 196:938–948

Taylor PL (2010) Overseeing innovative therapy without mistaking it for research: a function-based model based on old truths, new capacities, and lessons from stem cells. J Law Med Ethics 38(2):286–302

Research Ethics

16

Nir Lipsman and Mark Bernstein

16.1 Introduction

Research ethics deals with the ethical principles and challenges of conducting biomedical research (Weijer et al. 1997). Although spanning every part of the research process, from study design to publication of results, at the root of ethical research practice is the protection of the subject and of the population at large. To guide researchers, an influential report known as the Belmont Report was published in 1979, which outlined three basic principles of ethical research practice: beneficence, justice, and autonomy (Beauchamp 2004; Sims 2010). Autonomy means that the individual's ability to make free and informed decisions should be respected at all times and that as much information as necessary is provided prior to deciding to enroll in a study. Beneficence means that researchers should attempt at all times to maximize benefit to participants and minimize risk. Finally, justice means that research studies should not exclude populations from participation and should be as inclusive as possible, and the benefits of research should be evenly and widely, that is, fairly, distributed. These are all key components to value-based medicine.

Clinical neurosurgical research has many challenges, including complex populations, rare life-threatening illnesses, and clinical pictures that often fluctuate over time. Many of these practical challenges also translate into ethical challenges, wherein researchers attempt to balance their duties as clinicians with their duties as

N. Lipsman, MD
Division of Neurosurgery, University of Toronto, 399 Bathurst Street,
Toronto, ON M5T 2S8, Canada

Department of Surgery, University of Toronto, 399 Bathurst Street,
Toronto, ON M5T 2S8, Canada
e-mail: nir.lipsman@mail.utoronto.ca

M. Bernstein, MD, MHSc, FRCSC (✉)
Division of Neurosurgery, Toronto Western Hospital, University of Toronto,
399 Bathurst Street, Toronto, ON M5T 2S8, Canada
e-mail: mark.bernstein@uhn.ca

A. Ammar, M. Bernstein (eds.), *Neurosurgical Ethics in Practice: Value-based Medicine*, 181
DOI 10.1007/978-3-642-54980-9_16, © Springer-Verlag Berlin Heidelberg 2014

investigators, often treating patients and studying them at the same time (Bernstein 2003, 2006). The cornerstone of clinical research is trust: patients' trust that investigators will consider and respect their safety and well-being, investigators' trust in the validity of others' findings and their data, and society's trust that research resources will be properly allocated and findings used to benefit society at large (Council 2009).

To help understand the ethical challenges of clinical neurosurgical research, this chapter reviews important principles related to research practice in neurosurgical populations. We highlight the pertinent ethical challenges in the field that raise important questions about how to best safeguard patient and subject well-being. We begin by describing two cases that highlight key ethical principles and challenges that are common in neurosurgical practice and research.

16.2   Illustrative Cases

Case 1 (Conflict of Interest)

A neurosurgeon is interested in the complication rate associated with a cervical spine artificial disc that she has been using for the last 10 years. She intends to perform a retrospective chart review as well as informally assess patient attitudes toward the surgery when they are seen in clinic. Although the study is not industry sponsored, the neurosurgeon previously served as a consultant for the artificial disc manufacturer but is now no longer involved with the company. Is IRB approval required to perform this noninvasive study? Is there a possible conflict of interest (COI), and if so, how can it be managed?

Case 2 (Extremely Vulnerable Patient)

A therapy has been proposed for recurrent glioblastoma multiforme (GBM) that would see wafers containing a novel chemotherapy compound implanted into the intraoperative surgical bed following a subtotal resection. Investigators are hoping to recruit eight patients for a phase I pilot trial. Preclinical models identified only mild adverse events associated with the investigated compound, although its effects in humans are not known. While obtaining informed consent, the investigator is told by a patient, "I'm desperate! I'm willing to try any treatment that might work." Should this patient be enrolled in the study? What challenges to the consent process would a trial like this pose?

16.3   Approach to the Cases

Case 1

Although the study in question is technically "noninvasive" and will utilize only medical records and informal discussions with patients, it nevertheless necessitates institutional review board (IRB) approval. The IRB is an independent committee that regulates the ethical conduct of research and safeguards the privacy and safety of patients and caregivers. The neurosurgeon has a valid question related to outcomes of a novel surgical procedure that has the potential to change practice patterns. As a result, there is societal and academic validity to the question. Their previous involvement with the company, however, raises the possibility that a conflict of interest may be present that could influence their objectivity. The presence of COI requires careful management which begins with full and early disclosure. The surgeon should report any relationship, current or previous, with the company to the IRB and outline this involvement in the informed consent form. Further, the researcher should abstain from conducting patient interviews herself about the surgery, given the potential risk for more subtle COI related to her role as the clinician, which could influence patient responses. A third-party investigator or research assistant should conduct these interviews, which would ideally be formally structured and held at a different setting than the surgical clinic.

Case 2

The objective of a phase I trial is to establish the safety and tolerability of a novel intervention, not the establishment of efficacy. In the described study, preclinical evidence has suggested the compound's safety that now needs to be tested in humans. Provided proper IRB approval and oversight, such a study would be a critical first step in developing a new treatment. It is important, however, for patients to be aware that they are participating in research, not treatment. The therapeutic misconception is when patients believe that the investigations and interventions they will be or are receiving are designed specifically for as part of treatment, when in fact, they are enrolled in a structured clinical trial designed to answer a research question. The patient in this case should have the objectives of "treatment" and "research" explained to them and that they will be enrolling in the latter, not the former. The consent challenges in this case relate to the complexity of the trial, the futility of current treatments for a condition with universally poor prognosis, and the desperation of the patient. Careful communication, with no medical jargon and in the presence of a caregiver or family member, would help optimize the consent process.

16.4 Discussion

16.4.1 Societal and Academic Value of Research

Research is vital for the advancement of any field, and neurosurgery is a clear example. Advances in trauma, vascular, spinal, oncologic, and functional neurosurgery have all been made as a direct result of highly controlled and well-designed clinical studies. Examples include the use of temozolomide for glioblastoma multiforme (Stupp et al. 2005), the use of carotid endarterectomy in symptomatic carotid stenosis (Ferguson et al. 1999), and early surgery for traumatic spinal cord injury (Fehlings et al. 2012). Such trials have changed the practice of neurosurgeons and have added much to the field and to the treatment of neurosurgical patients globally.

Assessing the value of research is therefore an important component of ethical research practice, not least because patients can be exposed to significant risk (Emanuel et al. 2000; Bernstein 2006; Bernstein and Upshur 2003). As a result, a fundamental ethical principle for research in neurosurgery is that the research question being asked, or intervention being proposed, should be of some scientific and ultimately societal value. The role of the investigator, therefore, is in large part to clearly describe the objectives of the trial, both to the IRB and to eligible subjects. For example, phase I trials are designed to assess safety and feasibility and not to evaluate efficacy. Such trials recruit small numbers of patients, are open-label, and often have no placebo or control arm. The objectives of this type of study are very different from a phase III study, where the goal is to establish efficacy. These trials recruit large numbers of patients, involve a control arm with which to compare results, and can often involve multiple centers and treatment sites. Both types of trials are key to the treatment development process, but have very different objectives: safety and efficacy, respectively.

The societal value of research is fundamental to neurosurgical research because resources are also not equally distributed. Investigators must avoid unnecessary use of human and financial resources for research projects that would not add value to the scientific or clinical community. The balance between risk and potential benefit must consider both the individual and the community, and the value to the broader patient and medical community should be factored into the design of study protocols.

Two simple and similar frameworks for assessing the bioethical integrity of a neurosurgery clinical trial can be found in previous publications (Bernstein 2006; Emanuel et al. 2000). Below we discuss some of the more important elements of these frameworks.

16.4.2 Research Ethics Approval

An independent ethics review of a study protocol is a critical feature of good ethical practice and should be universally applied (Cook et al. 2013; Upshur 2011). The purpose of the Institutional Review Board (sometimes called Research Ethics Board) is to ensure the minimization of undue risk to subjects and to bring protocols and informed consent forms in line with universal ethical principles, such as patient autonomy and justice. By design, IRBs are multidisciplinary and are consisting of a committee of clinicians, allied health professionals, legal representatives, and community members. IRBs are typically affiliated with academic institutions, but their independence and separate oversight are fundamental to their role.

IRB review is often divided along two streams: a delegated, expedited stream and a "full-board," more comprehensive review. The former is reserved for studies that pose relatively low or no risk for study subjects, such as retrospective chart reviews, as well as some interview or survey studies. Often, a single or small group of ethics review professionals will review such studies and work closely with the investigator to ensure that both institutional and general ethical requirements are met. More comprehensive reviews, involving the entire IRB committee, are reserved for larger studies where there is more potential risk and/or features of a study that could in some way violate basic ethical principles of beneficence and/or nonmaleficence. Clinical trials, from phase I to III, will usually undergo a full review, a process that can take much time and effort on the part of both the IRB and the investigator. This is a critical component of neurosurgical research, as the IRB is the "gatekeeper" for potential ethical transgressions, whether intentional or unintentional. The IRB will ensure, among other things, that proper and understandable language is used in consent forms and may also, for example, request elimination of a placebo or control arm, if the scientific rationale is not provided.

It is important to recognize honestly that IRBs can produce obstacles for researchers. The initiation of the review usually is generally a complex online application; nowadays, the review generally takes several months irrespective of the complexity of the protocol, and many criticisms are a little too zealous, trivial, and/or inappropriate. IRBs mean well and perform a difficult and voluminous job, but there is substantial room for improvement to facilitate important research, instead of obstipating it, especially for more junior investigators who are less experienced with their institution's IRB (Burke 2005; Deslauriers et al. 2010; Stark et al. 2010).

> **Pearl**
> Because of the fundamental importance of IRB approval for research studies, most contemporary medical journals will not accept or publish manuscripts that do not explicitly state that IRB approval was obtained to conduct the reported research.

16.4.3 Informed Consent

There are three main components to the informed consent process, namely, voluntariness, capacity, and disclosure (Knifed et al. 2008; Lipsman et al. 2012). In general, these principles apply to the consent acquisition process prior to any medical or surgical intervention, whether it is for routine clinical management or prior to enrolment in a clinical trial. For the latter, it is the responsibility of the investigator to ensure that these principles are maintained. Voluntariness means that the decision to enroll in a clinical study was made free of coercion or undue influence. Sources of undue influence can range from a desire to please the investigator, family, or caregiver pressure, as well as the belief that not participating in the trial would in some way influence one's subsequent care. Disclosure means that the potential subject is provided with as much information as possible regarding the nature of the study, its risks, benefits, and rationale, prior to enrolment. The investigator, and their team if applicable, must ensure that the person enrolling in their trial has all of the information that a "reasonable person" would want or need prior to making the decision to enroll. Finally, capacity means that the patient is actually able to understand the details surrounding the trial.

In the context of neurosurgical clinical trials, these principles acquire a new dimension of complexity. Neurosurgical trials often involve serious, life-threatening pathology, where decisions are made rapidly, and situations where much of the details are not yet clear or still being determined. It has been argued that in these situations, and in similar ones in other clinical research domains, it may be impossible to achieve fully informed consent, but the investigator should instead strive to achieve as close as possible to this ideal (Bernstein 2005; Lipsman et al. 2012). For example, is it possible to truly know all of the risks associated with a given treatment? Can a "free and voluntary" decision really be made in the face of often universally poor prognoses with no treatment alternatives? Can patients with a terminal illness truly grasp the nuances of a phase I trial and distinguish its objectives from those of standard clinical management? All of these questions challenge disclosure, voluntariness, and capacity, respectively, and show that it is often not possible to achieve the "ideal" consent process. Investigators must therefore do their best to disclose as much information as they can and be as honest and forthright as possible regarding the objectives of the study and its risks. Reducing medical jargon, ensuring that consent is performed in the presence of a caregiver or family member, providing ample time to read the consent form and ask questions, and possibly even revisiting the consent process at subsequent visits will help to preserve the patient's ability to make a fully informed decision to participate.

> **Pearl**
> The universal components of informed consent are voluntariness, disclosure, and capacity. Although it may not be possible in some cases to get fully informed consent, the investigator must try to get as close as possible to this ideal.

16.4.4 Benefits and Risks

The objective of clinical neurosurgical research is to investigate questions that could be of value to patients and clinicians in the future. We want, as investigators, to benefit our patients and to avoid harm and undue risk. Importantly, it is not known at the beginning of a study who, if anyone, will benefit from a study and whether anyone will be harmed. The investigator must therefore make every attempt to consider all possible risks and benefits to eligible subjects prior to the enrollment of the first subject.

Potential benefits of a study are often straightforward to identify. For example, enrollment in a phase III trial will see the patient having multiple encounters with health-care professionals, be vigilantly followed, undergo screening examinations, and receive the type of attention that most patients in the community do not receive. Such "enhanced" care is a feature of many clinical trials and, indeed, may be part of the motivation for patients to participate in a trial. Benefit to society as well should be considered. For example, a small qualitative interview study about the consent process in neurosurgery patients may not benefit an individual participant, but the results may very much influence future consent discussions in a larger population of patients (Knifed et al. 2008).

In contrast to benefits, identifying potential risks of a clinical study can sometimes be challenging. In neurosurgical trials, some risks will be obvious, such as those related to a novel procedure or its postoperative course. Sometimes, however, there may be "hidden risks" that the investigator should try to identify. For example, there could be risks associated with screening and pre-intervention investigations, such as neuroimaging and bloodwork. In addition, the emotional toll of discussing a life-threatening diagnosis and the psychological consequences of a failed experimental treatment are factors that could negatively influence patients' experience and be considered risks of participation. Here, the IRB will work with the investigator to identify as best as possible these hidden risks, to disclose them to eligible subjects.

16.4.5 Therapeutic Misconception

When discussing study enrollment with eligible patients, it is imperative for investigators to clarify the difference between research and clinical practice. The therapeutic misconception is a term applied to the blurring of the line between treatment and research and is a frequent occurrence in clinical studies (Appelbaum et al. 2012). Subjects may, for example, believe that the investigations and interventions they will experience is an accepted part of the treatment of patients, designed to benefit them. Instead they have been enrolled in a trial, where investigations and interventions are experimental and have an unclear risk-benefit profile and where the overall objective is to further the development of scientific knowledge. This misconception is critical to address as it can significantly influence the experience of patients in a study as well as potentially their interest in participating (Lipsman et al. 2012). Sometimes, particularly in early phase clinical trials, it can be difficult to distinguish clinical management from experimental therapies, especially in conditions for which there are few effective therapy options. Honest and forthright communication with subjects is the best approach to avoid the therapeutic misconception.

> **Pearl**
> The enrolled subject must understand the distinction between research and clinical practice and that the former is designed to benefit society and the latter is designed to benefit the individual.

16.4.6 Conflict of Interest

Conflicts of interests (COI) can significantly influence clinical neurosurgical research (Bernstein 2003; Fisher et al. 2012; Lemmens and Singer 1998). There are several different types of COI, including financial, wherein investigators have a vested financial interest in the results or success/failure of a trial, and academic, where considerations such as authorship, intellectual property, and academic advancement factor into the design, execution, and analysis of study results. The first step in navigating COI ethical challenges is to disclose them completely and honestly at the start of any study. This is also typically a major component of most

REB submissions and subsequent deliberations. It is important to note that a COI does not automatically disqualify research projects from being valid, so long as COI are disclosed and properly managed. Managing COI involves several steps, including maintaining adequate distance between the involved party and the data, involving an independent data safety monitoring board (DSMB), employing an independent body for trial oversight, as well as keeping the investigator at arm's length from enrolled subjects if possible.

It is imperative for investigators to be aware that their presence can also exert subtle forms of pressure on potential study participants. There is therefore often a tension between one's role as a researcher and as a doctor, and COI between those roles can contaminate the validity of a study. Being aware of these issues, and fully disclosing them, is vital.

16.4.7 Placebo

The use of placebos in human subject research has generated much controversy and debate. Proponents of placebo-controlled studies argue that the presence of a clinical response in the absence of an active intervention (i.e., the "placebo effect") could at worst invalidate and at best contaminate the detection of a meaningful study effect. Using a design wherein deception or blinding procedures are employed would therefore control for this effect. Critics of placebos argue that any level of deception in the context of a clinical study, no matter how well intentioned or scientifically sound and even if the patient has consented to it, is still an act of deception, which contradicts the principle of nonmaleficence. The tension between benefit to the population and risk to the individual is thus expressed in the challenges surrounding placebo use. In neurosurgical trials, this question may arise in the context of procedures such as deep brain stimulation, where the possibility exists of blinding patients to device activation status. Some studies have also utilized sham surgery, although this remains relatively rare in a neurosurgical context (Kimmelman et al. 2009; LeWitt et al. 2011). The placebo issue may also arise in drug trials of neurotherapeutic agents, including trials of oncologic treatments.

As with the other challenges above, the onus is on the investigator to ethically justify the use of placebo in their study while being mindful of the risk-benefit balance. Any study intervention, including one that knowingly exposes subjects to a nil-treatment arm, that tips the scale toward risk and away from benefit should be viewed as not ethically sound.

Pearl
The use of placebos is controversial. Many argue that they are essential in some trials to ensure the research question is answered as definitively as possible, while many argue they are the ultimate deception of a patient.

Conclusion

A few frameworks have been published outlining factors critical to an ethically oriented design in clinical research (Emanuel et al. 2000; Bernstein 2006; Lipsman et al. 2010). These are important and valuable starting points to understanding the fundamental challenges of the field. With neurosurgical research, however, there is an added layer of complexity, stemming largely from pathology and conditions that are complex and sometimes life-threatening and sometimes alter the patients' cognition. Although the threshold for all clinical research in human subjects should always be high, clinical research in neurosurgery requires additional attention to the specific nuances of the highly delicate and unforgiving organ that we chose to investigate. Adhering to strict ethical principles and proactively addressing the ethical challenges we described will help ensure that clinical neurosurgical research proceeds with the interests of both subject and investigator safely guarded.

References

Appelbaum PS, Anatchkova M, Albert K et al (2012) Therapeutic misconception in research subjects: development and validation of a measure. Clin Trials 9(6):748–761

Beauchamp T (2004) The legacy and the future. 30 years after the Belmont report, Beauchamp sets the record straight. Prot Hum Subj Summer (10):1–3

Bernstein M (2003) Conflict of interest: it is ethical for an investigator to also be the primary care-giver in a clinical trial. J Neurooncol 63(2):107–108

Bernstein M (2005) Fully informed consent is impossible in surgical clinical trials. Can J Surg 48(4):271–272

Bernstein M (2006) Ethical guideposts to clinical trials in oncology. Curr Oncol 13(2):55–60

Bernstein M, Upshur REG (2003) Framework for bioethical assessment of an article on therapy. J Neurosurg 98:485–490

Burke GS (2005) Looking into the institutional review board: observations from both sides of the table. J Nutr 135(4):921–924

Cook AF, Hoas H, Joyner JC (2013) The Protectors and the protected: what regulators and researchers can learn from IRB members and subjects. Narrat Inq Bioeth 3(1):51–65

Council NR (2009) On being a scientist: a guide to responsible conduct in research, 3rd edn. The National Academies Press, Washington, D.C

Deslauriers C, Bell E, Palmour N et al (2010) Perspectives of Canadian researchers on ethics review of neuroimaging research. J Empir Res Hum Res Ethics 5(1):49–66

Emanuel EJ, Wendler D, Grady C (2000) What makes clinical research ethical? JAMA 283(20):2701–2711

Fehlings MG, Vaccaro A, Wilson JR et al (2012) Early versus delayed decompression for traumatic cervical spinal cord injury: results of the Surgical Timing in Acute Spinal Cord Injury Study (STASCIS). PLoS One 7(2):e32037

Ferguson GG, Eliasziw M, Barr HW et al (1999) The North American symptomatic carotid endarterectomy trial: surgical results in 1415 patients. Stroke 30(9):1751–1758

Fisher CG, DiPoala CP, Noonan VK et al (2012) Physician-industry conflict of interest: public opinion regarding industry-sponsored research. J Neurosurg Spine 17:1–10

Kimmelman J, London J, Ravina B et al (2009) Launching invasive, first-in-human trials against Parkinson's disease: ethical considerations. Mov Disord 24(13):1893–1901

Knifed E, Lipsman N, Mason W et al (2008) Patients' perception of the informed consent process for neurooncology clinical trials. Neuro Oncol 10(3):348–354

Lemmens T, Singer PA (1998) Bioethics for clinicians: 17. Conflict of interest in research, education and patient care. CMAJ 159:960–965

LeWitt PA, Rezai ARLeehey MA et al (2011) AAV2-GAD gene therapy for advanced Parkinson's disease: a double-blind, sham-surgery controlled, randomised trial. Lancet Neurol 10(4): 309–319

Lipsman N, Bernstein M, Lozano AM (2010) Criteria for the ethical conduct of psychiatric neurosurgery clinical trials. Neurosurg Focus 29(2):E9

Lipsman N, Giacobbe P, Bernstein M et al (2012) Informed consent for clinical trials of deep brain stimulation in psychiatric disease: challenges and implications for trial design. J Med Ethics 38(2):107–111

Sims JM (2010) A brief review of the Belmont report. Dimens Crit Care Nurs 29(4):173–174

Stark AR, Tyson JE, Hibberd PL (2010) Variation among institutional review boards in evaluating the design of a multicenter randomized trial. J Perinatol 30(3):163–169

Stupp R, Mason WP, van den Bent MJ et al (2005) Radiotherapy plus concomitant and adjuvant temozolomide for glioblastoma. N Engl J Med 352(10):987–996

Upshur RE (2011) Ask not what your REB can do for you; ask what you can do for your REB. Can Fam Physician 57(10):1113–1114

Weijer C, Dickens B, Meslin EM (1997) Bioethics for clinicians: 10 research ethics. CMAJ 156:1153–1157

Consent in Emergency Clinical Research

17

Erwin J.O. Kompanje and Mark Bernstein

17.1 Introduction

The need for medical research involving critically ill patients with severe neurological conditions is self-evident. Clinical trials in emergency and critical care settings frequently involve patients with acute catastrophic cerebral conditions causing loss of decision-making capacity and, given the emergency nature of the conditions, facing very short time frames. Examples of such conditions are severe traumatic brain injury, subarachnoid hemorrhage, spontaneous intracerebral hemorrhage, acute ischemic stroke, and secondary hypoxic brain injury after circulatory arrest. All clinical trials are subject to the ethical and juridical principles of good clinical practice and international and national guidelines and regulations.

The most important ethical principle underlying clinical trials is the respect for autonomy. Furthermore, protection against discomfort, harm, risk, and exploitation and of course the prospect of potential benefit are essential and core elements of value-based medicine. Specific ethical issues pertaining to clinical trials in acute severe neurological conditions include the emergency nature of research, the incapacity of subjects to consent, short therapeutic time windows, and a risk/benefit ratio based on the concept that in relation to the seriousness of the disease or trauma, significant adverse side effects may be acceptable for treatments with potential benefit.

E.J.O. Kompanje, PhD (✉)
Intensive Care Medicine, Erasmus MC University Medical Center,
Rotterdam, The Netherlands
e-mail: erwinkompanje@me.com; e.j.o.kompanje@erasmusmc.nl

M. Bernstein, MD, MHSc, FRCSC
Division of Neurosurgery, Toronto Western Hospital, University of Toronto,
399 Bathurst Street, Toronto, ON M5T 2S8, Canada
e-mail: mark.bernstein@uhn.ca

A. Ammar, M. Bernstein (eds.), *Neurosurgical Ethics in Practice: Value-based Medicine*, 191
DOI 10.1007/978-3-642-54980-9_17, © Springer-Verlag Berlin Heidelberg 2014

17.2   Illustrative Case (Research in a Severely Head-Injured Patient)

A 19-year-old man was admitted at 1:30 a.m. to the intensive care unit of a university hospital after he suffered a severe traumatic brain injury. He crashed his car at high speed. Emergency CT scan revealed a small subdural hematoma with severe swelling of the right cerebral hemisphere. There were no relatives present. In the hospital a multicenter placebo-controlled phase III trial was investigating the efficacy and safety of a single dose of a neuroprotective agent. The study protocol stipulates administration of the study drug within 4 h after injury. The IRB allows inclusion into the trial with deferred proxy consent. Two hours after the injury, the study drug was administered. The parents and sister of the man arrived in the hospital at 4:30 a.m. They were informed about the severity of the injuries, after which they visited the patient in the intensive care unit. In a second conversation, the relatives were told that the man had been randomized into a clinical trial, and they were asked their consent for continuation of the trial.

17.3   Approach to the Case

In this case, the main central issue relates to protection of the rights of an individual who cannot speak for himself. The principles of autonomy and nonmaleficence are paramount. Regarding the main ethical theories one might argue that utilitarian ethics and deontological ethics would clash on this case. Utilitarians would argue that the best outcome for the maximum number of people would be achieved by including the man in the trial, but deontologists might say that his rights and his dignity are being violated and that he is being used as a means to an end. Below several pivotal practical aspects of this scenario will be examined, with special attention to the various models of obtaining consent in neuro-emergency trials.

17.4   Discussion

17.4.1 Consent for Emergency Research

Informed consent in emergency situations can, given the emergency nature and severity of the neurological condition or due to medicinal sedation, seldom be obtained from patients themselves. Several solutions are internationally in use for obtaining consent in emergency situations: proxy consent, deferred proxy consent, deferred patient consent, consent by an independent physician, and waiver of consent.

17.4.1.1 Proxy Consent
In most international legislation, consent by legal representatives is considered valid and the most preferable and ethically valid alternative for patient informed consent in emergency neurosurgery clinical trials (Alves 2006). Proxy consent is

the substituted judgment by a close relative or legal representative about inclusion in a clinical trial. Theoretically, the proxy is supposed to act as the patient, if competent, would have decided. Proxy is essentially synonymous with substitute decision-maker and surrogate.

> **Pearl**
> Proxies are commonly recognized as the first party to represent an incapacitated patient in emergency situations but they do not always know the wishes of the incapacitated patient.

It is assumed that family members are best suited to make decisions that maximize the patient's best interest as proxies are supposed to know what is in the patient's best interest. Theoretically, this is an attractive alternative for patient informed consent, but practically there are some drawbacks. First, would the patient want to be represented by the particular relative? In one study only 41 % of 1,089 patients would want their spouse to be their representative, whereas 28 % wanted to be represented by the physician in charge for inclusion into the clinical trial (Roupie et al. 2000). A further question to ask is if legal representatives know the wishes of the now incapacitated patient. A particular proxy may know little about a patient's values and wishes for medical treatment in case of severe neurological conditions.

Agreement about health decisions between patients and their proxies varied between 57 and 81 % in one study (Sulmasy et al. 1994). Others found a false-positive consent rate up to 20 % in surrogate decision-making for critical care research (Coppolino and Ackerson 2001). Another found that no less than 45 % of the proxies refused consent in a study involving incapacitated patients (Mason et al. 2006). In the same study, in comparison, only 18 % of patients approached declined participation in the trial. Discrepancies between patient consent and proxy consent were found between 32 and 42 % in a study searching for the ability of family members to predict patient's consent to critical care research (Ciroldi et al. 2007). Significant discrepancy was found between patients and surrogates regarding consent for critical care research (Newman et al. 2012). In a systematic review evaluating the accuracy of surrogate decision-makers, accuracy was found between 61 and 72 % in consent for several critical interventions (Shalowitz et al. 2006). There was less effect of prior discussion of patient's treatment preferences and values (Ditto et al. 2001; Matheis-Kraft and Roberto 1997).

The process of obtaining proxy consent in an emergency situation contains three phases. First, information about the emergency critical care trial is provided. Second, the investigator or physician in charge asks the proxy for consent. Third, the proxy consents or refuses (Sugarman 2000). Several authors state that the emotional nature of the emergency situation limits the validity of surrogate consent. Given the complexities of informed consent documents, a larger proportion of proxies might fail to comprehend an actual protocol for an emergency trial (Hsieh et al. 2001). Given the time pressure and the emotionally charged situation, comprehension may be less than optimal (Kucia and Horowitz 2000). Patients enter critical care in physiologic crisis, whereas their relatives enter it in a psychological crisis (Woolley 1990). Uncertainty as to whether the patient will survive also has a profound influence on the proxy's reactions, actions, and strategies (Jansen et al. 2009). A questionnaire soliciting opinions rather than current practice mailed to 148 European Brain Injury Consortium-associated neurotrauma centers revealed that 48 % of the 78 respondents believe that relatives were not able to make a balanced decision under the emotional and stressful emergency conditions (Kompanje et al. 2005).

> **Pearl**
> Time pressures and overwhelming emotions may decrease the value of proxy consent in emergency situations. Deferred proxy consent is a more ethically and psychologically valid concept than proxy consent.

17.4.1.2 Deferred Proxy Consent

A solution to overcome some of the problems mentioned above is using deferred proxy consent. Deferred proxy consent, or retrospective proxy consent, is an alternative for informed patient consent and for prior proxy consent in the situation in which it is impossible to obtain consent from the patient, or from his/her representatives. Mostly this is due to extreme time pressure (Kompanje et al. 2007). Furthermore, proxies can be too overwhelmed to make a balanced decision. With deferred proxy consent, inclusion into the emergency research involves randomization at the discretion of the investigator or the physician in charge. After inclusion of the patient into the study and after starting the study procedures, the proxy is informed and subsequent consent for continuation in the study is requested.

Deferred proxy consent has been used in several randomized controlled neuro-emergency trails. The psychological distress may prohibit a valid understanding of the information about the trial, which is necessary for reliable consent by a surrogate. Relatives of a patient in a life-threatening condition can be temporarily incompetent. For this reason it has been proposed to approach relatives with information only when the physician in charge thinks it is ethically and psychologically valid to do so (Jansen et al. 2007, 2009). In order to prevent investigators abusing this ongoing circumstance, a time limit of 72 h after start of the study procedures for seeking consent is suggested (Kompanje et al. 2005).

> **Pearl**
> The physician in charge should judge if it is ethically valid to inform and ask the proxies for consent. In order to prevent investigators abusing this ongoing circumstance, a time limit of 72 h after start of the study for seeking deferred proxy consent is recommended.

17.4.1.3 Deferred Patient Consent

More ideal than deferred proxy consent, at least judged from a theoretical point of view, is deferred patient consent. Deferred patient consent, or retrospective patient consent, is an alternative for informed patient consent, for proxy consent, and for deferred proxy consent in the situation in which it is impossible to obtain consent from the patient ab initio. Inclusion in the emergency research involves randomization at the discretion of the investigator or the physician in charge. After inclusion of the patient into the study and after starting the study procedures, the patient is informed and subsequent consent for continuation in the study is requested. In theory, this approach is, judged from an ethical point of view, most ideal. However, in practice, it can seldom be achieved. Patients suffering from an acute and life-threatening neurological condition, who are included in an emergency trial, seldom reach a state in which they have full cognitive abilities of full comprehension. It is common that patients with acute neurological conditions face, after the first stabilization of the condition, cognitive impairment with aphasia, anosognosia, drowsiness, or coma that make the consent process impossible (Ciccone 2003). In the Third International Stroke Trial, in patients with dysphasia, 92 % were randomized into the trial with assent of a representative. However, 69 % of the patients with a motor deficit were able to consent themselves (Kane et al. 2005). Patients presenting in a coma seldom reach sufficient cognitive abilities for deferred patient consent within the time of the study procedures. Nevertheless, if possible, deferred patient consent must be sought, even after deferred proxy consent.

> **Pearl**
> Deferred patient consent must be sought, if possible, even if a proxy has already consented. In everyday practice, many patients with acute and severe neurological conditions will incur neurological deficits, prohibiting the cognitive ability to understand information and give a valid consent.

17.4.1.4 Consent by an Independent Physician

In some countries the primary approach to consent procedures in incapacitated patients in emergency research is randomization by an independent physician who has no involvement in the research and no vested interest in including patients in the clinical trial, even if proxy consent might be feasible. In other countries consent by an independent physician is only possible if a proxy is not available and deferred consent is not possible. As no attempt is made to respect the autonomy of the patient, consent by an independent physician is not equivalent to patient or proxy consent. It can, at best, only be seen as a justification for non-individual-based surrogate decision-making in the light of beneficence of a whole group of patients in an emergency situation. How do patients view this approach? One study investigated how patients included in an early phase acute myocardial infarction trial experienced the consent procedure (Ågård et al. 2001). The majority of the patients felt that the physician alone should be able to decide to include a patient with acute infarction in a trial when the patient is too ill to be asked for consent. Twenty-nine percent of patients in an emergency department stated that they want to be represented by the physician in charge of their care rather than by a surrogate (Roupie et al. 2000).

> **Pearl**
> Consent by an independent physician is never equivalent to patient or proxy consent.

17.5   Waiver of Consent

A waiver of consent relieves an investigator required to obtain consent for inclusion in a clinical trial from actually getting that consent. Waiving the requirement for obtaining informed consent means that the IRB has determined that investigators need not obtain consent. Waiver of consent has been used in several clinical trials in the USA in traumatic brain injury (Clifton et al. 2002) and stroke (Bateman et al. 2003).

In the USA, a number of federal agencies defined in 1996 "Exception from informed consent requirements for emergency research" (commonly referred to as Title 21, Code of Federal Regulations, Section 50.24, or CFR 50.24). The IRB responsible for review of a clinical investigation may approve a study without requiring informed consent if the following seven criteria are met:

1. The potential patient to be enrolled in the study is in an emergent, life-threatening situation, available treatment is unsatisfactory, and it is necessary to determine the safety and effectiveness of the proposed intervention.
2. Obtaining informed consent is not possible, because the patient cannot provide informed consent due to his/her medical condition, the intervention must be done before consent from a legally authorized representative is feasible, and there is no reasonable means to identify potential research subjects prospectively.
3. Participation in the study may benefit the patient directly, because he/she is in an emergent, life-threatening situation that requires intervention, appropriate preclinical studies have been carried out and the results indicate a potential direct benefit for the patient, and the risks associated with the intervention are reasonable in relation to what is known about the medical condition of the patient.
4. The clinical research cannot be carried out practicably without the exception to informed consent.
5. The research plan defines the duration of the therapeutic window, and the investigator will attempt to contact the legal representative within this window to obtain consent.
6. The IRB has approved the informed consent document and process to be used with the patient or their legal representative in situations where this is feasible. Furthermore, the IRB has approved the information and procedures to be used

when providing the opportunity for a family member to object to a patient's participation in the clinical study.

7. Additional efforts to ensure protection of the right and welfare of the patient will occur, at the minimum.

Waiver of consent is not possible in the European Union member states. In these countries consent is regulated in national laws and regulations based on the European Clinical Trial Directive 2001/20/EC.

17.6 Consent in the European Union Directive 2001/20/EC

In line with Article 3(2)a of the Charter of Fundamental Rights of the European Union, any intervention in the field of medicine and biology cannot be performed without free and informed consent of the person concerned. On April 4, 2001, the Directive 2001/20/EC of the European Parliament and of the council was published in the Official Journal of the European Communities (European Commission 2001). Article 4 of the Directive 2001/20/EC states that: "In the case of other persons incapable of giving their consent....the written consent of the patient's legal representative, given in cooperation with the treating doctor, is necessary before participation in any such clinical trial." The rules on the protection of subjects and on free and informed consent have been discussed extensively in the legislative process leading to Directive 2001/20/EC. The intent of this wording was to provide incapacitated subjects additional protection. It would appear likely that the population targeted primarily were chronic psychiatric patients. In practice the phrasing had direct adverse consequences for emergency research. Specifically the obligation to obtain written consent by the patient's legal representative has prevented much research in emergency settings. This has led to an outcry from the Emergency and Critical Care community (Liddell et al. 2006). Moreover, the use of the wording "legal representative" has created problems – in some countries this has been interpreted as requiring a court order as to who the legal representative is, and in others proxy consent was considered acceptable. From a practical perspective, many studies have replaced the terminology of legal representatives in their study protocols with legally acceptable representative, thus also including proxies. Concerns existed that the restriction in wording might end emergency research in acute life-threatening situations, and indeed substantial problems have ensued in some member states.

> **Pearl**
> In almost all of the European Union member states, prior consent by a legal representative is used as substitute for informed patient consent for nonurgent medical research. Deferred (patient and/or proxy) consent is accepted as substitute in acute emergency research in approximately half of the member states.

17.7   Consent in the Revised Proposal (July 2012), European Union

In July 2012, the EU Commission proposed a regulation which would replace the Directive 2001/20/EC (European Commission 2012). The rationale for revising this Directive is that the implementation of the legislation has resulted in unnecessary bureaucracy (Hartmann 2012). The proposed regulation from July 2012 does not, with the exception of the issue of clinical trials in emergency situations, substantially change the rules with respect to requirements for informed consent. In contrast to directive 2001/20/EC, the proposed regulation provides guidance for informed (deferred) consent in emergency situations. Informed consent may be obtained after the start of the clinical trial to continue the clinical trial, and information on the clinical trial may be given after the start of the clinical trial provided that five conditions are fulfilled. These conditions are as follows:

1. Due to the urgency of the situation, caused by a sudden life-threatening or other sudden serious medical condition, it is impossible to obtain prior informed consent from the subject and it is impossible to supply prior information to the subject.
2. No legal representative is available.
3. The subject has not previously expressed objections known to the investigator.
4. The research relates directly to a medical condition that causes the impossibility to obtain prior informed consent and to supply prior information.
5. The clinical trial poses a minimal risk to, and imposes a minimal burden on, the subject.

The conditions after inclusion in the clinical trial and start of the administration of the experimental agent and other study procedures are as follows:

1. The informed consent shall be obtained as soon as possible from the legal representative, and the information shall be given as soon as possible to the subject.
2. Informed consent shall be obtained as soon as possible from the legal representative or the subject, whichever is sooner, and the information referred to shall be given as soon as possible to the legal representative or the subject, whichever is sooner.
3. When informed consent has been obtained from the legal representative, informed consent to continue the trial shall be obtained from the subject as soon as it is capable of giving informed consent.

These provisions represent a substantial advance over the currently existing legislation, with specific recognition of the specific aspects of emergency research and research in incapacitated patients. It is good news that the principle of deferred consent in emergency situations is now acceptable. Despite these advances, some clouds remain on the horizon (Gamble et al. 2013; Matei et al. 2013; Perkins et al. 2013). Potential problems may result from the clause that demands minimal risk, interactions with European Data protection requirements, and the failure to explicitly recognize that capacity may be lost due to essential and unavoidable therapy as well as disease. But, deferred consent is now possible in the European member states.

Conclusion

1. In neuro-emergency trials patient informed consent is seldom possible.
2. Proxy consent by a relative or legal representative is most widely used as surrogate for informed patient consent.
3. In neuro-emergency trials, there is a conflict between the desire for early initiation of experimental treatment versus time required for following informed consent procedures.
4. In neuro-emergency trials, the conflict between the desire for following informed consent procedures and doubts about the validity of proxy consent in emergency situations is well recognized. Proxies are often too emotionally distressed and overwhelmed to give valid proxy consent.
5. Including patients in a neuro-emergency trial using deferred proxy consent is the best and most ethically valid solution available.
6. Waiver of consent can be used in neuro-emergency studies in the USA.
7. In almost all of the European Union member states, prior consent by a legal representative is used as substitute for informed patient consent for nonurgent medical research. Deferred (patient and/or proxy) consent is accepted as substitute in acute emergency research in approximately half of the member states.
8. Following the wording of the new proposal, in the European Union, emergency research is not possible and patients in life-threatening situations cannot be included in research when a proxy of the patient is present in the hospital and when there is no time to inform the overwhelmed relatives. Deferred consent is only possible when legal representatives are not available. This criterion will delay inclusion of patients in acute life-threatening conditions in short time frames.

References

Ågård A, Hermerén G, Herlitz J (2001) Patients' experiences of intervention trials on the treatment of myocardial infarction: is it time to adjust the informed consent procedure to the patient's capacity? Heart 86:632–637

Alves WM (2006) Ethical considerations in neuroemergency clinical trials. In: Alves WM, Skolnick BE (eds) Handbook of neuroemergency clinical trials. Elsevier Academic Press, Amsterdam, pp 257–273

Bateman BT, Meyers PM, Schumacher HC et al (2003) Conducting stroke research with an exception from the requirement for informed consent. Stroke 34:1317–1323

Ciccone A (2003) Consent to thrombolysis in acute ischaemic stroke: from trial to practice. Lancet Neurol 2:375–378

Ciroldi M, Cariou A, Adrie C et al (2007) Ability of family members to predict patient's consent to critical care research. Intensive Care Med 33:807–813

Clifton GL, Knudson P, McDonald M (2002) Waiver of consent in studies of acute brain injury. J Neurotrauma 19:1121–1126

Coppolino M, Ackerson L (2001) Do surrogate decision makers provide accurate consent for intensive care research? Chest 119:603–612

Ditto PH, Danks JH, Smucker WD et al (2001) Advance directives as acts of communication: a randomized controlled trial. Arch Intern Med 161:421–430

European Commission (2001) Directive 2001/20/EC of the European Parliament and of the Council of 4 April 2001 on the approximation of the laws, regulations and administrative provisions of the Member States relating to the implementation of good clinical practice in the conduct of clinical trials on medicinal products for human use. Off J European Comm L 121:34–44

European Commission (2012) Proposal for a regulation of the European Parliament and of the Council on clinical trials on medicinal products for human use, and repealing Directive 2001/20/EC. http://ec.europa.eu/health/files/clinicaltrials/2012_07/proposal/2012_07_proposal_en.pdf

Gamble C, Woolfall K, Williamson P et al (2013) New European Union regulation of clinical trials is conflicting on deferred consent in emergency situations. BMJ 346:f667

Hartmann M (2012) Impact assessment of the European Clinical Trials Directive: a longitudinal, prospective, observational study analyzing patterns and trends in clinical drug trials applications submitted since 2001 to regulatory agencies in six EU countries. Trials 13(53):1–10

Hsieh M, Dailey MW, Calloway CW (2001) Surrogate consent by family members for out-of-hospital cardiac arrest research. Acad Emerg Med 8:851–853

Jansen TC, Kompanje EJO, Bakker J et al (2007) Deferred consent in emergency intensive care research: what if the patient dies early? Use the data or not? Intensive Care Med 33:894–900

Jansen TC, Kompanje EJO, Bakker J (2009) Deferred consent in emergency critical care research: ethically valid and practically feasible. Crit Care Med 37(Suppl):S65–S68

Kane I, Lindley R, Lewis S et al (2005) Impact of stroke syndrome and stroke severity on the process of consent in the third international stroke trial. Cerebrovasc Dis 21:348–352

Kompanje EJO, Maas AIR, Hilhorst MT et al (2005) Ethical considerations on consent procedures for emergency research in severe and moderate traumatic brain injury. Acta Neurochir (Wien) 147:633–640

Kompanje EJO, Maas AIR, Slieker FJA et al (2007) Ethical implications of time frames in a randomized controlled trial in acute severe traumatic brain injury. Prog Brain Res 161:243–250

Kucia AM, Horowitz JD (2000) Is informed consent to clinical trials an 'upside selective' process in acute coronary syndromes? Am Heart J 139:94–97

Liddell K, Kompanje EJO, Lemaire F et al (2006) Recommendations in relation to the EU Clinical Trials Directive and medical research involving incapacitated adults. Wien Klin Wochenschr 118:183–191

Mason S, Barrow H, Phillips A et al (2006) Brief report on the experience of using proxy consent for incapacitated adults. J Med Ethics 32:61–62

Matei M, Kompanje EJO, Maas AIR et al (2013) Clinical research into the ICU: clouds at the horizon, once again. Intensive Care Med 39:1479–1480

Matheis-Kraft C, Roberto KA (1997) Influence of a values discussion on congruence between elderly women and their families on critical health care decisions. J Women Aging 9:5–22

Newman JT, Smart A, Reese TR et al (2012) Surrogate and patient discrepancy regarding consent for critical care research. Crit Care Med 40:2590–2594

Perkins GD, Bossaert L, Nolan J et al (2013) Proposed revisions to the EU clinical trials directive – comments from the European Resuscitation Council. Resuscitation 84:263–264

Roupie E, Santin A, Boulme R et al (2000) Patient's preferences concerning medical information and surgery: results of a prospective study in a French emergency department. Intensive Care Med 26:52–56

Shalowitz DI, Garett-Mayer E, Wendler D (2006) The accuracy of surrogate decision makers. Arch Intern Med 166:493–497

Sugarman J (2000) Is the emperor really wearing new clothes? Informed consent for acute coronary syndromes. Am Heart J 140:2–3

Sulmasy DP, Haller K, Terry PB (1994) More talk, less paper: predicting the accuracy of substituted judgments. Am J Med 96:432–438

Woolley N (1990) Crisis theory: a paradigm of effective intervention with families of critically ill people. J Adv Nurs 15:1402–1408

Neuroethics

18

Adefolarin O. Malomo and Mark Bernstein

18.1 Introduction

The actual and potential applications of neuroscience are so profound in human self-understanding, that the exploration of their ethical implications is a major concern and justification of the relatively new bioethical field called neuroethics (Farah 2010; Illes and Sahakian 2011). The practice of neuroethics focuses on the ethics of neuroscience (Racine and Illes 2008). It concerns the ethical, legal, and social impact of the neurosciences, including ways in which neurotechnology can or could be used to predict or alter human behavior (Roskies 2002). Neuroethics has been defined as "the ethics of neuroscience and the neuroscience of ethics" (Roskies 2002), but clearly the former constitutes the major and important part of neuroethics. With rapid advances in our technological ability to investigate and alter brain function, this field will gain more relevance and importance in the future (Lipsman and Bernstein 2009, 2011) for all neurosurgeons and especially functional neurosurgeons. Value-based medicine can help inform neuroethics debates.

A.O. Malomo, MB, BS, MHSc, FWACS
Departments of Surgery and Human Anatomy, University of Ibadan, Ibadan, Nigeria

Department of Neurological Surgery, University College Hospital, Ibadan, Nigeria
e-mail: ademalomo@yahoo.com

M. Bernstein, MD, MHSc, FRCSC (✉)
Division of Neurosurgery, Toronto Western Hospital, University of Toronto,
399 Bathurst Street, Toronto, ON M5T 2S8, Canada
e-mail: mark.bernstein@uhn.ca

A. Ammar, M. Bernstein (eds.), *Neurosurgical Ethics in Practice: Value-based Medicine*,   201
DOI 10.1007/978-3-642-54980-9_18, © Springer-Verlag Berlin Heidelberg 2014

18.2 Illustrative Case (Seeking Information About Contracting a Degenerative Brain Disease)

John Curious is a 59 year old Associate Professor of African Literature born of a British mother and an African father. He lives in the United States of America. His mother suffered from severe depression and later died of disseminated malignancy at the age of 69. His elder brother has suffered from epilepsy of unknown cause since he was 30 years old. His father succumbed from dementia, probably of Alzheimer type. John has followed developments in the neurosciences in the media and he recently saw advertisements for noninvasive brain scans like fMRI and genetic tests which might help define his neurological genetic, structural, and functional status. He decides to get the tests and awaits the results with guarded anticipation. What are the ethical implications of this situation?

18.3 Approach to the Case

Respecting John's autonomy would clearly suggest that it is his right to undertake whatever tests he wishes and to seek whatever information about himself he wishes to, as long as the risk/benefit ratio of the tests is acceptable. Against this is the potential societal harm if everyone knew about various conditions he/she might have or have the potential to develop. This knowledge could lead to the consumption of limited health-care resources needed by people with actual diseases and thus pose a threat to justice and an ethical challenge in the realm of priority setting (resource allocation). And what if the test reveals something unexpected and devastating like an existing glioblastoma multiforme or a predisposition to develop one? What would be the duty of disclosure and by whom? What about the reliability of the tests – has there been sufficient preclinical data to demonstrate sufficient accuracy of the results? At the bottom line, is society ready for its citizens to have access to finding out information about themselves that was just not meant to be found in this way or that society at large is not prepared to handle?

> **Pearl**
> Neuroethics is a fairly new subdivision of bioethics focusing mainly on the ethical issues raised by advances in the neurosciences. To date its main areas of application are the ethical uses of fMRI, pharmacological enhancement, and "psychosurgery."

18.4   Discussion

18.4.1   Neuroethics of Enhancement

By enhancement is meant adding to what is normally considered adequate or normal. Medical norms are usually statistically derived from a population of those considered healthy. Can we, however, derive "ought" from "is" in medicine? The validity of this empirical "is" and empirical "ought" is confirmed by the balance, harmony, and homeostasis maintained, but do we know that the present balance and homeostasis are the only possible homeostasis complex possible or are they relative? We cannot be sure. Many average parameters in many societies have altered without any ill effects; however, other changes have been attended with disequilibrium, and so the need for caution remains.

Human history is full of examples of technological advancements being greeted with horror, going through acceptance to desire and high demand. Also, devices and methods that are developed for one purpose become adapted and improved to cater to a wider range of challenges (Arras et al. 1999). In all of these, world views, goals, and values seem to be elastic in ultimately adjusting to the new scopes of reality and possibility. History has also shown that more is not always better.

18.4.1.1   Pharmacological Enhancement

Examples of relevant neuropharmacological agents used for enhancement include selective serotonin reuptake inhibitors (SSRI) that can make nondepressed persons feel even better with side effects that can be mitigated by yet other drugs, methylphenidate and amphetamines that can increase attention focus and sustenance in persons without attention-deficit hyperactive disorder (ADHD), ampakines that can further improve normal memory, modafinil that can increase wakefulness in persons without narcolepsy, and sildenafil that improves sexual performance in some normal males (Farah 2002).

Issues of ethics abound in all these uses. Chemically altering and then readjusting our internal environment has biological implications in the long run. Functional costs sometimes exist, as in the case of memory expanders that tend to reduce capacity for generalization in reasoning. On the other side, it may be paternalistic to disallow adults to choose for themselves. Also temporary enhancement may be required in unusual circumstances such as combat situations. What must be advocated, however, is that proper cost-benefit analyses be undertaken before those saddled with the responsibilities present these as options to potential users especially for enhancement purposes. Society should also be educated to know that medicine as a whole and psychiatry in particular are imprecise sciences. In psychiatry, mind parameters are dynamic with the environment and advertisements and other social pressures are some of the relevant factors in self, need, and mood perceptions.

In many countries, enhancement medicines are now consumerism driven, yet drugs that have been so offered are sometimes found dangerous years later. Examples include SSRI that are now regarded as dangerous decades later and benzodiazepines which now have problems of epidemic iatrogenic addiction. Often, somehow, some of these challenges become well known only after drug patents have expired (Pieters and Snelders 2009). Obviously increased stringency in the conditions of making enhancement drugs available and education to make the public more wary are important responsibilities of all concerned.

At social levels, it can be argued that wariness over the advantages of these forms of enhancement is inconsistent with the usual practice of other ways of enhancing opportunities, for instance, by getting the best school possible for children and a regular workout regime that builds one's body. These methods that enhance through natural mechanisms can usually be differentiated from those that are imposed by the use of chemicals or technology from without because unlike the latter, the former are harmonious and enduring forms of gain in the body.

Would enhancement not make the strong relatively stronger and the weak relatively weaker in society? It likely would but that in itself would not be unethical unless it gets to a point when socially desirable goals are missed demonstrably because of it or socially undesirable states occur because of it. Normally, enhancement is a product of affluence (Elliott 2004). The wealthy also should not be punished just for being so; wealth may have a price which the poor are "unwilling" (Granat 2003) or unable to pay. In any case these social issues raise ethical issues mostly when advantages taken are undue, the process or outcome of enhancement endangers others, or resource allocation is unacceptably skewed.

18.4.1.2 Surgical Enhancement and Psychosurgery

One of the most relevant applications of neuroethics in the world of the neurosurgeon relates to the growing specialty of altering abnormal and normal states with the use of psychosurgery or deep brain surgery. The advent of deep brain stimulation (an impermanent treatment), as opposed to lesion making (a permanent treatment), has made it easier for surgeons to recommend and patients to accept surgical treatment that alters neurophysical and psychological functions. Society is still appropriately mindful of functional neurosurgery and its abuses decades ago (Freeman 1958). The question we all must ask is: Is society ready for increasingly sophisticated interventions which may soon be able to alter normal functions or alter states of mind? Recent qualitative research has shed some light on this issue. A number of studies have shown that both patients and surgeons will accept deep brain surgery for pathological states such as depression or eating disorders, but find ethically dubious its use for enhancement of normal states (Mendelshon et al. 2010, 2013 Lipsman et al. 2011). In another study, patients were willing to accept treatments that may alter identity if it was the only response to threat to life, but they considered procedures to alter a normal state as ethically dubious (Lipsman et al. 2009). All these ethical issues are compounded by additional challenges like informed consent, which in this setting will often be required to be obtained from patients who are cognitively and/ or psychiatrically compromised (Grant et al. 2013; Lipsman et al. 2010). Such professional and scientific investigation will go a long way in reassuring society that due diligence is being done to ensure that mistakes of the past are not repeated.

This confirms the caution that neurosurgeons must exercise when neuroenhancing surgical procedures become available. Being an artificial person or getting a new personhood as an adult should not be put in the same category as cosmetic surgery such as rhinoplasty and breast augmentation and getting eye glasses to improve vision. It is, however, worth underscoring that the above mentioned responses by surgeons and patients are good to know, but will require efforts at implementation, considering the usually indistinct borders between normalcy and abnormality in mental states and the fact that in some chronic subtle conditions, "previous personality" might in fact refer to abnormal states undetected. Ethics vigilance should never be relaxed; the stains of abuses are very hard to remove from any profession's perception in society, and patients may be unduly harmed if vigilance is relaxed.

Pearl
Qualitative research indicates that deep brain stimulation (DBS) is seen by patients and surgeons to be ethical for pathological conditions such as depression and eating disorders, but not for enhancement of normal states. These views are fairly universal. Therefore, there may not be an "ethical marketplace" for such procedures.

18.4.2   Functional Magnetic Resonance Imaging (fMRI)

18.4.2.1   General Aspects of fMRI
Increased electrical activity and metabolism in the brain cause an increased flow of oxygenated blood to the area of interest through autoregulatory mechanisms. Inflow of oxygenated hemoglobin causes the fMRI signal emanating from the area of interest to increase. This is the basis of blood oxygenation level-dependent (BOLD) fMRI. Signal is captured by detectors and calibrated into digital forms. Data processing involves the subtraction of study data from control averages, and products are presented as pictures superimposed on static brain images. Images seen are therefore products of background assumptions, models, statistically processed data, and inferences. From basic and functional neuroanatomy, active areas can be correlated with known functions, or if it is function that is being localized, regions affected by function can be known. It is important to note that the pictures are derived, but not directly; they are indeed direct measurements of event-related increased blood flow, not neuronal activities nor thoughts. Drugs, seizures, or structural abnormalities of the brain can affect and confound results. Some functions are not yet fully localized to agreed defined regions, but the interobserver correlation, sensitivity, and specificity of fMRI continue to improve. All these are important for lay members of society in considering such studies especially under direct to consumer advertisements (DTCA) and self-referrals. Functional MRI is noninvasive and is safe from a physical risk point of view, and its imitations are not usually mentioned during advertisements, and therefore it is easy for people to accept and even seek out fMRI.

18.4.2.2 Lie Detection by fMRI

Conscious lying involves more areas of the brain than truth telling. These areas can be detected by fMRI and can be differentiated from mistaken or false memories (Illes 2004). Such studies do not show what would happen with spontaneous big lies or "white lies" or in normal persons versus sociopaths. Programs for detecting lying by fMRI are now available. They require comparison with baselines and their reliability depends on questions being used, the actual events being detected, and discrimination between baseline and actual events. More data are required especially if this is to be used outside research settings. It is more promising than old polygraphy (testing skin conductance, sweating, respiration and heart rates, blood pressure) and event-related potentials on electroencephalogram. Furthermore, a lot of cooperation is required both in responding and in staying still for about 10 min (Langleben 2008). A new set of guidelines and safeguarding policies will be required when these become better validated and are to be used on suspected criminals. The threshold of reliability that may be legally acceptable will be another aspect to be considered. The fundamental question is: "Is it ethical to subject an accused to a test which can look into his brain and detect something which is beyond his/her control of divulging voluntarily?" Even criminals and sociopaths have rights, and we must all be wary that the invasion of privacy represented by fMRI may erode bigger societal issues than the positive value of confirming the guilt of one criminal.

18.4.2.3 Brain Privacy, Confidentiality, and fMRI

The lie detection fMRI process described above is not capable of intrusion into personality. There is no doubt, however, that ongoing efforts will move fMRI to the point when better cognition and disposition definition will be very reliable. That would mean information beyond that immediately relevant to the particular situation might be detectable. One could imagine the implications if care providers, employers, insurance companies, visa officers, police, and other law enforcement agents were able to fairly accurately categorize citizens and see misdeeds or other behaviors in their futures. It would be a different world, with marked increased individual vulnerability. Confidentiality, that privilege of no intrusion, and confidentiality which involves "secret keeping" will assume different dimensions especially in situations where danger to a third party may be involved. Court and tribunal evidences and testimonies about character would be of a different dimension (Roskies et al. 2013). The ethical challenges would be formidable and it is this kind of possible technological development that ought to make us ask if we should pursue all that we may and if we should do things just because we can. An ethical assessment of the potential of new technologies should be performed by researchers and societies before they become a clinical reality, if possible.

Similar problems occur with other neurodiagnostic imaging modalities such as PET scanning (The neuroscientist who discovered he was a psychopath 2013).

18.4.2.4 Misapplication of fMRI

Functional MRI like all significant developments offers great opportunities for abuses. We have mentioned some social and ethical ones related to them.

Scientific misuse would involve overstating the sensitivity, specificity, and reliability of this technology.

A bigger concern is that scientists might extrapolate conclusions beyond what data, design, method, and other scientific premises allow. Reductionism, that over-enthusiastic translation of one paradigm, theory, interpretation, and conclusion into a completely different set, is a dangerous intellectual behavior (Harris and Schaffner 1992). Ordinary empirical projections of data and its implicational meaning, for instance, blood flow and neuronal activity, should be acknowledged not to represent mechanical models of metaphysical entities like life, mind, personhood, and so on. Absolute reductionism and fatalism could have serious consequences (Illes and Racine 2005). Finally, whereas it is desirable that entrepreneurs should optimize the gains of science and technology, excesses can occur when facilities are pressed for uses in areas where reliability has not been sufficiently established in the usual scientific manner (Farah 2004; Illes et al. 2006; Racine et al. 2006).

> **Pearl**
> Neuroscience holds a lot of promise for basic and translational research and clinical care. Premature applications, overenthusiasm, as well as unjustified fears are all unethical and can only cause needless private and public pains.

18.4.3 Neuroethics of Neurotechnology

Since the dawn of industrialization, science has been tempted to serve technology, technology industry, industry business, and business. It is therefore expected that neuroscience will yield neurotechnology which is the interphase between basic neuroscience, medical and surgical neurology, and advanced technology. Neurotechnological successes include cochlear implants and artificial retina which transduce sound and light respectively, neuromotor devices that transduce brain signals into signals that can operate various devices like computers, deeply implanted electrodes for deep brain stimulation to control abnormal movements and compulsive and emotional disorders (discussed above), and the more short-lived effects of transcranial magnetic stimulation for various psychiatric disorders. The new field of nanotechnology may provide more innovative brain-machine interfaces (Lee et al. 2013). There have even been applications of technologies like spinal cord stimulation to impossible challenges like chronic vegetative state (Della Pepa et al. 2013).

Issues related to these technologies involve the principles of respect for persons, contextual cost-benefit analysis, and justice. Experimental treatments require policies that increase openness, accountability, and formal oversight of interactions. Many of these are resource intensive, and the issue of ethical priority setting (resource allocation) and overall social justice would be more relevant here than in most routine therapy situations. Also, the conditions usually treated by these measures are often physically, emotionally, and socially challenging. Centers that undertake these levels of care usually are mindful of the complications both of the disease process and treatment measures and adopt a scientific approach.

> **Pearl**
> There is no substitute for continuing research and cautious application in maximizing the value and minimizing the pains of innovations in neuroscience.

18.4.4 Neuroethics and Developing Societies

Developing societies can be affected by innovative developments in neuroscience and neurotechnology partly because travel makes it possible for practitioners and patients from these societies to take advantage of them (Malomo and Bernstein 2011). fMRI and deep brain stimulation surgery may not be widely available yet in most of Africa, for example, but the world is getting smaller every day from an information transfer perspective and patients may hear about these opportunities and pursue them. Conversely, some developing societies do have access to such technologies, but ethical infrastructure may not be as well developed and these technologies may be even more subject to potential abuse in these settings where people are even more vulnerable.

> **Conclusion**
> Neurosurgeons are fortunate to be at the forefront of developments in the neurological sciences. We will be consistently challenged by technological innovations and the application of older and new techniques to treat conditions not previously considered treatable by surgical intervention. These situations will tax our skill and our judgment. We would be wise to embrace and engage in neuroethics discussions along with philosophers, bioethicists, psychiatrists, neurologists, and neuroscientists, so that we are part of the decision-making and not passive recipients of decisions which could relegate us to be technicians. A working understanding of neuroethics will help us embrace the future of the sciences and practice of our specialty.

Acknowledgement We thank Sylvia O. Malomo and A. D. Faraye for their suggestions.

References

Arras JD, Steinbock B, London AJ (1999) Moral reasoning in the medical context. In: Arras JD, Steinbock B (eds) Ethical issues in modern medicine, 5th edn. Mayfield Pub. Co, Houston

Della Pepa GM, Fukuya C, LaRocca G et al (2013) Neuromodulation of vegetative state through spinal cord stimulation: where are we now and where are we going? Stereotact Funct Neurosurg 91:275–287

Elliott C (2004) Better than well: American medicine meets the American dream. WW Norton and Company, New York

Farah MJ (2002) Emerging ethical issues in neuroscience. Nat Neurosci 5(11):1123–1129

Farah MJ (2004) Neuroethics: a guide for the perplexed. Cerebrum 6(4):32

Farah MJ (2010) Neuroethics: an overview. In: Farah M (ed) Neuroethics, an introduction with readings. MIT Press, Cambridge, MA

Freeman W (1958) Prefrontal lobotomy: final report of 500 Freeman and Watts patients followed for 10 to 20 years. South Med J 51(6):739–745

Granat P (2003) Unjust self-administration of enhancements even more common among the poor. http://www.bmj.com/cgi/eletters/327/7414/567#36307. Last accessed 9 Aug 2013

Grant RA, Halpern CH, Baltuch GH et al (2013) Ethical considerations in deep brain stimulation for psychiatric illness. J Clin Neurosci 21(1):1–5

Harris HW, Schaffner KF (1992) Molecular genetics, reductionism, and disease concepts in psychiatry. J Med Philos 17(2):127–153

Illes J (2004) A fish story? Brain maps, lie detection, and personhood. Cerebrum 6(4):73–80, http://www.dana.org/news/cerebrum/detail.aspx?id=1200. Last accessed 9 Sept 2013

Illes J, Racine E (2005) Imaging or imagining? A neuroethics challenge informed by genetics. Am J Bioeth 5(2):5–18

Illes J, Sahakian BJ (2011) The Oxford handbook of neuroethics. Oxford University Press, Oxford

Illes J, Racine E, Kirschen MP (2006) In: Illese J (ed) A picture is worth 1000 words, but which 1000? Neuroethics: defining the issues in theory, practice, and policy. Oxford University Press, New York, p 161

Langleben DD (2008) Detection of deception with fMRI: are we there yet? Leg Criminol Psychol 13(1):1–9

Lee B, Liu CY, Apuzzo ML (2013) A primer on brain-machine interfaces, concepts, and technology: a key element in the future of functional neurorestoration. World Neurosurg 79(3–4):457–471

Lipsman N, Bernstein M (2009) Ethical challenges for the future. In: Lozano AM, Gildenberg PL, Tasker RR (eds) Textbook of stereotactic and functional neurosurgery, 2nd edn. Springer, Heidelberg

Lipsman N, Bernstein M (2011) Ethical challenges in functional neurosurgery: emerging applications and controversies. In: Illes J, Sahakian BJ (eds) Oxford handbook of neuroethics. Oxford University Press, Oxford/New York

Lipsman N, Zener R, Bernstein M (2009) Personal identity, enhancement and neurosurgery: a qualitative study in applied neuroethics. Bioethics 23(6):375–383

Lipsman N, Bernstein M, Lozano AM (2010) Criteria for the ethical conduct of psychiatric neurosurgery clinical trials. Neurosurg Focus 29(2):E9

Lipsman N, Mendelsohn D, Taira T et al (2011) The contemporary practice of psychiatric surgery: results from a survey of North American functional neurosurgeons. Stereotact Funct Neurosurg 89:103–110

Malomo AO, Bernstein M (2011) On neuroethics. Arch Ibadan Med 11(1):9–14

Mendelshon D, Lipsman N, Bernstein M (2010) Neurosurgeons' perspectives on psychosurgery and neuroenhancement: a qualitative study at one center. J Neurosurg 113:1212–1218

Mendelsohn D, Lipsman N, Lozano AM et al (2013) The contemporary practice of psychiatric surgery: results from a global survey of functional neurosurgeons. Stereotact Funct Neurosurg 91:306–313

Pieters T, Snelders S (2009) Psychotropic drug use: between healing and enhancing the mind. Neuroethics 2(2):63–73

Racine E, Illes J (2008) Neuroethics. In: Singer PA, Viens AM (eds) The cambridge textbook of bioethics. Cambridge University Press, Cape Town, pp 495–504

Racine E, Bar-Ilan O, Illes J (2006) Brain imaging: a decade of coverage in the print media. Sci Commun 28(1):122–142

Roskies A (2002) Neuroethics for the new millennium. Neuron 35:21–23

Roskies AL, Schweitzer NJ, Saks MJ (2013) Neuroimages in court: less biasing than feared. Trends Cogn Sci 17(3):99–101

The neuroscientist who discovered he was a psychopath (2013). Available at: http://www.salon.com/2013/11/23/this_neuroscientist_discovered_he_was_a_psychopath_partner/

Training of Neurosurgeons

19

George M. Ibrahim and Mark Bernstein

19.1 Introduction

Patients undergoing neurosurgical procedures are often faced with the added stresses of navigating health-care systems. Since neurosurgical conditions are usually complex and affect multiple organ systems, patients with such diagnoses often meet numerous specialists that may be involved to varying extents in their care. Additionally, given that a large proportion of neurosurgical care occurs in large tertiary and quaternary teaching centers, patients are likely to interact with trainees during the course of their clinical care. These interactions have been the subject of considerable recent interest and research.

While trainees play a significant role in their care, patients are often uncertain about their roles and responsibility. This raises ethical concerns regarding informed consent, adequate disclosure, and truth-telling, as it pertains to the patients' rights to self-determination and autonomy. Furthermore, conflicts may arise if patients are hesitant toward the involvement of trainees in their care, which raises questions regarding the rights of trainees as both practitioners and learners and can erode the practice of value-based medicine. The most responsible or senior surgeon must often balance seemingly competing obligations as the patients' primary care giver and the trainees' teacher or mentor. These ethical tensions in neurosurgery training have been articulated before (Bernstein and Knifed 2007). The current chapter explores the interaction between patients and trainees, particularly pertaining to the

G.M. Ibrahim, MD
Division of Neurosurgery, Department of Surgery, Institute of Medical Science,
University of Toronto, 399 Bathurst Street, Toronto, ON M5T 2S8, Canada
e-mail: george.m.ibrahim@gmail.com

M. Bernstein, MD, MHSc, FRCSC (✉)
Division of Neurosurgery, Toronto Western Hospital, University of Toronto,
399 Bathurst Street, Toronto, ON M5T 2S8, Canada
e-mail: mark.bernstein@uhn.ca

A. Ammar, M. Bernstein (eds.), *Neurosurgical Ethics in Practice: Value-based Medicine*, 211
DOI 10.1007/978-3-642-54980-9_19, © Springer-Verlag Berlin Heidelberg 2014

rights of each party in the setting of a teaching hospital. The relevant literature is reviewed and an approach for ethical conflict resolution is presented.

19.2   Illustrative Case (Patient's Request for Resident Not to Operate)

A patient with a newly diagnosed brain tumor presents to the clinic and is seen by a staff neurosurgeon and a resident. Following a thorough discussion of the risks and benefits of surgery, the patient agrees to undergo awake craniotomy with intraoperative mapping for maximal safe tumor resection. The resident is particularly interested in learning intraoperative mapping methods. Before the patient signs the consent form, she asks whether the resident will also be involved in the operating theater. The patient is apologetic, yet adamant that she does not want "students" to be involved during the procedure. How do the neurosurgeon and resident respond to the patient? Who should be involved in the patient's care going forward?

19.3   Approach to the Case

Patients have an inalienable right to autonomy and self-determination during their clinical care. Surgical treatment can only proceed with their informed consent, which requires capacity, voluntariness, and a lack of undue influence. In contemporary health-care systems, physicians have a responsibility not only to state the risk and benefits of procedures but also to speak truthfully. Truth-telling encompasses directness and clarity regarding all aspects of the patient's care, including disclosure of those individuals who are expected to be involved. Neurosurgeons also have a fiduciary obligation to ensure that the procedure is performed safely and without unnecessary risk to patients.

These aforementioned goals must also be achieved without compromising trainee education. Societies have a moral obligation to train competent surgeons for the care of future patients, and technical expertise is best acquired through practice. Although good patient care and resident training are rarely dichotomous goals, the illustrative case demonstrates an instance where a conflict emerges between the rights of patients and the rights of trainees.

It has been previously shown that patients do not often understand or appreciate the role of trainees in the day-to-day operation of a neurosurgical service (Knifed et al. 2008a). The majority of conflicts between the rights of patients and those of trainees arise from failures to effectively communicate, evidenced by the fact that residents often believe that patients are not well informed about their role in their care (Knifed et al. 2010). Since patients are more accepting of trainees if they are better informed of their role and involvement earlier in their care, the attending neurosurgeon should introduce the importance of the residents' responsibilities during presurgical consultations. Even the most hesitant patients often understand that surgery cannot be performed without a team of dedicated health-care workers, including trainees and surgical assistants.

> **Pearl**
> Good patient care and trainee education are rarely dichotomous goals. The majority of conflicts between the rights of patients and those of trainees arise from failure to effectively communicate.

19.4 Discussion

19.4.1 Rights of Patients

The recognition of the rights of patients to make their own decisions regarding their care has evolved significantly over the last several decades. Currently, patient rights comprise an important area of medical bioethics and are enshrined in laws, policies of professional societies, and hospital codes of conduct. The current discussion will focus on three central aspects of patient rights in relation to their interaction with trainees. First, we review the concept of autonomy, a central principal of medical bioethics. This pertains to patients' right to directly consent to their care and play an active role in all aspects of their treatment. Second, we provide a discussion of truth-telling and the rights of patients to not be deceived. Finally, the right of patients to receive high-quality care and evidence surrounding trainee safety are reviewed.

19.4.1.1 Autonomy: Relational Rather than Absolute

In 1947, the Nuremburg trial established that patients must consent to procedures being performed on their person and established autonomy as one of the major pillars of contemporary medical bioethics (Shuster 1998). Autonomy refers to the right of a capable individual to make decisions regarding their care free of coercion or influence. The concept of autonomy is essential to the practice of medicine and the conduct of surgical procedures.

A traditional view of autonomy holds that capable individuals should be informed of all options, alternatives, and perceived benefits and risks, thereby allowing them to reach informed decisions regarding their personal care. Practically speaking, this discussion is affected by cultural, social, and personal considerations. For instance, some patients do not wish to be informed of material risks associated with a given neurosurgical procedure.

A "relational" view of autonomy has been proposed, whereby the treating surgeon must acknowledge and take into consideration the patient's internal moderating factors that affect his/her autonomy (Sherwin 1988). While a capable patient has the right to make decisions regarding his/her personal care, various moderating variables may affect this decision. For instance, numerous factors may be involved in a patient's reluctance to include trainees in their medical care. Preoperative stress about the surgical procedure may make the patient hesitant about the involvement of less experienced individuals, previous encounters with medical errors may render the patient more suspicious of medical systems, or the patient may originate from a country or region with a strict hierarchical health-care system where being treated exclusively by a senior surgeon is highly desirable. Alternatively, a lack of knowledge about the integral role of trainees in the daily operation of hospitals may result in a belief that their presence is superfluous or that they are only there to learn, rather than contribute to the patient's care.

Indeed, many of these factors are related to socioeconomic, cultural, and geographic factors beyond the information received by the patient, irrespective of how adequate or comprehensive. A patient from a rural setting, for example, may have had less exposure to trainees and may be unfamiliar with their role in clinical care. Attitudes toward trainees may also differ by culture and age. The level of knowledge of resident involvement in clinical care is low among patients in general to start with (Knifed et al. 2008a). Interestingly, residents themselves have also reported feeling as though patients were rarely well informed about their roles (Knifed et al. 2010). The partnership between the neurosurgeon and the patient may therefore have a role in affecting the individual patient's autonomous decision to have trainees involved in his/her care. Information presented to patients regarding the involvement of trainees in their care should be placed within the individual patient's contextual and relational understanding.

> **Pearl**
> A "relational view" holds that many moderating factors affect patients' ability to reach a decision autonomously. Information given to patients regarding the involvement of trainees in their care should be presented in the context of their internal moderating factors.

19.4.1.2 Truth-Telling: A Bidirectional Process

Although the concept of truth-telling has evolved over the last several decades, it is a self-evident statement that patients deserve to be told the truth. Deception, however, often occurs in clinical settings, although the vast majority of deceptive acts are not self-serving (Everett et al. 2011; Yu and Bernstein 2011). For example, a substantial proportion of medical residents were found to be willing to deceive insurance companies for additional patient benefits (Everett et al. 2011). Germane to the current discussion, it has been previously found that surgeons do not often voluntarily inform patients about the involvement of residents in their operation (Knifed et al. 2008b).

Truth-telling is a bidirectional process aimed at empowering patients to navigate their illness. The evolution of truth-telling is perhaps most apparent in the field of neuro-oncology. Whereas in 1961, most physicians did not reveal a cancer diagnosis to patients (Oken 1961); by 1979, only 2 % reported that they would withhold such information (Novack et al. 1979). Patients are also increasingly empowered to play an active role in directing their medical treatment. The globalization of information and greater awareness of the organization and hierarchical structure of hospital-based medicine, via the internet, or even medical dramas on television, have provided patients with greater insight into the involvement of trainees in routine care. Greater dissemination of information has also empowered patients to critically appraise all aspects of their care, including the involvement of trainees.

The question remains to what extent disclosure of trainees' roles to patients is important, as it has been previously deemed inconsequential by treating physicians. A qualitative study of patients undergoing brain tumor surgery demonstrated that patients generally prefer to know exactly what the physician knows, even if it may be seemingly inconsequential to their care (Yu and Bernstein 2011). As a component of truth-telling, it should be explained to patients that trainees play an important role in their surgical and postsurgical care. Their involvement throughout the patient's illness should be emphasized to facilitate the strengthening of the therapeutic resident-patient relationship. This is particularly relevant as it has been previously shown that patients consider direct communication with the surgeon postoperatively as very important (Rozmovits et al. 2010) and patients are likely to frequently encounter trainees in their postoperative care.

19.4.1.3 Safety: An Uncompromising Necessity

One uncompromising feature of health-care systems is to deliver the highest quality care. Certainly, the foremost concern for patients is their underlying diagnosis and its safe treatment. Conflicts may arise between patients and trainees if the former view the latter as a threat to their safety. Patients who hold such views are, however, a small minority. Studies have consistently shown that patients generally view the care provided by trainees favorably (Resnick et al. 2008; Stewart et al. 2011). In fact, patients often perceive trainees as reliable sources of information and have problematic relationships with residents if they are perceived as inaccessible or lacking communication skills (Boutin-Foster and Charlson 2001; Ruiz-Moral et al. 2006).

Mounting evidence indicates that trainees performing a procedure under appropriate supervision do not adversely affect patient outcomes (Freiberg et al. 1997; Wachter et al. 1998). Although neurosurgery-specific data are more limited, it has been previously reported that good outcomes for procedures performed by supervised trainees are possible (Woodrow et al. 2005). In this study, the authors performed a review of 167 intracranial aneurysm clipping surgeries, arguably one of the least forgiving procedures in neurosurgery. Although neurosurgical trainees performed over 90 % of the procedures under supervision, patient outcomes were comparable to historical data. The sharing of such information with patients is valuable to dispel false beliefs regarding trainees as a threat to safety. Furthermore, additional studies to evaluate the effect of neurosurgical trainee involvement on patient outcomes are necessary to inform evidence-based and pragmatic presurgical discussion.

> **Pearl**
> Patients have a right to be told the truth, including the fact that trainees may be involved in their care.

> **Pearl**
> The view that trainee involvement is a threat to patient safety has been largely dispelled by a body of evidence indicating favorable patient outcomes with trainee involvement.

19.4.2 Rights of Trainees

Trainees in teaching hospitals provide valuable service to patients. They are often the point of first contact and the first to respond to patient concerns throughout their hospital admission. During their education, trainees are also entitled to certain rights. Societies have an obligation to train competent surgeons for the care of future patient populations. This obligation may fall under the tenet of justice, a central principle of medical bioethics. In the subsequent section, we explore impediments and ethical approaches to the teaching of surgical competence, including the concept of graduated responsibility and the establishment of a strong therapeutic resident-patient alliance.

19.4.2.1 Surgical Competence: A Necessity for the Service of Future Patients

Basic competencies for neurosurgical residents have been defined as follows: (1) patient care, (2) medical knowledge, (3) practice-based learning and improvement, (4) interpersonal and communication skills, (5) professionalism, and (6) system-based practice (Heros 2003). Inherent to practice-based learning is the acquisition of technical neurosurgical skills that will allow trainees to safely and confidently transition to independent practice. As a society, we have an ethical obligation to adequately equip trainees with the knowledge and technical skills to serve future patients.

Increasingly, surgical educators are evaluating novel methods to benchmark surgical competency (Gonzalez et al. 2012). While educators generally agree that competency-based training is more effective than traditional models, various challenges exist to the acquisition of technical skills. These include systemic changes, such as the limitation of the number of consecutive hours that trainees may work, thereby limiting the time available to acquire technical skills. Although various innovators are devising novel and laudable methods to teach neurosurgical skills, such as virtual reality simulators (Alaraj et al. 2013; Ferroli et al. 2010; Ganju et al. 2013; Marcus et al. 2013), and mobile technology (Gonzalez et al. 2012), the fact remains that trainees must acquire technical skills through patient encounters. This fact has been recognized in legal rulings. In one seminal case, the staff surgeon was not found guilty of negligence by allowing residents to operate unsupervised in a case in which a devastating complication was caused by the residents. The judge recognized that this form of graded responsibility was necessary for the training of competent surgeons (Ginsberg 1994).

The hesitation of patients to undergo procedures by trainees is therefore an important impediment to the education of competent surgeons. In a survey of 202 emergency department patients, the majority of patients did not realize they may be the first person on whom the trainee is performing a given procedure (Santen et al. 2004). Interestingly, while the majority were uncomfortable being the first patient, the discomfort increased with the perceived difficulty or invasiveness of the procedure. For example, fewer patients were willing to be the first for a lumbar puncture (15 %) compared to suturing (49 %). Furthermore, patients felt they had a right to be informed if the trainee was performing the procedure for the first time, particularly if the procedure was perceived as being more difficult or invasive.

The conflict between the ethical duty to train competent surgeons and the fiduciary responsibility to speak truthfully and respect patient autonomy may be mitigated in several ways. First, as previously mentioned, effective communication is essential to explain the importance of the role of trainees to patients, particularly during early presurgical discussion. Second, the enforcement of a teaching model of graduated responsibility may allow trainees to eventually transition to independent practice, while mitigating patients' discomfort that invasive procedures are being performed on them by trainees. Finally, emphasis of the therapeutic resident-patient relationship in surgical training may align the potentially competing rights of trainees and patients. These solutions are explored further below.

> **Pearl**
> Societies have an ethical obligation to train competent surgeons. The hesitation of patients to undergo procedures by trainees may be an impediment to the training of surgically competent surgeons, but this hesitation may be mitigated by effective communication, enforcement of a therapeutic resident-patient relationship, and emphasizing graduated autonomy for trainees.

19.4.2.2 Graduated Autonomy

It is important for surgical trainees to learn to operate autonomously. Surgeons have previously reported that they are comfortable allowing residents to operate independently with graduated responsibility (Knifed et al. 2008b); however, a large survey also found that there was less satisfaction among residents with responsibility, specifically in performing cases as the primary surgeon (Bernstein et al. 2006). A review of case logs of junior neurosurgical residents has also shown that they are readily comfortable with simple procedures such as cerebrospinal fluid diversion and evacuation of subdural hematoma (Fallah et al. 2010), but are less comfortable with more complex neurosurgical procedures.

Graduated autonomy implies that trainees incrementally expand the scope of their responsibilities until they are able to practice independently. This approach has been advocated by numerous educators as it increases trainee independence without compromising patient safety. It is therefore an ethical way to justify trainee involvement in a given procedure. While graduated autonomy represents a departure from the medical axiom of "see one, do one, teach one," the approach is endorsed by regulatory bodies, including the American Council for Graduate Medical Education (ACGME).

It should also be noted that trainees have an ethical responsibility to avoid performing procedures independently if they have not yet achieved competence in doing so. The recognition of one's limitations is important in patient care to uphold the values of beneficence and nonmaleficence as well as professionalism. While it is important to note that patients typically understand that errors may occur irrespective of the skill or experience of the surgeon or trainee (Holliman and Bernstein 2012), they also value trust in their surgeons. Under normal circumstances, performing procedures without adequate training can at best be viewed as a form of deception and at worst, a violation of the patient's person.

An important negative element in resident training is the "rich get richer and poor get poorer" dilemma. Residents who are skilled surgeons get more responsibility bestowed upon them by the consultant and are allowed to do more surgery, for obvious reasons. Residents who are less skillful technically will get more supervision and less autonomy, perhaps being relegated to assistant with the consultant or perhaps a clinical fellow as first surgeon. There are many obvious reasons for this like peace of mind for overworked consultants, time management issues (e.g., getting all three cases done instead of being stopped after two because of slower surgery), and concerns for patient safety by the consultant. These are real-life issues which consultants must recognize and mitigate as best as possible so justice prevails and all residents get equal access to education and operative experience. This issue may become even more problematic as work hours for residents are on the decline which makes it more urgent for residents to get as much experience as possible during less time and with presumably less cases to work on (Miulli and Valcore 2010). Mentoring of residents is important to their success, and this access to mentoring should be egalitarian and in fact not inversely proportionate to one's need.

19.4.2.3 Resident-Patient Relationship

The doctor-patient relationship is at the center of any therapeutic interaction between physicians and the individuals in their care. The "resident-patient relationship" is perhaps a special case of this. Like the doctor-patient relationship, the resident-patient relationship is nearly universally asymmetric with greater vulnerability on the side of patient. This relationship is, however, unique to that cultivated by attending or consultant surgeons in many ways. First and foremost, residents rarely follow patients longitudinally in the long-term or see them in preoperative consultations. This may create a challenge in forging a strong therapeutic relationship and educating patients about the role of residents in their care. Second, although patients are admitted under a single consultant, they may interact with numerous residents at varying stages of their training, thereby potentially contributing to confusion regarding their role and experience. Finally, residents are less knowledgeable than consultants, raising concerns among patients as to whether they are competent sources of information and technical skills.

Despite these differences, residents have previously reported that they felt they are generally successful at building these relationships (Knifed et al. 2010). Trainees often manage the day-to-day issues of patients, providing ample opportunities to build trust and reassure patients of their competence. Furthermore, residents are typically the first individuals to address concerns raised by patients. Effective communication may therefore allow residents to establish trust and build an effective therapeutic alliance with patients, which may dispel concerns related to their involvement.

19.5 Recommendations

In the setting of an academic teaching hospital, patients have a right to autonomy in making treatment decisions, as well as a right to receive the highest possible quality of care. Physicians must, therefore, ensure that they are truthful in disclosing information, including about trainee involvement to patients, as well as creating a safe environment for both trainee education and patient care. Conversely, trainees in the same setting have a right to learn technical skills that are relevant to transition to an independent practice. Early disclosure of trainee involvement emphasizing the importance of their role for patient care and establishing a therapeutic resident-patient relationship are important steps to mitigate conflicts that may arise between the rights of patients and the rights of trainees.

Conclusion

In the context of a teaching hospital, patients and trainees are entitled to certain rights. Patient rights pertain to self-determination, being informed truthfully of trainee involvement, and undergoing surgical procedures safely by competent and skilled individuals. Trainees have a right to progress along a trajectory that will allow them to practice independently. Although the realization of these end points is rarely dichotomous, ethical conflicts that may arise between the rights of trainees and the rights of patients are often resolved through effective communication. The education of patients on the relevant role of trainees as well as the disclosure of trainee involvement early on during their care may mitigate such conflicts. Furthermore, establishing a system of graduated autonomy for residents and cultivating a therapeutic resident-patient alliance may establish trust and confidence between both parties.

References

Alaraj A, Charbel FT, Birk D et al (2013) Role of cranial and spinal virtual and augmented reality simulation using immersive touch modules in neurosurgical training. Neurosurgery 72(Suppl 1): 115–123

Bernstein M, Knifed E (2007) Ethical challenges of in the field training: a surgical perspective. Learn Inq 1:169–174

Bernstein M, Hamstra SJ, Woodrow S et al (2006) Needs assessment of neurosurgery trainees: a survey study of two large training programs in the developing and developed worlds. Surg Neurol 66:117–124

Boutin-Foster C, Charlson ME (2001) Problematic resident-patient relationships: the patient's perspective. J Gen Intern Med 16:750–754

Everett JP, Walters CA, Stottlemeyer DL et al (2011) To lie or not to lie: resident physician attitudes about the use of deception in clinical practice. J Med Ethics 37:333–338

Fallah A, Ebrahim S, Haji F et al (2010) Surgical activity of first-year Canadian neurosurgical residents. Can J Neurol Sci 37:855–860

Ferroli P, Tringali G, Acerbi F et al (2010) Brain surgery in a stereoscopic virtual reality environment: a single institution's experience with 100 cases. Neurosurgery 67:79–84

Freiberg A, Giguere D, Ross DC et al (1997) Are patients satisfied with results from residents performing aesthetic surgery? Plast Reconstr Surg 100:1824–1831

Ganju A, Aoun SG, Daou MR et al (2013) The role of simulation in neurosurgical education: a survey of 99 United States neurosurgery program directors. World Neurosurg 80(5):e1–e8

Adams v Ginsberg (1994) OJ No. 2673 (QL) (Ct J(GD))

Gonzalez NR, Dusick JR, Martin NA (2012) Effects of mobile and digital support for a structured, competency-based curriculum in neurosurgery residency education. Neurosurgery 71:164–172

Heros RC (2003) Neurosurgical education: the "other" competencies. The 2003 presidential address. J Neurosurg 99:623–629

Holliman D, Bernstein M (2012) Patients' perception of error during craniotomy for brain tumour and their attitudes towards pre-operative discussion of error: a qualitative study. Br J Neurosurg 26:326–330

Knifed E, July J, Bernstein M (2008a) Neurosurgery patients' feelings about the role of residents in their care: a qualitative case study. J Neurosurg 108:287–291

Knifed E, Taylor B, Bernstein M (2008b) What surgeons tell their patients about the intraoperative role of residents: a qualitative study. Am J Surg 196:788–794

Knifed E, Goyal A, Bernstein M (2010) Moral angst for surgical residents: a qualitative study. Am J Surg 199:571–576

Marcus H, Vakharia V, Kirkman MA et al (2013) Practice makes perfect? The role of simulation-based deliberate practice and script-based mental rehearsal in the acquisition and maintenance of operative neurosurgical skills. Neurosurgery 72(Suppl 1):124–130

Miulli DE, Valcore JC (2010) Methods and implications of limiting resident duty hours. J Am Osteopath Assoc 110(7):385–395

Novack DH, Plumer R, Smith RL et al (1979) Changes in physicians' attitudes toward telling the cancer patient. JAMA 241:897–900

Oken D (1961) What to tell cancer patients. A study of medical attitudes. JAMA 175:1120–1128

Resnick AS, Disbot M, Wurster A et al (2008) Contributions of surgical residents to patient satisfaction: impact of residents beyond clinical care. J Surg Educ 65:243–252

Rozmovits L, Khu KJ, Osman S et al (2010) Information gaps for patients requiring craniotomy for benign brain lesion: a qualitative study. J Neurooncol 96:241–247

Ruiz-Moral R, Perez Rodriguez E, Perula de Torres LA et al (2006) Physician-patient communication: a study on the observed behaviours of specialty physicians and the ways their patients perceive them. Patient Educ Couns 64:242–248

Santen SA, Hemphill RR, McDonald MF et al (2004) Patients' willingness to allow residents to learn to practice medical procedures. Acad Med 79:144–147

Sherwin S (1988) A relational approach to autonomy in health-care. In: Sherwin S, Feminist healthcare network (eds) The politics of women's health: exploring agency and autonomy. Temple University Press, Philadelphia, pp 19–44

Shuster E (1998) The Nuremberg code: hippocratic ethics and human rights. Lancet 351: 974–977

Stewart EA, Marzio DH, Guggenheim DE et al (2011) Resident scores on a patient satisfaction survey: evidence for maintenance of communication skills throughout residency. J Grad Med Educ 3:487–489

Wachter RM, Katz P, Showstack J et al (1998) Reorganizing an academic medical service: impact on cost, quality, patient satisfaction, and education. JAMA 279:1560–1565

Woodrow SI, Bernstein M, Wallace MC (2005) Safety of intracranial aneurysm surgery performed in a postgraduate training program: implications for training. J Neurosurg 102:616–621

Yu JJ, Bernstein M (2011) Brain tumor patients' views on deception: a qualitative study. J Neurooncol 104:331–337

Part V

Neurosurgeons and Society

Conflict of Interest

20

Patrick McDonald

20.1   Introduction

Conflicts of interest are encountered in all aspects of life, both professional and personal. For the purposes of physicians involved in clinical care and/or research, a conflict of interest is defined as "a set of conditions in which professional judgment concerning a primary interest tends to be unduly influenced by a secondary interest." (Thompson 1993). In the case of a neurosurgeon in practice, the primary interest is usually the welfare of an individual patient, but secondary competing interests may be financial gain, the integrity and validity of a research project, or the teaching of residents, medical students, and other trainees. Although most people think of financial gain as the most likely secondary interest, other interests can serve in that role, including academic advancement, prestige, both personal and institutional, and promotion. Personal factors can also serve as a secondary interest, such as spending time with family, hobbies, and the need for rest. The dual loyalties of a surgeon-scientist can be particularly difficult to navigate (Bernstein 2003), where the primary interest in patient care and outcomes can be tested by a surgeon's role in an ongoing research project.

Institutions such as hospitals and universities can also have conflicts of interest where the primary interest in patient care or knowledge acquisition and dissemination are in conflict with secondary interests relating to funding and competition for patients, among other things.

The mere presence of a conflict of interest, however, does not necessarily indicate immoral or unethical behavior; in fact, it is impossible not to have conflicts of

P. McDonald, MD, MHSc, FRCSC
Section of Neurosurgery, Department of Surgery, Winnipeg Children's Hospital,
University of Manitoba, Manitoba Institute of Child Health,
GB-138, 820 Sherbrook Street, Winnipeg, MB R3A 1R9, Canada
e-mail: pmcdonald@hsc.mb.ca

A. Ammar, M. Bernstein (eds.), *Neurosurgical Ethics in Practice: Value-based Medicine*,   225
DOI 10.1007/978-3-642-54980-9_20, © Springer-Verlag Berlin Heidelberg 2014

interest of one form or another (Bernstein 2003; Emanuel and Thompson 2008). It is how one acts in the context of a particular situation that may be cause for concern (Lemmens and Singer 1998).

Although some talk of potential or perceived conflict of interest versus actual ones, a conflict of interest refers to a tendency, not an actual occurrence – "it exists if the individual or institution is making decisions under circumstances that, based on past experience, tend to lead to distortions in judgment" (Emanuel and Thompson 2008).

At the heart of discussions of conflict of interest is the concern that poorly managed, they can erode the trust the public in general and patients specifically have in the care they are given and the integrity of scientific research. The bioethical underpinning of concerns regarding conflicts of interest stems from the principle of nonmaleficence, which is central to value-based medicine. If secondary interests are allowed to supersede the primary interest of patient care, there can be a significant risk of harm to the patient.

> **Pearl**
> Conflicts of interest are ubiquitous and unavoidable. The presence of a conflict of interest does not necessarily mean immoral or unethical behavior as long as it is dealt with properly.

20.2 Illustrative Case (Financial Enticement to Try New Spine Instrumentation)

As a busy neurosurgeon with a subspecialty interest in spinal neurosurgery, you are invited to a symposium by a device manufacturer who is developing a new product for minimally invasive spinal fusion. At the symposium, a prominent colleague, who was involved in the design of the device, speaks eloquently on the possible merits of the device relative to the current standard of care and presents preliminary data suggesting high fusion rates, low complications, and shorter hospital stays. You are asked if you would be willing to participate in a trial of the new device, where you will be taught how to use the new system and enroll patients in the proposed trial, with the ultimate goal of regulatory approval of the device. For each patient you enroll, you will receive $6,000.00 to support the hiring of a research assistant and other infrastructure costs of participation. It is suggested that you could also be an author on a publication that may result from the trial.

20.3 Approach to the Case

The first step to managing a conflict is awareness of its presence, and the illustrative case above presents a number of examples where a conflict exists. First, does the invitation to the symposium come with a monetary benefit such as travel expenses, accommodation, meal, and an honorarium for participation? Second, what is the relationship between the speaker(s) and the device manufacturer – do they receive financial compensation in any way or stand to benefit from the success of the device? This can include honoraria, consulting fees, royalties, or an equity or ownership stake in the company. Third, is the per patient enrollment fee excessive, that is, is it likely to exceed the actual cost of hiring a research assistant and maintaining a research infrastructure? Fourth, who controls the data derived from the study, how is it analyzed, who decides whether or not it is published, and is there an independent review of adverse events? Finally, does your participation in the trial warrant authorship?

In general, when a conflict of interest is present, it can be managed by a variety of means, ranging from voluntary disclosure to authorization by a third party to prohibition. Disclosure means making potentially interested parties aware of the conflict. This may include patients or research participants, Institutional Review Boards or IRBs (also known as Research Ethics Boards or REBs), journal editors when papers are submitted for publication, and your own hospital or university. Authorization by a third party can often follow disclosure, where the policies of an IRB, hospital, government agency, or university determine whether the conflict is allowed. Prohibition, the most extreme approach to conflicts of interest, prohibits certain relationships between industry and physicians.

20.4 Discussion

20.4.1 Industry and Neurosurgery

Although there are many sources of conflicts of interest encountered by neurosurgeons, it is the relationship between industry and neurosurgery that is most likely to introduce bias and undermine patient and public trust in our specialty. Nowhere does that relationship play a larger role than in the interactions between neurosurgeons and industry in research.

Funding from industry plays an increasingly important role in biomedical research. Industry-sponsored research now accounts for over half of all funding at over $60 billion per year (Moses and Martin 2001). The percentage of industry funding as a percentage of total research funding increased from 27 % in 1977 to 58 % in 2008 (Raad and Appelbaum 2012). There are concerns that the abundance of industry-funded research leads to bias – industry-sponsored research is more likely to yield positive "pro-industry results" (Bhandari et al. 2004), and there are examples where negative results have been suppressed or attempts made to suppress them (Moynihan 2010). A 2003 review of studies on the relationship between industry and medical research showed that 25 % of investigators had industry affiliations and two-thirds of academic institutions had an equity interest in companies that sponsored research at their institution (Bekelman et al. 2003).

In 2008, the president of the American Association of Neurological Surgeons (AANS) devoted his entire Presidential Address at the Annual AANS meeting to concerns about the relationship between industry and neurosurgery (Robertson 2008).

He highlighted the role and conflict present in industry-funded continuing medical education but devoted most of his address to industry-sponsored research in neurosurgery and the relationship between industry and neurosurgical researchers.

> **Pearl**
> Industry involvement in neurosurgery, through continuing medical education, research funding, and device development, introduces many opportunities for conflicts of interest.

20.4.2 Disclosure

Voluntary disclosure is the most common approach to dealing with conflicts of interest. In neurosurgical research, the Journal of Neurosurgery Publishing Group, like most journals, requires that authors of submitted papers to disclose the source of funding (be it government and not-for-profit funding agencies or industry funding) as well as any other financial conflicts, including consulting fees, royalties, stock holdings, or ownership stakes in device manufacturers or pharmaceutical companies (Journal of Neurosurgery Publishing Group 2008). These constitute what is known as "simple disclosures" where the actual dollar amount involved is not indicated. Disclosure of conflicts of interest allows reviewers and ultimately readers of journal articles to decide if the nature of the conflict of interest is strong enough to bias the results of the study. Review of disclosure rates in the Journal of Neurosurgery in 2011 revealed that 35 % of published papers disclosed some type of conflict of interest.

At present, there is no mechanism for disclosure of conflicts of interest to patients outside the context of research. Many surgeons, including neurosurgeons, receive royalties, honoraria, and consulting fees from device manufacturers and some have stock or ownership stakes in the same companies (Chimonas et al. 2010). As a result, a surgeon may benefit financially every time a device is used – something that ethical purists would say should be disclosed to patients.

20.4.2.1 Problems with Disclosure: Compliance

Although it is hoped that most conflict of interest disclosures are complete, there is evidence to suggest this is not the case. A study comparing voluntary disclosure by authors with company payment data in the orthopedic literature found that only 50 % of authors disclosed payments of one form or another from orthopedic device manufacturers (Chimonas et al. 2010). All the more alarming was the fact that the authors of this study only studied payments greater than $1 million. Even with this large amount of money, disclosure was only made in half the papers published.

The limitations of voluntary disclosure can also be seen in the recent controversy surrounding published industry-sponsored trials of recombinant human bone morphogenic protein-2 also known as rhBMP-2 marketed under the trade name INFUSE (Caragee et al. 2011; Meier and Wilson 2011; Spengler 2011). In the 2000s, a number of industry-sponsored trials were published using rhBMP-2 as an adjunct to stimulate spinal fusion. The results were notable in that not a single adverse event was reported with rhBMP-2 use. After publication of these studies, rhBMP-2 use increased from 0.7 to 25 % of all spinal fusions in the United States in a 5-year period ending in 2006 (Caragee et al. 2011). Many of these fusions were "off-label" uses, that is, used in fusions for which the product had not been specifically approved by the US Food and Drug Administration (FDA).

In a systematic review of the 13 original industry-sponsored studies (Carragee et al. 2011) coupled with a review of adverse events made available to the FDA, the actual number of adverse events was estimated to be 10–50 times greater than the original estimates. In addition, it was found that many of the authors of the original studies had significant financial ties to the company which sponsored the trials and manufacturers INFUSE. Some researchers received up to $20 million in royalty payments from the company.

In an unprecedented move, The Spine Journal devoted an entire issue to the topic with the lead editorial stating "It harms patients to have biased and corrupted research published," and "it harms patients to have unaccountable special interests permeate medical research" (Carragee et al. 2011). The Finance Committee of the United States Senate investigated the company's influence on INFUSE studies (United States Senate Finance Committee 2013). They found that the company had paid almost $210 million to physician authors and that an employee of Medtronic recommended against publishing a list of adverse events. The Committee recommended the implementation of "more stringent disclosure policies that detail industry funding to physician authors."

In 2013, the Physician Payment Sunshine Act of 2009, sponsored by Senator Charles Grassley, a senior member of the Senate Finance Committee, came into effect. The Sunshine Act requires that all payments to both physicians and institutions in the United States greater than $10 must be reported and available on a searchable Internet database. Fines for noncompliance start at $10,000.

20.4.2.2 Problems with Disclosure: Professional and Public Perceptions

It is clear that disclosure of conflicts, whether voluntary or mandatory, is not a panacea. Most conflict disclosures, both at scientific meetings and in medical journals, simply state a relationship with industry but fail to include the amount of monies received. As stated above, in some cases, the amount of money involved can be significant, even in the tens of millions of dollars (Carragee et al. 2011; Chimonas et al. 2010; Spengler 2011). It has been argued that "the greater the value of the secondary interest - the larger the financial gain, the more likely its influence on researchers judgment" (Emanuel and Thompson 2008). As such, simple conflict disclosures without dollar amounts are not enough. There is some evidence that surgeons are more likely to accept these simple conflict declarations as adequate compared to internists and learners (de Gara et al. 2013). A survey of surgeons, internists, and learners showed that 71 % of surgeons will accept a simple declaration compared to only 35 % of internists and 39 % of learners. This may be an example of the so-called halo effect where an audience is less likely to consider bias as evident simply because the author or speaker disclosed a conflict of interest (Lowenstein and Sah 2012).

Despite concerns regarding the potential bias that industry-supported research can create, the public considers it valuable for patients. A survey of persons visiting the SpineUniverse website (SpineUniverse website) indicated that 82 % felt industry-sponsored research was valuable (Fisher et al. 2012). Most (71 %) felt that such research should be regulated by a combination of government, hospitals or universities, company representatives, and doctors.

20.4.3 Management

A second way to approach conflicts of interest is by management, usually through a combination of regulation, review, and policy (Emanuel and Thompson 2008; Lemmens and Singer 1998; Raab and Appelbaum 2012). IRB's and REB's are tasked with determining whether industry involvement in a research trial creates too great a risk of bias by either not approving or suggesting alterations to the relationship, such as the formation of an independent data and safety monitoring board (DSMB). Hospitals and universities may limit the amount of compensation a researcher can receive from industry and limit any other financial interests.

20.4.4 Prohibition

In some circumstances, the potential bias resulting from a conflict of interest or the concern regarding the erosion of public trust in the integrity of research or an institution may be so significant that the only way to address the conflict is to prohibit it from occurring. Some have argued that members of drug or device regulatory agencies, for example, should not be allowed to own stock in pharmaceutical companies or device manufacturers (Lexchin and O'Donovan 2010). The US National Institutes of Health prohibits employees from receiving any monies from drug or device manufacturers (Raad and Appelbaum 2012). Although there are no examples of prohibition specific to neurosurgery, concerns have been raised about neurosurgeon-owned private, for-profit specialty hospitals (Babu et al. 2011).

> **Pearl**
> There are several ways to deal with conflicts of interest including disclosure, management, and prohibition.

20.4.5 Nonfinancial Conflicts of Interest

Besides financial conflicts of interest, there are other more subtle and harder to detect forms. A common one is the conflict of interest experienced by a neurosurgeon who wants a patient to undergo an operation not only because he/she feels it is the right thing, but to increase the neurosurgeon's numbers and experience. Perhaps the increased numbers will enable him/her to gain recognition and even fame. Similarly neurosurgeons who are clinical investigators will want a patient to enroll in the study so the study will be completed earlier, mainly for the altruistic reasons that the neurosurgeon wants to find the answer to the question so other patients can be benefited in the future. But he/she may also want the study to be completed as soon as possible so it can be published and again possibly bring recognition, promotion, and other nonfinancial rewards to the neurosurgeon (Bernstein 2003). Another situation may be that there is an observer at the neurosurgeon's center who has come a distance to observe a specialized procedure like awake craniotomy with cortical mapping. The case that is booked that day is not an ideal candidate for awake craniotomy but you consider doing it that way so that you do not disappoint the observer. These conflicts of interest are normal and are not unethical. It is only unethical if these conflicts are not recognized by the neurosurgeon and/or lead to his/her making treatment decisions for the wrong reasons.

> **Pearl**
> Nonfinancial conflicts of interest are very common in everyday practice and especially in the setting of clinical research. Neurosurgeons should be on the alert to recognize these conflicts and make certain to not let them alter their judgment and/or disadvantage the patient in any way regarding their correct clinical care.

20.5   Recommendations

This chapter focused primarily on the conflicts of interest arising from industry relationships with neurosurgeons. Neurosurgeons encounter many other conflicts that can impact their primary role – the provision of excellent patient care. Examples of other conflicts that can serve as secondary interests include work/life balance, academic advancement, teaching responsibilities, and roles as administrators. Similar principles to those outlined for industry relationships can be also be applied to these on a daily basis by neurosurgeons: awareness of the conflict, disclosure, management, and, where required, prohibition.

> **Conclusion**
> Conflicts of interest are encountered regularly in neurosurgery – as part of clinical practice, research, and the rigors of an academic career. Although the presence of a conflict does not necessarily mean the behavior is unethical, when improperly addressed, they have the potential to erode patients' confidence in the care they are provided as well as society's confidence in the integrity of neurosurgical research. Public and media concerns regarding

conflicts of interest in medicine are increasing and governments and other regulatory agencies will likely play a more prominent role in addressing these concerns in the future.

References

Babu MA, Rosenow JM, Nahed BV (2011) Physician-owned hospitals, neurosurgeons, and disclosure: lessons from law and the literature. Neurosurgery 68:1724–1732

Bekelman JE, Yan L, Gross CP (2003) Scope and impact of financial conflicts of interest in biomedical research. JAMA 289:454–465

Bernstein M (2003) Conflict of interest: it is ethical for an investigator to also be the primary caregiver in a clinical trial. J Neurooncol 63:107–108

Bhandari M, Jonsson A, Buhren V (2004) Association between industry funding and statistically significant pro-industry findings in medical and surgical randomized trials. CMAJ 170:477–480

Caragee EJ, Hurwitz E, Weiner BK (2011) A critical review of rhBMP-2 trials in spinal surgery: emerging safety concerns and lessons learned. Spine J 11:471–491

Carragee EJ, Ghanayem AJ, Weiner BK et al (2011) A challenge to integrity in spine publications: years of living dangerously with the promotion of bone growth factors. Spine J 11:463–468

Chimonas S, Frosch Z, Rothman DJ (2010) From disclosure to transparency: the use of company payment data. Arch Intern Med 171:81–86

de Gara CJ, Rennick KC, Hanson J (2013) Perceptions of conflict of interest: surgeons, intensivists and learners compared. Am J Surg 205:541–546

Emanuel EJ, Thompson DF (2008) The concepts of conflicts of interest. Oxford textbook of clinical research ethics. Oxford University Press, Oxford

Fisher CG, DiPoala CP, Noonan VK et al (2012) Physician-industry conflict of interest: public opinion regarding industry-sponsored research. J Neurosurg Spine 17:1–10

Journal of Neurosurgery Publishing Group (2008) Policy on conflict of interest. J Neurosurg Pediatr 1:110–111

Lemmens T, Singer PA (1998) Bioethics for clinicians: 17. Conflict of interest in research, education and patient care. CMAJ 159:960–965

Lexchin J, O'Donovan O (2010) Prohibiting or "managing" conflict of interest? A review of policies and procedures in three European drug regulation agencies. Soc Sci Med 70:643–647

Lowenstein G, Sah SC (2012) Viewpoint: the unintended consequences of conflict of interest disclosure. JAMA 307:669–670

Meier B, Wilson D (2011) Spine experts repudiate Medtronic studies. New York Times, June 28

Moses H, Martin JB (2001) Academic relationships with industry: A new model for biomedical research. JAMA 285:933–935

Moynihan R (2010) Rosiglitazone, marketing and medical science. BMJ 340:1848

Physician Payments Sunshine Act of 2009, S.301, 111th Congress, 2009–2010. Available at: http://www.govtrack.us/congress/bills/111/s301

Raad R, Appelbaum PS (2012) Relationships between medicine and industry: approaches to the problem of conflicts of interest. Annu Rev Med 63:465–477

Robertson JH (2008) Neurosurgery and industry. J Neurosurg 109:979–988

Spengler DM (2011) Resetting standards for sponsored research: do conflicts influence results? Spine J 11:492–494

SpineUniverse website. Available at: www.spineuniverse.com

Thompson DF (1993) Understanding financial conflicts of interest. N Engl J Med 329:573–576

United States Senate Finance Committee (2013) Staff report on Medtronic's influence on INFUSE clinical studies. Int J Occup Environ Health 19:67–76

Priority Setting

21

George M. Ibrahim and Mark Bernstein

21.1 Introduction

Priority setting, formerly known as rationing or resource allocation, is necessary to ensure that health-care systems function fairly and effectively while protecting patient safety (McKneally et al. 1997). Clinicians constantly exercise priority setting in their day-to-day care of patients. For example, a surgeon may cancel or delay a scheduled operation in order to accommodate a sicker patient. It is important to realize that priority setting is grounded in the ethical tenet of justice, or fairness, a central guiding force in value-based medicine. Justice implies the fair distribution of available resources; however, one person's idea of what is fair may differ from that of another. For a neurosurgical center to function effectively, systems-level decisions need to be made between many different individuals or stakeholders. Such decisions may be complex as the individual stakeholders have different and often competing priorities.

Accountability for reasonableness (A4R) is a modern framework that has been proposed to increase fairness in systems-level priority setting (Daniels and Sabin 1998, 2002). It is based on the premise that individuals may disagree about the results of decisions made; however, consensus exists that the process itself should be unbiased and ethical. Here, the application of A4R for neurosurgical priority setting is demonstrated through an everyday real-life example, the prioritization of elective OR's when cancellations can occur due to inadequate inpatient beds

G.M. Ibrahim, MD
Division of Neurosurgery, Department of Surgery, Institute of Medical Science,
University of Toronto, 399 Bathurst Street, Toronto, ON M5T 2S8, Canada
e-mail: george.m.ibrahim@gmail.com

M. Bernstein, MD, MHSc, FRCSC (✉)
Division of Neurosurgery, Toronto Western Hospital, University of Toronto,
399 Bathurst Street, Toronto, ON M5T 2S8, Canada
e-mail: mark.bernstein@uhn.ca

A. Ammar, M. Bernstein (eds.), *Neurosurgical Ethics in Practice: Value-based Medicine*,   233
DOI 10.1007/978-3-642-54980-9_21, © Springer-Verlag Berlin Heidelberg 2014

(Ibrahim et al. 2013), but countless other examples exist which would benefit from application of this approach. A4R is superior to "reactive" decision-making and bestows benefits to patients, surgeons, and health-care systems. It can provide a framework for neurosurgeons and their institutions to ethically tackle the problem of allocating resources within a fixed resource package. Although we mostly discuss the application of A4R in systems-level decision-making, it may also be applied to inform personal or individual everyday priority setting.

> **Pearl**
> Priority setting, formerly known as rationing or resource allocation, is necessary to ensure that health-care systems function fairly and effectively and that limited resources are optimally and ethically used.

21.2 Illustrative Case (Which Surgeon Gets Priority in OR if Inpatient Beds Are Short)

It is Tuesday morning and a busy night on call has filled the neurosurgical inpatient beds at your institution. Eight surgeries are schedule in your department today among three surgeons – one is already an inpatient and two are outpatient procedures. This leaves five beds needed and your administrator tells you there are only three available. There are some discharges today, but at 8:00 a.m. it is not certain how many. Which surgeons and, therefore, which patients get the available beds so surgery can proceed? How do we handle such an occurrence today and in the future?

21.3 Approach to the Case

A system adopted at one neurosurgical center addresses these problems using the A4R (Ibrahim et al. 2013). All the neurosurgeons have previously agreed that an adaptive, versatile, and ethically justifiable process for such decision-making should be utilized and have therefore adopted A4R. On the day prior to every elective OR date, all neurosurgeons and appropriate anesthetists, nurses, and administrators receive an e-mail from an assigned delegate, outlining the resource allocation strategy for that particular day (Table 21.1). Typically, all first cases are scheduled to proceed, as usually there are adequate resources to allow this or beds will be found during the course of the day. The prioritization of second and subsequent cases in the event of unforeseeable cancellations is outlined in the correspondence. Factors that are used in the prioritization algorithm are included in the e-mail, and the neurosurgeons are encouraged to contest the prioritization decisions, should they have compelling reasons to do so.

Table 21.1 Example of the actual e-mail correspondence sent to all stakeholders at a teaching hospital every day for the following OR day (surgeons' names have been changed to letters herein). Elective ORs are prioritized in the event of cancellations due to insufficient resources (i.e., beds). Factors taken into consideration for prioritization decisions are included in the e-mail, and all stakeholders are encouraged to appeal the decisions

Start all first cases. After that:

Dr. X 2nd case
Dr. Y 2nd case
Dr. Z 2nd case
Dr. X 3rd case

Please feel free to challenge any of this. Transparency and opportunity to appeal are 2 of the 4 key elements of the modern boiethics framework for priority setting know as the *accountability for reasonableness*.

If there are extenuating circumstances (e.g. case is fairly urgent; patient was previously cancelled; etc) please let me know the day before.

DSU cases and inpatients in Neuro do not get prioritized. Inpatients needing an upgrade from medical or Neuro ward to NCCU or ICU enter the prioritization ladder with high priority.

Some of the factors used in prioritizing
Urgency of case
Patient was previously cancelled
Expected timing of end of first cases
Whether surgeon OR time has recently been affected
Surgeons' use of day surgery for eligible cases
Stereotactic case when frame has been put on in the morning
Extraneous funding does not affect resources available for others
Total cases that will get done given different prioritization schemes

Every morning, the neurosurgeons refer to the correspondence to determine who will proceed with their elective cases. Documentation of those surgeons affected by cancellations is made for future reference in order to minimize repeated cancellations to the same group of individuals. A monthly audit of surgeon cancellation is performed and the process is reviewed. With each iteration, more items are added to the list of possible factors that may influence priority setting.

> **Pearl**
> Priority setting may not be relevant in circumstances where hospital resources are essentially unlimited, such as in some private hospitals. On the other hand, priority setting in very low resource settings, including many developing countries, is associated with additional challenges. These include availability of drugs, equipment, and ICU beds.

21.4 Discussion

21.4.1 OR Cancellations: An Everyday Challenge for Neurosurgeons

All health-care systems must find solutions to challenges that arise as a result of resource limitations. One very common example in neurosurgery is the cancellation of elective ORs, which may occur for a variety of reasons, including facility limitations, overrun of previous surgeries, or patient- and surgeon-related factors. This problem has been described in multiple health-care systems in all parts of the world (Argo et al. 2009; Chiu et al. 2012; Garg et al. 2009; Gonzalez-Arevalo et al. 2009; Haana et al. 2009; Kumar and Gandhi 2012; Lau et al. 2010; McIntosh et al. 2012; Mesmar et al. 2011; Schofield et al. 2005). Some authors have reported cancellation rates in excess of 30 % on the day of surgery. Although various studies have attempted to design more effective OR schedules to minimize cancellations (Pandit and Carey 2006; Pandit and Tavare 2011), the majority have not been found to be effective, as cancellations are typically very difficult to predict (Tung et al. 2010). Neurosurgeons, therefore, continue to struggle with how best to address elective OR cancellations. A mechanism to inform and guide such decision-making is therefore highly valuable.

21.4.2 Accountability for Reasonableness: An Ethical Approach to Systems-Level Decision-Making

A4R was introduced by Daniels and Sabin as a framework for ethical priority setting (Daniels and Sabin 1998, 2002). It is based on the premise that individuals unanimously agree that the decision-making process should be fair and ethically justified, although they may disagree on what factors are important to consider when constructing prioritization algorithms. This framework asserts that reasonable decision-making mechanisms should satisfy four primary conditions: relevance, publicity/transparency, revision/challengability, and enforcement/oversight (Table 21.2). This creates a tool by which decisions may be held accountable to the standard of reasonableness.

This framework may be applied to systems-level neurosurgical priority setting in order to render the process more fair and ethically justifiable. This may bestow benefits to patients, surgeons, and hospital administrators. No one likes bad news, but surgeons and patients can accept decisions that negatively affect them if they believe some thought, preparation, and ethical consideration went into the decision. In other words, most mature people can accept bad results as long as they know that the process leading to that outcome was fair and no one got special treatment. In the subsequent sections, we outline how the conditions of A4R may be satisfied in order to achieve an improved priority setting process for elective OR cancellations.

Table 21.2 Conditions of accountability for reasonableness as applied to OR prioritization decisions

Framework expectation	Explanation	Application to OR prioritization decisions
Relevance	The process is based on factors that the stakeholders predetermine to be relevant	All surgeons agreed that A4R should be adopted to inform ethical prioritization decisions The list of factors used in the decision-making are deemed relevant
Publicity/transparency	Distribution of the decisions as well as the factors involved in the decision-making process to all stakeholders	OR prioritization decisions are distributed to all stakeholders well in advanced of the day of OR Factors used in determining prioritizations are also distributed
Revision	Opportunities to challenge the decisions are offered	All stakeholders are invited to appeal the decision should they have compelling reasons to challenge it
Enforcement/oversight	A mechanism is in place to ensure that the three prior conditions are met	Oversight of the process occurs, for example, by auditing the decisions are predefined time intervals

Pearl

The modern bioethical framework for assessing ethical priority setting is called the accountability for reasonableness. Its four elements are relevance, transparency, challengability, and oversight.

21.4.2.1 Relevance

The relevance condition of A4R states that under a given circumstance, decisions should be based on factors that stakeholders have predetermined to be relevant, in other words, good reasons. As applied to elective OR cancellations, all neurosurgeons in the previously described scenario recognized the need for the application of a fair mechanism for priority setting. This is important to establish formally, as it ensures that the individual neurosurgeons are committed to upholding the conditions of the framework.

At most neurosurgical centers, a single person is charged with prioritization of elective ORs in cases where cancellations may be encountered, and it is usually done in real time as opposed to in advance. Usually, this is the OR manager or Division Head. This is typically achieved using unclear, inconsistent, or arbitrary considerations. Furthermore, the process is typically "reactive," that is, considered

Table 21.3 Factors that may be used in priority setting

Categories	Relevant factors
Case-specific factors	Urgency of case
	Extraneous funding available, which would not interfere with resources for other patients
	Expected length of case (i.e., maximum number of cases that could get completed given different prioritization schemes)
	Special surgical circumstances (i.e., stereotactic neurosurgery case where frame has already been placed on patient)
Patient-specific factors	Patient was previously cancelled
	Patient traveled a long distance to reach OR
	Other unique patient circumstances
Surgeon-specific factors	Surgeon OR time recently affected
	Surgeon's history of use of OR time
	Other agreed-upon factors

only when a cancellation is imminent. This is problematic as it may not result in fair or reasonable prioritization algorithms.

If asked, surgeons can agree on the factors that should be considered important when establishing prioritization schemes. Many of these are intuitive. For example, patients with more urgent conditions should have higher prioritization (e.g., cervical myelopathy trumps cervical radiculopathy, brain tumor with midline shift trumps small tumor with no mass effect). Furthermore, patient-specific considerations are taken into account. For example, most reasonable people would agree that those patients who were previously cancelled should be prioritized higher than those who were not previously cancelled, or patients who have come from a great distance might be prioritized over local patients. Other hospital- and system-specific factors may also be considered. For example, if the hospital receives incremental or additional funding for a certain subgroup of patients, they may be prioritized, providing that their care does not affect that of urgent patients. A list of sample factors that may be considered is presented in Table 21.3. Although these factors may differ from center to center, they should be unanimously deemed relevant by the stakeholders given the individual institution's circumstances.

21.4.2.2 Publicity/Transparency

The second expectation of A4R is that of transparency. This is achieved in the above scenario by distribution of the prioritization decisions, as well as the factors taken into consideration to all stakeholders in advance of the OR date. This provides an opportunity for all surgeons to evaluate the decisions and propose amendments should they have compelling reasons to put forth a challenge. To meet this condition, there must be well-delineated definitions of who the stakeholders are. The individual neurosurgeons involved are certainly among the stakeholders, but depending on the health-care system and institutional policies, it may be appropriate to also involve OR managers, anesthetists, nursing staff, or other health-care professionals.

This may be important as OR managers, for instance, may challenge the OR prioritization based on factors that are not known to the surgeons. Some groups may also view the patients themselves as stakeholders in the process. Ethical purists would suggest the patients, who are the ultimate stakeholders, should be privy to the prioritization, but most surgeons and administrators would likely be uncomfortable with that level of transparency. Certainly, on a personal level surgeons should exercise transparency to patients with messages like: "I'm so sorry your meningioma operation has to be cancelled tomorrow – I was on call on the weekend and several urgent cases were admitted. We'll get yours done soon." This kind of honesty and transparency reinforces patients trust in their surgeon and in the system.

Patient involvement in systems-level decisions pertaining to their care is increasingly recognized and promoted (Neil et al. 2004; Oakley 2009), as well as ethically justified by the ethical tenets of autonomy and informed consent. While it may be very reasonable for some institutions to distribute the prioritization lists to patients, it should also be recognized that it may also adversely affect their care, for instance, by increasing anxiety prior to surgery. We would suggest that the individual neurosurgeons act as advocates and that distribution of the prioritization list to the patients themselves is not advisable.

21.4.2.3 Appeals/Challengability

Challenges and appeals to the prioritization algorithm constitute the third element of A4R. In order to maintain legitimacy, it is important to allow revisions to the decisions through a fair appeals process. This may be problematic in neurosurgery, as decisions must often be made quickly with little time for deliberation. Indeed, as we have previously described, in the absence of such a formalized decision-making process, "reactive" decisions rarely allow time for reasonable appeals. In the scenario above, the prioritization list is distributed to the stakeholders in advance of the OR date, allowing time to consider challenges to the decisions. Each stakeholder knows to look for the prioritization e-mail the afternoon before any given OR day. Furthermore, with each iteration of the process, new challenges emerge that may expand the list of factors on which prioritization decisions are established. In fact, a "case law" can emerge from multiple iterative processes of decisions and appeals (Hasman and Holm 2005).

21.4.2.4 Enforcement/Oversight

The final expectation of A4R is oversight, which ensures that the former three expectations are met. In previous studies, it has been shown that oversight is the least met condition of A4R (Reeleder et al. 2005; Martin et al. 2003). Furthermore, oversight processes may exist, but may not be well known to stakeholders. Various methods for oversight may be implemented. For example, there may be a rotating schedule, whereby different individuals are responsible for creating the prioritization algorithm. Also, a third party (or parties) may periodically review the decisions at predefined time intervals to ensure that the process is functioning effectively and fairly. In the current system described, data are studied each month to make sure the OR cancellations are not unfairly borne by a small number of surgeons – this is a simple form of oversight.

Pearl

Priority setting is based around one of the four dominant principles guiding bioethics – fairness (also known as justice).

21.5 Recommendations

Although we used elective OR cancellations as an example to demonstrate the benefits of A4R, it may be applied in numerous scenarios where systems-level decision-making is necessary. Additional examples of systems-level decisions where A4R may be applied include the prioritization of funding allocation for the purchase of equipment (e.g., an additional OR microscope versus a new surgical navigation system) and the hiring of hospital staff, fair access to ICU beds, and many more. Since A4R holds decision-makers accountable for the reasonableness of their decisions, it is very versatile and may be implemented in multiple different contexts. It is beneficial for surgeons, as all stakeholders have equality of opportunity; for patients, as individuals are prioritized if their surgery is more urgent or they were previously disadvantaged; and for hospital administrators, as precious OR time is not wasted in deliberations. Its adoption, therefore, serves to mitigate conflicts and guide ethical allocation of limited resources.

Although we described the application of A4R in systems-level decision-making (i.e., decision-making between a group of people or more than one stakeholder), it can also be applied to inform the priorities of an individual person. For example, if a surgeon is faced with OR cancellations and must prioritize his/her patients accordingly, relevant factors may be applied to guide the decision-making process. The relevance requirement may be met by consensus between individuals or may be what the surgeon deems appropriate under the circumstances. He/she may disseminate the priorities to the patients, who may be permitted to appeal the process if they have legitimate reasons to do that are not known to the surgeon. It therefore provides a versatile framework to address the challenges of resource allocation across multiple levels.

Several previous studies have applied A4R in multiple different contexts (Kapiriri et al. 2009). One challenge to its implementations that has been previously identified relates to existing power imbalances within a system's organizational hierarchy (Gibson et al. 2005). Asymmetries in power may hinder the process' ability to function effectively by decreasing the opportunity for appeals and biasing oversight. Some authors have suggested that a fifth expectation be added to the framework, empowerment (Gibson et al. 2005), which would require mitigation of hospital-based power imbalances.

A4R may also be relevant for other domains of health policy, where inequities in opportunity exist. For example, one may apply this framework to evaluate which patients should receive an intervention if it provides a greater benefit to those who are already better off (Daniels and Sabin 2008). For example, surgical strategies to treat epilepsy may bestow a large net benefit on those who are least adversely affected by epilepsy, while providing incremental benefit for those who are most severely affected (Ibrahim et al. 2011). A "double jeopardy" may occur when those with a lower initial quality of life have a lower priority placed on treatments that can improve their lives (Harris 1987, 1988; Ibrahim et al. 2012). A4R may therefore provide a human rights approach to health care, particularly when evaluating prioritizations for vulnerable patient populations (Gruskin and Daniels 2008).

Conclusion

Hospitals are increasingly faced with constraints imposed by resource limitations. As a result, decision-makers are increasingly scrutinized for the reasonableness of their decisions. Through the example of the prioritization of elective ORs in circumstances where cancellations are necessary, it is evident that A4R is a versatile, adaptable, and effective framework to inform fair and ethically justifiable decision-making. It provides benefits to patients, surgeons, and health-care systems by mitigating conflicts, optimizing resource usage, and providing equality of opportunity. Its application to novel facets of health policy is an emerging area of applied ethics research.

References

Argo JL, Vick CC, Graham LA et al (2009) Elective surgical case cancellation in the veterans health administration system: identifying areas for improvement. Am J Surg 198:600–606

Chiu CH, Lee A, Chui PT (2012) Cancellation of elective operations on the day of intended surgery in a Hong Kong hospital: point prevalence and reasons. Hong Kong Med J 18:5–10

Daniels N, Sabin J (1998) The ethics of accountability in managed care reform. Health Aff (Millwood) 17:50–64

Daniels N, Sabin J (2002) Setting limits fairly: can we learn to share scarce resources? Oxford University Press, Oxford

Daniels N, Sabin JE (2008) Accountability for reasonableness: an update. BMJ 337:a1850

Garg R, Bhalotra AR, Bhadoria P et al (2009) Reasons for cancellation of cases on the day of surgery-a prospective study. Indian J Anaesth 53:35–39

Gibson JL, Martin DK, Singer PA (2005) Priority setting in hospitals: fairness, inclusiveness, and the problem of institutional power differences. Soc Sci Med 61:2355–2362

Gonzalez-Arevalo A, Gomez-Arnau JI, delaCruz FJ et al (2009) Causes for cancellation of elective surgical procedures in a Spanish general hospital. Anaesthesia 64:487–493

Gruskin S, Daniels N (2008) Process is the point: justice and human rights: priority setting and fair deliberative process. Am J Public Health 98:1573–1577

Haana V, Sethuraman K, Stephens L et al (2009) Case cancellations on the day of surgery: an investigation in an Australian paediatric hospital. ANZ J Surg 79:636–640

Harris J (1987) QALYfying the value of life. J Med Ethics 13:117–123

Harris J (1988) Life: quality, value and justice. Health Policy 10:259–266

Hasman A, Holm S (2005) Accountability for reasonableness: opening the black box of process. Health Care Anal 13:261–273

Ibrahim GM, Fallah A, Snead OC et al (2011) Ethical issues in surgical decision making concerning children with medically intractable epilepsy. Epilepsy Behav 22:154–157

Ibrahim GM, Barry BW, Fallah A et al (2012) Inequities in access to pediatric epilepsy surgery: a bioethical framework. Neurosurg Focus 32:E2

Ibrahim GM, Tymianski M, Bernstein M (2013) Priority setting in neurosurgery, as exemplified by an everyday challenge. Can J Neurol Sci 40:378–383

Kapiriri L, Norheim OF, Martin DK (2009) Fairness and accountability for reasonableness. Do the views of priority setting decision makers differ across health systems and levels of decision making? Soc Sci Med 68:766–773

Kumar R, Gandhi R (2012) Reasons for cancellation of operation on the day of intended surgery in a multidisciplinary 500 bedded hospital. J Anaesthesiol Clin Pharmacol 28:66–69

Lau HK, Chen TH, Liou CM et al (2010) Retrospective analysis of surgery postponed or cancelled in the operating room. J Clin Anesth 22:237–240

Martin DK, Singer PA, Bernstein M (2003) Access to intensive care unit beds for neurosurgery patients: a qualitative case study. J Neurol Neurosurg Psychiatry 74:1299–1303

McIntosh B, Cookson G, Jones S (2012) Cancelled surgeries and payment by results in the English national health service. J Health Serv Res Policy 17:79–86

McKneally MF, Dickens BM, Meslin EM et al (1997) Bioethics for clinicians: 13. Resource allocation. CMAJ 157:163–167

Mesmar M, Shatnawi NJ, Faori I et al (2011) Reasons for cancellation of elective operations at a major teaching referral hospital in Jordan. East Mediterr Health J 17:651–655

Neil DA, Clarke S, Oakley JG (2004) Public reporting of individual surgeon performance information: United Kingdom developments and Australian issues. Med J Aust 181:266–268

Oakley J (2009) Surgeon report cards, clinical realities, and the quality of patient care. Monash Bioeth Rev 28:21.1–21.6

Pandit JJ, Carey A (2006) Estimating the duration of common elective operations: implications for operating list management. Anaesthesia 61:768–776

Pandit JJ, Tavare A (2011) Using mean duration and variation of procedure times to plan a list of surgical operations to fit into the scheduled list time. Eur J Anaesthesiol 28:493–501

Reeleder D, Martin DK, Keresztes C et al (2005) What do hospital decision-makers in Ontario, Canada, have to say about the fairness of priority setting in their institutions? BMC Health Serv Res 5:8

Schofield WN, Rubin GL, Piza M et al (2005) Cancellation of operations on the day of intended surgery at a major Australian referral hospital. Med J Aust 182:612–615

Tung A, Dexter F, Jakubczyk S et al (2010) The limited value of sequencing cases based on their probability of cancellation. Anesth Analg 111:749–756

Medicolegal Issues

Ahmed Ammar

22.1 Introduction

Neurosurgeons, like other medical and surgical practitioners, have the duty to provide ethical medical care for their patients without compromise and to practise truly value-based medicine. The patient is entitled to be treated according to the recognized standard of care. In cases of discontentment of a patient with the medical care provided by the practitioner, or any complications from procedures incurred due to negligence, patients have the right to complain and file a medical malpractice lawsuit against the treating practitioner.

Medical malpractice is professional negligence by an act of omission or commission by a healthcare provider in which the treatment provided falls below the accepted standard of practice in the medical community and results in injury to the patient. Cases of medical litigation are increasing annually in different places in the world (Jena et al. 2011; Nahed et al. 2012; Rovit et al. 2007; Sandor 1957). Medical malpractice is defined in one jurisdiction as a failure of a physician, hospital, or employee of a hospital in rendering services to use reasonable care, skills, and knowledge (Nevada Revised Statutes (NRS) Chapter 41A.015 2011). Similarly, professional negligence has also been defined as "negligent act or omission of act" by the provider of healthcare in rendering professional service, wherein "act" or "omission" is the proximate cause of a personal injury or wrongful death of the patient". The term does not include services that are outside the scope of services for which the healthcare provider is licensed or services for which any restriction has been imposed by the applicable regulatory board or healthcare facility.

A. Ammar, MBChB, DMSc, FICS, FACS, FAANS
Department of Neurosurgery, King Fahd University Hospital, Dammam University,
40121, Al Khobar, 31952, Saudi Arabia
e-mail: ahmed@ahmedammar.com

A. Ammar, M. Bernstein (eds.), *Neurosurgical Ethics in Practice: Value-based Medicine*, 243
DOI 10.1007/978-3-642-54980-9_22, © Springer-Verlag Berlin Heidelberg 2014

Neurosurgeons may find themselves involved in one of three different phases of the medicolegal system:
1. Expert witness. The practitioner states his/her professional opinion in a litigation case.
2. Defendant. The practitioner defends and justifies his/her practice, decision, skills, and medical performance in a medical litigation case.
3. Claimant. This is extremely rare.

22.2 Discussion

22.2.1 The Neurosurgeon as Expert Witness

22.2.1.1 Illustrative Case (Request to Be an Expert Witness)
Lawyers for the local court sent official letters to four different neurosurgeons from three different hospitals for an expert opinion. The case was a patient who died after a neurosurgical operation. The three experts received a full copy of the patient's file and a form containing the following questions: Was the qualification of the practitioner suitable to perform such surgery? Was the preoperative preparation of the patient accurate? Was the operation performed in accordance to national and international standards? Was the patient aware of the practitioner's qualifications, and had he/she signed a consent? Was the risk of death or serious complication included in the consent, and was it explained to the patient? Was there any negligence? Were the instruments or techniques used on the procedure new? Did the practitioner make necessary consultations? Did the patient receive the correct management after the surgery? The expert witness has to answer clearly these two questions: (1) Does he/she think that the practitioner who operated on the deceased patient is responsible for his poor outcome? (2) To what extent is he responsible?

One consultant apologized because he knew the case and did not want to be involved. Another said he was too busy to take on the case. A third accepted to be an expert witness – he knew the case and his opinion would be based according to what he believed were the facts. The fourth accepted the request, and he had no knowledge of the case.

22.2.1.2 Approach to the Case
There are four elements that must be proven:
1. The duty of care was owed to the patient by the physician.
2. The physician violated the applicable standard of care.
3. The patient suffered a compensable injury.
4. The injury was caused by, and proximately due to, substandard conduct.

In a malpractice lawsuit, the burden of proving these elements is on the plaintiff. The evidence must satisfy the burden of proof which is called the "balance of probabilities" in civil law. This means that there should be a greater than 50 % chance that the harm is due to the substandard care provided by the physician.

There is evidence showing the number of malpractice lawsuit cases has increased in different parts of the world (Jena et al. 2011). The courts are always asking for professional expert witnesses. The report of the expert witness has direct impact on the decision which the court may take in any medical litigation case. The expert witness is obliged to be honest, objective, and professional in writing the required report. Many neurosurgeons may feel uncomfortable to be an expert witness, especially if the defendant of the case is one of their colleagues, but it is the neurosurgeons' duty and honour to help "police" their own profession. They should also consider accepting cases both for the claimant and the defendant, not just the defendant.

22.2.1.3 The Expert Witness' Duties

A medical expert witness is a qualified medical expert who is fully licensed by legal authority. He/she should be active in the practice of the same field of specialty related to the subject of the claim for malpractice and should have a practical (professional) degree in that specialty. His/her academic degree and his/her involvement in research related to the disease, including publication record, should also be considered in his/her qualifications.

Citizens, in any country, have the duty and responsibility to support the legal system of courts. Therefore, neurosurgeons should not refuse the court's request to be an expert witness. It has been the practice in some countries that attorneys' offices hire experienced medical practitioners in different subspecialties to be part of their defence strategy. These practitioners work for them as private and independent experts who act as expert witnesses, to any party, in cases of lawsuit against medical practices. Neurosurgeons and other medical practitioners are in need to have guidelines how to write an honest, fair, and professional testimony. The courts in some countries have special offices that determine which medical experts are appropriate according to the presented medical malpractice case (Brent 1982). Several NGO committees share in that effort as well. Guidelines have been issued for expert witness testimony in medical practice (Guidelines for Expert Witness Testimony in Medical Malpractice Litigation. Committee on Medical Liability. American Academy of Pediatrics 2002).

Most neurosurgeons who receive an invitation to stand as a medical expert witness will contemplate these questions: "Shall I accept the request to be the expert witness in that particular case or not? Do I have time? I know the neurosurgeon; will that affect my judgement?" There are a limited number of neurosurgeons in an area or community, and most know each other. Patients may have had consultations or been seen by several neurosurgeons within this community before they are treated at a particular clinic. Therefore, a requested expert witness may have examined the patient previously and have formed a personal opinion which may result in a potential risk of bias; in this situation, the surgeon should decline the case.

The role of official guidelines and formats should help the expert to focus on the factual testimony or "balance of probabilities" (Andrew 2006; Slovenko 1993). Figure 22.1 summarizes the questions the expert should answer before accepting to write the report. Writing a medical testimony is a complex task and involves several stages, but it requires foremost diligence and honesty (Maggiore et al. 2011).

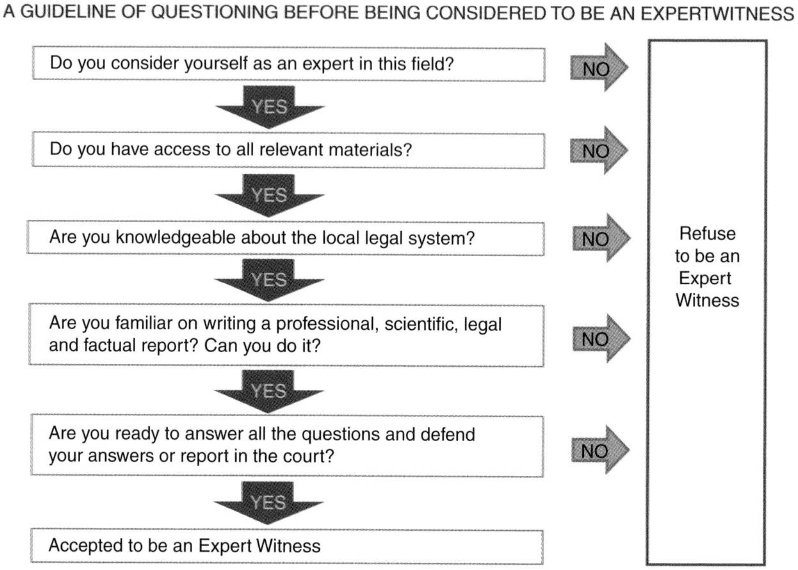

A GUIDELINE OF QUESTIONING BEFORE BEING CONSIDERED TO BE AN EXPERTWITNESS

Fig. 22.1 Questions a neurosurgeon should ask him-/herself before being an expert witness

Nowadays neurosurgical expert witnesses advertise on the internet which may be an unfortunate commentary on the whole medicolegal situation (JurisPro Expert Witness Directory).

Pearl

Medical expert testimony is crucial in medical malpractice litigation and is a very important part of the legal system. The testimony should be undertaken with a great degree of integrity and fairness. In order to avoid any possible bias, certain guidelines should be followed to guide the witness to focus on the questions of liability. He/she should stick to the available evidence and offer his/her personal opinions if asked. The expert witness should be chosen with special care and according to special criteria.

22.2.1.4 Preparatory Stage

A neurosurgeon who takes on the responsibility to be an expert witness should focus on the evidence, circumstances, nature of treatment, and the standard of care. Therefore, it is mandatory that the expert witness have access to all the case-related information such as the patient's file, investigations, reports of the treating neurosurgeon, and other witness reports. Sometimes the expert is not supplied with original imaging, only reports – in this case the expert must insist that the lawyer obtain the raw imaging. The expert witness must support his/her testimony with appropriate literature and research. It is important that he/she understands the circumstances, general medical environment, and the standard of care provided by the hospital and the treating neurosurgeon. Furthermore, the accepted guidelines of the concerned court and the instructions should be studied judiciously and should support the preparations and writing of his testimony.

22.2.1.5 Writing the Testimony

The testimony should present facts and opinions. The standard of performance of the alleged malpractice case should be compared and weighed to the accepted standard of that specialty and in that local area of practice.

In determining any breach of duty of care, falling below the accepted standard of care which would be considered negligent, it is important to take into consideration the standard of care at the time the alleged negligence occurred because it may differ from the practice at the time of litigation due to new techniques, understanding, and technology (Bolam v Friern Hospital Management Committee 1957). Standard practice should be deemed reasonable and not "best practice" since every doctor or hospital cannot provide or meet the best standard of care (i.e. there is always someone somewhere who can "do it better" than any given neurosurgeon).

The expert witness has to state the facts clearly and candidly. The medical terms used should be written in full, detailed, and explained. The testimony has to be signed and dated. Whilst writing the report, the expert has to mentally prepare him/herself to answer any questions related to his/her testimony the court might ask.

22.2.1.6 Wrongful Claim Review

The possibility of "wrongful claim review" may occur and expose the expert witness to legal consequences. The medical expert will be held responsible if he/she retains any information or falls short in stating the medical malpractice committed by the defendant neurosurgeon. He/she will also be responsible if he/she omits any available evidence that will prove the defendant guilty.

Unfortunately, some medical experts' credibility is not always accurate, honest, and unbiased (Brent 1982; Sloan et al. 1989). These surgeons may be making their living being expert witnesses, and their testimonials may be contaminated by their personal opinions and are not based on factual evidence but on unreasonably high expectations of average neurosurgeons. There is often difficulty distinguishing between personal opinion based on personal experience and medical evidence based on well-known and established scientific evidence which follows accepted and reasonable standards of care.

> **Pearl**
> Neurosurgeons have a duty to serve the legal system. They should accept to write expert witness testimony if they have the skills, ability, and the expertise to do so. The report they present must clearly identify the areas of failure, in accordance with the standard of treatment. The report must be authentic, accurate, and not misleading. The expert witness should separate his/her own opinion from the evidence and focus on the facts, but his/her expert opinion is also valued.

22.2.2 The Neurosurgeon as Defendant

It is accepted that patients and families have the right to file complaints and sue any member of the treating team. However, medical litigation is a nightmare for any neurosurgeon – it is not only devastating psychologically, but it consumes a great deal of time the surgeon would prefer to be spending helping other patients and other constructive pursuits (Charles 1999). Furthermore, it is not optional like accepting to be an expert witness; a sued neurosurgeon must comply. Most neurosurgeons may also consider these cases as threatening to their career and damaging to their reputation. Therefore, the defendant neurosurgeon may show signs of emotional disturbance, which in some cases reflects negatively on his/her practice and family life. The careers of some sued neurosurgeons have been altered as a direct result of medical litigation. It is important for any neurosurgeon who faces such a situation to hold and stick to his/her practice and other regular activities. He/she may be well advised to speak to senior colleagues, hospital leaders, friends, and counsellors for words of wisdom and support.

22.2.2.1 Illustrative Case (Neurosurgeon Sued for Post-operative Respiratory Death)

A 57-year-old senior consultant neurosurgeon received a notification from the court that he was being sued by the son of a 74-year-old patient who passed away 15 days after successful anterior cervical discectomy. The patient suffered respiratory complications 3 days after surgery, and medical treatment in the intensive care unit failed to cure his lung problem, and he succumbed.

22.2.2.2 Approach to the Case

There is no doubt that filing a malpractice lawsuit is one of the patient's rights. The patient's families also have rights to file a complaint against the treating teams. Neurosurgeons should consider the risk to be sued as one of the facts of medical practice, which every neurosurgeon should be prepared for and know how to deal with ethically and professionally. There are several steps that should be taken in dealing with any medical litigation case such as:

1. Read carefully the court notification and analyse the complaint.
2. Go back to the case and review the details and collect and review all the facts, investigations, admission notes, progress notes, and operative notes.
3. Seek professional legal advice and obtain an attorney who specializes in these cases (most neurosurgeons pay yearly dues to a medical protective organization, and a lawyer will be provided for him/her).
4. Prepare an honest, detailed, and comprehensive report about the case; any lapses in care or mistakes should be acknowledged.
5. The attorney or legal consultant should review and study this report carefully.
6. The attorney should be consulted about every step in court.
7. In court, the defendant neurosurgeon should be absolutely honest and keep a high level of professionalism.

8. The defendant neurosurgeon should not consider the malpractice lawsuit filed
   against them as a personal attack or an event which will damage their reputation.
   The court reached a decision that the neurosurgeon was not guilty in this case.

22.2.2.3 How at Risk Are Neurosurgeons from Litigation?

In one study, across specialties, 7.4 % of physicians annually were sued (Jena et al.
2011). There was significant variation across specialties in the probability of facing
a claim, ranging annually from 19.1 % in neurosurgery, 18.9 % in thoracic-
cardiovascular surgery, and 15.3 % in general surgery to 5.2 % in family medicine,
3.1 % in paediatrics, and 2.6 % in psychiatry. In an attempt to repeat the study in
Eastern Province, Saudi Arabia, the total number of litigations in Saudi Courts during 2003–2012 was found to be 641, of which 13 (2 %) were neurosurgical cases.
Of these neurosurgical cases, three neurosurgeons were found guilty. The obstetri-
cians and paediatricians were the most exposed to litigation. Some litigation is
driven by lawyers either because they truly believe they are crusaders against patient
injury by doctors or for more crass motives (Saxton and Finkelstein 2007).

Neurosurgeons are at true risk to face a malpractice medical litigation once or
more during their years of practice (Emery et al. 2013; Zhang et al. 2013).
Neurosurgeons should be prepared for such a risk and learn how to deal with it.
Neurosurgeons are widely different in reacting to medical lawsuit cases. Some consider the medical litigation as a direct and personal threat to their career. However,
others may consider such litigation as an occupational hazard and another challenge
they have to get through. The support of friends, family, colleagues, and hospital
administration is badly needed. The defendant neurosurgeon needs legal advice and
a professional attorney to build up the strategy to defend him/her in the court. The
defendant and his/her attorney should adhere to medical ethics and be honest and
acknowledge any mistakes or errors.

> **Pearl**
> The best strategy to deal with a malpractice case is with honesty and profes-
> sionalism and to try to not take it personally. Legal consultation is a must and
> support from colleagues very valuable.

22.2.3 Does Medicolegal Litigation Help or Hinder Progress in Medical Care?

Recent studies demonstrate a rise in medical litigation cases against medical
practitioners. In some of these studies, neurosurgeons top the list (Carrier et al.
2010; Danzon 1986; Jena et al. 2011; Mello et al. 2003; Mohr 1992). Discussing
the subject of medical malpractice may send a chill down every neurosurgeon's
spine. Neurosurgery is one of the most rapidly growing subspecialties; what
was considered standard a few years ago is by no means standard practice today.

The impact of new technology is enormous in the rapid development of neurosurgery. With every application of new technology or method, there is a learning curve which is associated with some risk of unexpected complications. How can neurosurgery grow as a speciality and neurosurgeons obtain new skills to climb their learning curve whilst minimizing the risk of complication and the threat of potential medico-legal consequences?

22.2.3.1 Illustrative Case (Neurosurgeon Sued for Not Recommending a Futile Operation)

A 62 year-old patient, with a known case of diabetes and hypertension, suffered a massive left (dominant) cerebral infarction. The patient was in a coma with Glasgow Coma Scale (GCS) of 5. He was referred to a neurosurgical centre with a recommendation for decompression craniectomy. The patient arrived at the neurosurgical centre 38 h after the stroke. Examination upon arrival showed the patient was in deep coma; GCS was 4. Pupils were dilated and sluggishly responsive to light stimulation. The neurosurgeon strongly recommended against decompressive craniectomy because she believed it was too late for the patient's condition to undergo the procedure and that if he survived the outcome would be unacceptable to the patient. Instead, he was treated conservatively in the ICU. Five days later the patient died. A few months later the neurosurgeon was sued for not operating on the patient.

22.2.3.2 Approach to the Case

The illustrative case presented above shows conflict between different ethical principles: autonomy, the patient's (or family's) right to choose the method of treatment, and beneficence and maleficence in which the neurosurgeon considers the expected outcome of a procedure according to the patient's condition based on his/her accumulated experiences and the evidence available. The patient has the right to choose the method of treatment, within limits. Exposing the patient to an unnecessary procedure disregards the patient's interest and benefits and violates the principle of nonmaleficence. When the neurosurgeon reflected on this case, she did wonder if she might have done a better job of explaining clearly to the family why she was so against operating.

The case remained in the court for nearly 2 years, and in the end, the court found the neurosurgeon not guilty.

Pearl

Incomplete neurosurgical information may cause a lot of confusion and unwanted conflict. It is important to provide the patient and family with a complete background of scientific facts concerning the medical problems, so they are in a position to make the "right" decision.

22.2.3.3   Analysis of the Current Reality

Many qualified and competent neurosurgeons, who are sincere in giving their utmost to help their patients, ask themselves before taking the decision to operate on serious cases how to protect themselves against the risk of litigation. Unfortunately, this worry has forced several very good neurosurgeons to adapt the policy of "defensive medicine", even changing the nature of their practice and which cases they will accept. This has recently become a huge problem in the USA costing billions of dollars and resulting in a reduction in the quality of care due partly to more ordering of tests.

In many cases, neurosurgeons refuse to operate on patients and decide to transfer them to other hospitals out of fear of litigation. This is a sad, unfortunate current reality. In addition, the patient loses the chance to receive immediate treatment at a nearby facility and is transported to more distant hospitals for an operation which could very possibly have been performed closer to home. Once a neurosurgeon loses incentive to take risks, he/she loses the ability to innovate and make progress in medicine. The system and the country lose billions of dollars which are being spent on unnecessary investigations and transportation of patients abroad for treatment. This situation puts patients at risk and diminishes the chance to develop excellent treatment centres.

The impact of medical litigation on medical practitioners, particularly neurosurgeons, is huge and takes several forms (Studdert et al. 2005; Thorpe 2004; Zuckerman et al. 1990). There is a large amount of money involved in medical litigation cases. In most western countries, insurance companies have increased their fees for medical malpractice substantially in the last 10 years.

> **Pearl**
> Medical litigation should not hinder progress in medical practice. It serves to help provide protection of patients' rights. Neurosurgeons must do their best to help their patients irrespective of the threat of lawsuits. Every neurosurgeon can help protect him/herself by making good decisions, executing impeccable care, documenting things well, and, of course, having medical liability insurance.

22.2.3.4   What Is Defensive Medicine?

Defensive medicine is the changing of medical practice based on the fear of litigation. In one definition it was described as the practice of diagnostic or therapeutic measures conducted primarily not to ensure the health of the patient but as a safeguard against possible malpractice liability (Anderson 1999).

The impact of defensive medicine is unfavourable on patients and on neurosurgeons. Defensive medicine may take several forms including delayed decision-making by engaging the patient in a series of investigations, tests, and consultations which are not necessary. In some cases, neurosurgeons may refuse to operate on certain risky cases and refer them to another centre, which is called "avoidance behaviour". At times, the neurosurgeon may present the informed consent discussion with exaggeration of the risk of certain procedures in the hopes that the patient declines the procedure. The delay of surgery may sometimes endanger the life of the patient or at least delay the recovery. The neurosurgeon likewise suffers as this behaviour may have a negative impact on their learning curve and their academic progress. It may also impact their earnings. Defensive medicine which is a direct result of medical litigation has a harmful impact on all parties. The question is whether it is actually unethical or simply a behavioural adaptation. Manipulation and misuse of the informed consent process as alluded to above is definitely ethically dubious.

22.2.3.5 Does the System Need Adjusting for Medical Litigation Cases?

It has been reported that the majority of cases of in-hospital patient complaints may be solved in the offices of the hospital administration. The most common cause of complaint is related to poor communication between the patient and family on one side and the treating team (doctors and nurses) on the other side. The second most common cause is unexpected complications. Most hospitals have an office where patients can complain, and if handled well only a small minority of these complaints will proceed to legal action. The role of the administration and hospital legal team should be emphasized, and these offices should take more responsibility and authority to help solve these complaints.

The legal system in many countries causes medical litigation cases to run in the court for years (often 2–4 years). Prolonging the case in court has a negative impact on the patient, the patient's family, and the neurosurgeon. It may damage, sometimes beyond repair, the professional image of the neurosurgeon, both from outside and from within. In the majority of the cases, the final verdict finds the neurosurgeon neither guilty nor accountable. However, nothing can compensate the neurosurgeon for this ordeal. There should be a way to reduce the period spent examining the case in court.

22.2.3.6 Some Practical Tips to Avoid/Manage Legal Actions

1. The patient has the right to receive the best possible medical treatment.
2. Neurosurgeons should establish excellent communication with the patients and their families and make themselves available and accessible to chat.
3. Neurosurgeons have a duty to do their best and to continually update their knowledge and skills in order to provide the best possible care.
4. Neurosurgeons should honestly disclose errors and complications that occur.
5. Neurosurgeons should not work under the stress or fear of possible litigation.
6. The natural history of some neurosurgical diseases is poor (e.g. malignant glioma). This fact should be explained to the patient and families very well. Well-informed consent must be obtained before every surgery. This is the right thing to do and may also decrease the incidence of medicolegal actions.
7. The patient has to understand that neurosurgeons can only do their best but cannot guarantee a cure or a perfect outcome.
8. The public and the media have to be professional and unbiased in dealing with cases of suspected malpractice. They have to present the facts honestly.

9. Hospitals and administrations should play a stronger role in helping their medical staff, not serving a role of punition if a surgeon errs and/or is sued, but one of support.

10. If a neurosurgeon is sued, he/she must work closely with the lawyer and must try not to take it personally and let it affect his/her day-to-day life.

Conclusion

Neurosurgeons and lawyers become professional allies in two situations: (1) when a lawyer is a patient and (2) when a lawyer engages with a neurosurgeon to defend him/her in suit or request him/her to be an expert witness. Being sued is an ever-present dread of any clinician but when/if it happens, the neurosurgeon must try not to take it personally and should follow the simple tips outlined in this chapter. Similarly when a neurosurgeon is asked to be an expert witness, even though many may find this work distasteful and/or too time-consuming, the neurosurgeon should take this request seriously and try to comply. An everyday neurosurgeon's input (as opposed to professional expert witnesses) is likely to be more honest and helps us regulate our noble profession.

References

Anderson RE (1999) Billions for defense: the pervasive nature of defensive medicine. Arch Intern Med 159(20):2399–2402

Andrew L (2006) Expert witness testimony: the ethics of being a medical expert witness. Emerg Med Clin North Am 24:715–731

Bolam v Friern Hospital Management Committee (1957) http://oxcheps.new.ox.ac.uk/casebook/Resources/BOLAMV_1%20DOC.pdf

Brent RL (1982) The irresponsible expert witness: a failure of biomedical graduate education and professional accountability. Pediatrics 70:754–762

Carrier ER, Reschovsky JD, Mello MM et al (2010) Physicians' fears of malpractice lawsuits are not assuaged by tort reforms. Health Aff (Millwood) 29:1585–1592

Charles SC (1999) How to handle the stress of litigation. Clin Plast Surg 26(1):69–77

Danzon PM (1986) The frequency and severity of medical malpractice claims: new evidence. Law Contemp Probl 49:57–84

Emery E, Balossier A, Mertens P (2013) Is the medicolegal issue avoidable in neurosurgery? A retrospective survey of a series of 115 medicolegal cases from public hospitals. World Neurosurg 81(2):218–222

Guidelines for Experts Witness Testimony in Medical Malpractice Litigation. Committee on Medical Liability. American Academy of Pediatrics (2002) Pediatrics 109:974–979

Jena AB, Seabury S, Lakdawalla D et al (2011) Malpractice risk according to physician specialty. N Engl J Med 365:629–636

JurisPro Expert Witness Directory. http://www.jurispro.com/category/neurosurgery-s-481/

Maggiore WA, Kupas D, Glushak C, National Association of EMS Physicians (2011) Expert witness qualifications and ethical guidelines for emergency medical services litigation: resource document for the National Association of EMS Physicians position statement. Prehospital Emerg Care 15:426–431

Mello MM, Studdert DM, Brennan TA (2003) The new medical malpractice crisis. N Engl J Med 348:2281–2284

Mohr JC (1992) The emergence of medical malpractice in the United States. Trans Stud Coll Physicians Phila 14:1–21

Nahed BV, Babu MA, Smith TR et al (2012) Malpractice liability and defensive medicine: a national survey of neurosurgeons. PLoS One 7(6):e39237

Nevada Revised Status NRS (2011) http://www.leg.state.nv.us/NRS/NRS-041A.html

Rovit RL, Simon AS, Drew J et al (2007) Neurosurgical experience with malpractice litigation: an analysis of closed claims against neurosurgeons in New York State, 1999 through 2003. J Neurosurg 106(6):1108–1114

Sandor AA (1957) The history of professional liability suits in the United States. J Am Med Assoc 163:459–466

Saxton JW, Finkelstein MM (2007) How a successful litigator decides whether or not to sue you. J Med Pract Manag 23(2):90–93

Sloan FA, Mergenhagen PM, Burfield WB et al (1989) Medical malpractice experience of physicians: predictable or haphazard? JAMA 262:3291–3297

Slovenko R (1993) Expert testimony: use and abuse. Med Law 12:627–641

Studdert DM, Mello MM, Sage WM et al (2005) Defensive medicine among high-risk specialist physicians in a volatile malpractice environment. JAMA 293(21):2609–2617

Thorpe KE (2004) The medical malpractice 'crisis': recent trends and the impact of state tort reforms. Health Aff (Millwood) Suppl Web Exclusives:W4-20

Zhang ZY, Yao Y, Zhou LF (2013) To err is human-medicolegal issues and safe care in neurosurgery. World Neurosurg 81(2):244–246

Zuckerman S, Bovbjerg RR, Sloan F (1990) Effects of tort reforms and other factors on medical malpractice insurance premiums. Inquiry 27:167–182

Neurosurgeons and the Media

23

Tania DePellegrin and Mark Bernstein

23.1 Introduction

The media has been an integral source in developing public awareness of medical/ethical issues that doctors are faced with daily (Rosenfeld 1999; Garcia et al. 1997; Grilli et al. 2000, 2002). The media is literally defined as "the main means of mass communication" (Oxford Dictionary 2013). It is often criticized in medical circles for creating erroneous or simplified reports of complex medical and bioethical events (Daoust and Racine 2014; Gilbert and Ovadia 2011), including even being blamed for hindering the procurement of organs for donation because of its reporting of brain death in one jurisdiction (Kleindienst et al. 1999). Factors pertaining to the nature of the reporter's job regularly create barriers to optimal reporting of medical stories (Leask et al. 2010). The media's need to create an abbreviated synopsis of complicated neurosurgical events can result in reports that focus on sensational aspects rather than the more instructive and germane elements of the case and the medical and ethical reasoning used in the decision-making process. The media's interaction with clinicians and vice versa can help promote value-based medicine or, if mishandled, set it back (Stamm et al. 2003).

Herein we discuss how a mutually supportive relationship between the media and the neurosurgical community can help clarify vital details in medically complicated and ethically challenging stories and in doing so aim to strengthen the public's confidence in their own medical system.

T. DePellegrin, MHSc (✉)
Joint Center of Bioethics, University of Toronto, Toronto, ON, Canada
e-mail: tdepellegrin@gmail.com

M. Bernstein, MD, MHSc, FRCSC
Division of Neurosurgery, Toronto Western Hospital, University of Toronto,
399 Bathurst Street, Toronto, ON M5T 2S8, Canada
e-mail: mark.bernstein@uhn.ca

A. Ammar, M. Bernstein (eds.), *Neurosurgical Ethics in Practice: Value-based Medicine*, 255
DOI 10.1007/978-3-642-54980-9_23, © Springer-Verlag Berlin Heidelberg 2014

23.2 Illustrative Case (Media Frenzy over a Wrong-Site Surgery)

Early Thursday morning news reports are screaming about a serious wrong-site surgery made by neurosurgeon A. The patient is in the ICU. Every television, radio, and print reporter is calling to ask neurosurgeon B for an interview. Social media is now posting questions online. Neurosurgeon C at another local hospital is faced with a reporter's first barrage of questions which include the following: "How could such an error have been made? Is this a mistake you could have made yourself? How should this doctor be disciplined? Do you think this type of error is a result of long work hours or a general lack of safety precautions? Who should pay the additional costs due to this error?" How should neurosurgeons handle this situation?

23.3 Approach to the Case

The initial reaction to a request for a media interview, especially for a surgeon who is new at this, is the fear that they will get tongue-tied or cornered and end up looking bad. Once they get over this fear, and decide to do the interview, the neurosurgeon should seek and receive permission from his/her hospital to speak on this topic. He/she would clarify in detail what he/she is legally and ethically able to address in an interview (e.g. factors possibly leading to this type of error, surgical checklists, work hours, and mandatory time outs). After first confirming that this case does fall within his/her area of expertise, he/she would then gather as much information about the case as possible like description of the surgery performed and condition of the patient prior to and after surgery.

Understanding his/her rights as a doctor versus the rights of the media, he/she would set up his/her own boundaries. The interview would take place in the privacy of his/her office with just one reporter at a time, if multiple interviews are requested. Prior to the interview, he/she would discuss with the reporter that he/she does not have knowledge of the specific events leading to this error and would ask what questions he/she would like answered. The neurosurgeon being interviewed would develop solid answers to address difficult questions, avoid personal attacks, and create a "main message" that he/she would like conveyed regarding medical error in general. This message should be one that speaks to the case without discussing specific details, addressing both public concern and methods to avoid such adverse outcomes in the future. The message should be clear and concise. For example, he/she might say: "Medical error is a serious problem which hurts patients, costs money, and erodes the trust between patients and doctors. Health-care professionals have an ethical duty to provide a level of patient safety that ensures safety checklists are met and that there is disclosure and apology when mistakes are made. New policies may still be needed".

> **Pearl**
> Some hospitals may have policies that restrict neurosurgeons from speaking directly to the media, reserving all comments for a hospital administrator or public relations representative. In these cases, the neurosurgeon's knowledge of the procedure and his/her expertise would still be invaluable in assisting the hospital spokesperson in preparing a strong medical/ethical response to difficult questions.

23.4 Discussion

23.4.1 Engaging with the Media

The tendency for many doctors when dealing with a complicated ethical case is to completely avoid the media. However, a physician's participation in accurately communicating medical/ethical events of a story to the mass public can greatly contribute to a better-informed and less anxiety-provoked society (Doyle 2003).

Media reports can influence health behaviour and policies and health-care utilization, and in many populations, mass media is named as the main source of medical knowledge (Grilli et al. 2002; Alaqeel et al. 2014). In fact, a US national poll by the National Health Council found that of those surveyed, the primary sources for their health news were television (40 %), doctors (36 %), magazines or journals (35 %), newspapers (16 %), and the Internet (2 %). (Note: These add up to more than 100 % as participants could list more than one preference.) Fifty-eight% of respondents said they have taken some kind of action or changed their behaviour as a result of a medical or health news story learned from the media (National Health Council 1997).

Doctors and journalists are two different groups, often with different values and consistently different goals. When these diverse cultures interact, there is frequently a chance for confusion and misunderstanding (Nelkin 1996). In challenging cases such as the above scenario, a neurosurgeon's involvement with the media could help clarify for both the reporter and the general public what may have gone wrong and inform them about the safeguards that neurosurgeons should routinely use to prevent such events (Cohen et al. 2010). It is here that the surgeon being interviewed can provide assurance to the general public that despite the seriousness of this case, they still have a health-care system that they can trust.

Without a physician's input on this case, the reporter's story could end up taking an angle that focuses on the negligent actions of the surgeon and a pending lawsuit rather than potential errors that could occur with this type of surgery, the possibility of new guidelines, and the policy changes that may prevent adverse outcomes in the future (Clary 1995).

Table 23.1 Questions a neurosurgeon should ask the reporter before starting

1. What is your name?
2. What is the name of your publication or programme, and who is its target audience?
2. What is your deadline?
3. Is the interview live or taped? When will it air?
4. What aspects of the case exactly would you like me to comment on?
5. Who else will you be interviewing?
6. What time do you need me and for how long?
7. Could you give me your number? I will call you right back

Before engaging with the media, the neurosurgeon should ask the journalist a few pertinent questions listed in Table 23.1.

The answers to a few preliminary questions will help give the neurosurgeon an opportunity to calmly collect his/her thoughts, liaise with his/her hospital's legal team and public affairs representative, decide if this case falls within his/her sphere of expertise (i.e. comfort zone), and then prepare for the interview.

Given our scenario, the reporter would likely use this initial conversation to ask if there is a patient who has also suffered a wrong-site surgery who would be willing to be interviewed. From a reporter's perspective, a personal account of how an individual was impacted by a wrong-site surgery would make the story more compelling to the average person. Though a neurosurgeon's thought process may be focused on the issues of patient consent and confidentiality, including a patient's personal story would likely help the issue gain further public attention. Studies on this topic have also recommended telling the patient that agreeing or refusing to participate would not have any affect on their future care (Farberman 1999).

23.4.2 Working Effectively with the Media Means Understanding the Media

23.4.2.1 Different Types of Media, Different Needs

Several different types of media exist that affect the public's perception of any given health-care story, each type having different needs. One of the simplest and safest methods is neurosurgeons offering their opinions on important medical issues by submitting short pieces for publication in the letters or op-ed page of printed newspapers and/or electronic newspapers (Bernstein 2003, 2009). Many of these are extremely personal, selfless, and inspiriting to other readers within our profession (Kalanthi 2014). It is also important to note that public advertising of equipment and/or expertise in the media does happen, and while there may be no law against this, it often results in false or misleading claims and should be frowned upon (Linskey 2000).

However this chapter focuses on the more timely and interactive ways neurosurgeons can engage with the media. Considering our case, a reporter working for a print publication may ask for a taped telephone interview from which the neurosurgeon could offer more details on this type of procedure, surgical checklists, and how or when a mistake could have been made that led to this error. Print journalists are sometimes allowed more space than other types of media to include background information and relevant statistics (e.g. number of wrong-site surgeries recorded in the last 10 years).

A radio news reporter may only have enough time for a very brief phone interview as they frequently file several stories over the course of the day. Radio news reports are usually no longer than 15 s or 30 s for a big story. The result is often a very short clip from the surgeon which may not include everything the doctor had wanted to express. This is a perfect example of when a previously prepared "main message" statement could be used.

A television news reporter would ask for a videotaped interview involving a camera crew coming into the surgeon's hospital, shooting the interview and likely extra footage for editing purposes. Broadcast stories, although brief, can vary in length from approximately 1.5 to 3.5 min depending on the programme and news outlet. Most television news reporters have to file their story for the same-day news broadcast. In this scenario, the surgeon's physical appearance and the background are both important points to consider in addition to the message being communicated. Visual aids or, if available, a previously taped video of the procedure in question would be a helpful tool to provide the broadcast journalist for editing of the final piece.

The rise of social media offers new opportunities and complexities to the field of health news reporting. Medical professionals now have a direct route to comment on issues via blogging and Twitter (Leask et al. 2010). In our given case, a neurosurgeon could use social media to communicate an unfiltered statement on medical error, the procedure that was performed, and the ethical issues at the core of this case. For the health reporter, social media is yet another tool for collecting information on their given story. Social media sites like Facebook are a useful means of locating family and friends of those affected by a health-care story, and it is an effective way to reach people and receive information, but it needs to be treated with respect, and everything must be verified.

Physicians should exercise caution when replying to questions posted on social media sites. Unlike mainstream media, there are no governing bodies overseeing the content and accuracy of the independent social media writer. Sharing credible health information and resources may be helpful to the general public. Conversely, physicians should avoid writing about specific patients and remember to protect the patient's identity (Chretien and Kind 2013).

23.4.2.2 Similar Constraints Among the Media

Despite the varying needs of each type of media, many of them share similar constraints. All journalists are faced with strict deadlines. Most reporters are assigned a story during a morning news meeting and often the angle that it should take. One study exploring how journalists select and construct health news stories found that between 10:00 a.m. and 2:00 p.m. was usually the only time reporters were given to educate themselves with background information and technical aspects of the case, find and conduct interviews, write, and then review the accuracy of their scripts

(Leask et al. 2010). Given the tight time frame that reporters are given to produce their story and that most reports have a same-day deadline, a physician's cooperation in being both accessible and prompt in returning reporters' calls is crucial.

Journalists are often faced with restrictions on the length of their story. Producers and editors are always pushing for something shorter that can still manage to capture the audience's attention and inform the public on the issue being discussed. Having a medical professional who can explain a complicated case in simple, clear, and concise terms allows the journalist more space to include other important points in the story. It also avoids forcing the journalist to condense the statement and unintentionally distort the message.

The constraints of deadlines and restricted story lengths may result in news story content being sacrificed. News people are forced to make quick judgements from imperfect information and deliver their product at a set time, ready or not (Meyer 1990). The content of any given news story always challenges the journalist in several ethical categories including truthfulness, fairness, and standards of decency (Hanson 2014). Health-care professionals have an underlying concern that the content of a medical story will be sensationalized by the journalist in an effort to make the news item more appealing to the public (Leask et al. 2010). Competition among news organizations and even between reporters on the same staff can occasionally result in a blurring of the facts. Journalists fighting for their story to be "the lead" may sometimes overstate or slightly dramatize certain aspects of a medical event while still keeping within the boundaries of truth. Other constraints may be specific to certain cultures and societies (Riaz 2008). By getting involved with the media, neurosurgeons can help uphold a level of accuracy with health news stories and the way they are expressed to the public.

> **Pearl**
> Media content can be affected by factors outside of media organizations including economic policies, advertisers, and government influence. These issues are often prevalent in developing countries that rely on outside funding to keep their media institutions in operation.

23.4.3   Getting Ready and the Interview

23.4.3.1   Setting Up Boundaries

Before agreeing to participate in the interview, the neurosurgeon must find out what he/she is legally and ethically able to discuss. This includes notifying department heads, legal teams, and public relations representatives. It is also wise to advise any assistants that the interview is taking place and request that there are no interruptions. In our illustrative case, the neurosurgeon would also inform the journalist that he/she has no specific knowledge of the details of this case and will not speak to them.

Table 23.2 Basic rules for engaging in an interview with the media

1. Speak clearly.
2. Avoid fidgeting.
3. Look at the reporter, not the camera in broadcast interviews.
4. Nothing is off the record. The interview is ongoing until the journalist has left.
5. Record your interview and get a copy of the final news piece. If in the future legal action is taken, it is advisable to have a record of what was said.

The doctor should request a one-on-one interview in a location where he/she feels comfortable. For a phone interview, it must be somewhere quiet with little distraction. For a television interview, a visually dynamic location is preferable (e.g. an operating room).

23.4.3.2 Language and Presentation

It is imperative that doctors use clear language easily understood by the layman. Physicians should not expect the reporter or the public to have any science background and should avoid giving complicated statements filled with medical jargon. That being said, specialist health and medical reporters usually have a stronger technical understanding and are therefore better able to deliver an accurate and comprehensive news story (Johnson 1998).

The neurosurgeon's language should be simple, short, and strong. As previously mentioned, a "main message" helps keep the interview focused and directs the journalist and ultimately the public to the most important issues. As part of the interview preparation, these key points should be written down and rehearsed on one's own and, if possible, with a colleague. The interview should never be the first time the surgeon's "main message" is heard. Doctors should avoid responding to difficult questions with "no comment" as it usually makes one look defensive. Instead, they should try guiding the conversation back to the "main message".

The doctor being interviewed should remember some basic rules listed in Table 23.2.

23.4.3.3 Tricky Questions and the Hostile Reporter

Our case scenario has the potential to develop into a confrontational interview. Personal questions such as "Is this a mistake you could have easily made?" should be redirected by saying "It is not about me. The main message here is…". Questions like "How should this doctor be disciplined?" and "Is this a factor of long work hours or defective systems?" could both be addressed with this reply: "I can't speak directly to this case as we don't have all of the facts. However, in this hospital, safety checklists including preoperative reviews, proper marking of incision sites, and mandatory timeouts are routine for this type of procedure". When dealing with a hostile reporter, doctors may be interrupted, rushed, or bombarded with multi-part questions. The response should be calm and always on message (Table 23.3).

Many of the issues in Table 23.3 could be most easily dealt with if they are previously anticipated. As part of the preparation for the interview, the neurosurgeon

Table 23.3 Tips when dealing with a hostile reporter

1. Do not play tug of war to gain control of the interview. If you are interrupted, wait until the reporter has finished speaking, and then calmly answer the question
2. Do not rush your answers
3. Answer only what you know and move on
4. Do not offer personal opinions or speculate by answering "What if…?" or "Would you…?" style questions. This kind of questioning could create an ethical or legal dilemma for the neurosurgeon
5. Do not be surprised if you are asked the same question twice – the journalist may be looking for a different or shorter response
6. Side step accusatory questions by bringing the conversation back to your previously prepared main message

should try to think like a reporter and anticipate the questions a reporter would ask. In our illustrative case scenario, the big questions would likely all be around the issue of accountability (i.e. Who is to blame for the patient's pain and suffering?).

23.4.3.4 Seeking Help

Before the interview, the neurosurgeon should request the opinion of the hospital's legal team, public affairs, and work colleagues. In addition, if he/she feels that he/she may be asked to participate in interviews regularly, it would be wise to seek some assistance with formal media training.

> **Pearl**
> When asked to engage with the media, the neurosurgeon should always alert and consult the hospital public relations department and/or the physician and administrator he/she reports to.

23.5 Recommendations

The guidelines discussed in this chapter on how to deal with the media can be applied to many different scenarios. The more complicated the case, the more imperative it is that doctors get involved with the media and help the public better understand complex issues that arise in their health-care system. In an effort to bridge the gap between the two professions, there are international organizations whose purpose is to minimize the constraints that journalists face by compiling accurate, newsworthy, medical stories, useful background information, and a list of professionals who can speak on health-related issues (Science Media Centre). Physicians can also play an active role by providing background information to the journalist prior to the interview, thereby increasing the reporter's knowledge base and understanding of the medical topic. Moving forward, medical professionals should consider taking a proactive approach by contacting the media first. Establishing a contact list of local health and medical specialist reporters will enable the neurosurgeon – and other doctors alike – to form an ongoing relationship with the media. This association is mutually beneficial, and once established, the neurosurgeon can begin to trust that the health news reports are both ethically and medically accurate.

Conclusion

Neurosurgeons have the opportunity to make a difference in the way challenging health news is covered. By getting involved in the process and following these aforementioned guidelines, health news stories will hopefully contain fewer mistakes and more pertinent information. Neurosurgeons and journalists must share the responsibility for accurate communication of both positive stories and negative medical events such as wrong-site surgery. Higher-quality medical news coverage ultimately creates a more informed society with improved trust in their health-care system.

Pearl

Interaction with the media can be unnerving for neurosurgeons. However, this can ultimately lead to improved communication between the medical profession and a more educated and trusting public. This learning experience can also prove to be gratifying for individual neurosurgeons.

References

Alaqeel A, AlAmmari A, Alsyefi N et al (2014) Stroke awareness in the Saudi community living in Riyadh: prompt health measures must be implemented. J Stroke Cerebrovasc Dis 23(3):500–504

Bernstein M (2003) Digging out after the SARS storm. The Toronto Star, April 18, p A25

Bernstein M (2009) Intolerable resource shortages in health care. Toronto Sun, February 26, p 17

Chretien KC, Kind T (2013) Social media and clinical care: ethical, professional, and social implications. Circulation 127:1413–1421

Clary M (1995) String of errors put Florida hospital on the critical list. Los Angeles Times, April 14

Cohen FL, Mendelsohn D, Bernstein M (2010) Wrong-site craniotomy: analysis of 35 cases and systems for prevention. J Neurosurg 113:461–473

Daoust A, Racine E (2014) Depictions of 'brain death' in the media: medical and ethical implications. J Med Ethics 40(4):253–9

Doyle J (2003) SARS coverage fuels fear instead of calming it. Globe and Mail, April 28th

Farberman RK (1999) What the media need from news sources. Psychology and the media: a second look, 1st edn. American Psychological Association, Washington, DC, pp 9–23

Garcia VD, Goldani JC, Neumann J (1997) Mass media and organ donation. Transplant Proc 29:1618–1621

Gilbert F, Ovadia D (2011) Deep brain stimulation in the media: over-optimistic portrayals call for a new strategy involving journalists and scientists in ethical debates. Front Integr Neurosci 5:16

Grilli R, Freemantle N, Minozzi S et al (2000) Mass media interventions: effects on health services utilization. Cochrane Database Syst Rev (2)

Grilli R, Ramsay C, Minozzi S (2002) Mass media interventions: effects on health services utilization. Cochrane Database Syst Rev (1)

Hanson RE (2014) Mass Communication:Living in a Media World. CQ Press, SAGE Publications, Washington, DC, Chpt 14

Johnson T (1998) Medicine and the media. N Engl J Med 339:87–92

Kalanthi P (2014) How long have I got left? New York Times, New York, http://www.nytimes.com/2014/01/25/opinion/sunday/how-long-have-i-got-left.html?

Kleindienst A, Haupt WF, Hildebrandt G (1999) Brain death and organ donation in Germany: analysis of procurement in a neurosurgical unit and review of press reports. Acta Neurochir (Wien) 141(6):641–645

Leask J, Hooker C, King C (2010) Media coverage of health issues and how to work more effectively with journalists: a qualitative study. BMC Public Health 10:535

Linskey ME (2000) Stereotactic radiosurgery versus stereotactic radiotherapy for patients with vestibular schwannoma: a Leksell Gamma Knife Society 2000 debate. JNS 93(Suppl 3):90–95

Meyer P (1990) News media responsiveness to public health. In: Atkin C, Wallack L (eds) Mass communication and public health: and conflicts. Sage, Newbury Park, pp 52–59

National Health Council report (1997) Americans talk about science and medical news. Roper Starch Worldwide, New York

Nelkin D (1996) An uneasy relationship: the tension between medicine and the media. Lancet 347:1600–1603

Oxford Dictionary (2013) Oxford University Press, New York

Riaz S (2008) Agenda setting role of mass media. Glo Media J 1(2), Pakistan Edition

Rosenfeld A (1999) The journalist's role in bioethics. J Med Phil 24:108–129

Science Media Center. http://www.sciencemediacentre.ca/smc/

Stamm K, Williams JW, Noel P et al (2003) Helping journalists get it right. A physician's guide to improving health care reporting. J Gen Intern Med 18:138–145

International Neurosurgery Collaborations

24

Mark Bernstein

24.1 Introduction

Interest in making contributions to medical practice in developing countries and resource-poor settings has become increasingly popular and prevalent. This stems from doctors in resource-rich settings wishing to help level the playing field for patients who are so unfortunate on many levels, including the medical care they can expect to receive. It is essentially a virtuous and beneficent activity. Most recognizable has been the primary care and preventative health measures applied toward maternal and child health, vaccination strategies for infectious diseases, and targeting the HIV/AIDS pandemic. These activities embody the spirit of value-based medicine on a more global scale.

In recent years, more attention has addressed surgical disease, which is a significant burden in resource-poor counties (Mathers and Loncar 2006; Tollefson and Larrabee 2012; Weiser et al. 2008). Although typically dominated by individual missions or groups, there is now a more concerted effort with surgical care being included in the comprehensive primary health-care plan set by the World Health Organization (2008). In neurosurgery the need is great (El Khamlichi 2001). The main organizations involved in facilitating international neurosurgical exchange and education are FIENS (Ablin et al. 1999; Bagan 2010) and the WFNS (World Federation of Neurosurgical Societies 2012). With the significant activity with these much-needed surgical initiatives, health-care teams now more than ever need to openly reflect on and discuss the ethical issues inherent in international surgery.

M. Bernstein, MD, MHSc, FRCSC
Division of Neurosurgery, Toronto Western Hospital, University of Toronto,
399 Bathurst Street, Toronto, ON M5T 2S8, Canada
e-mail: mark.bernstein@uhn.ca

A. Ammar, M. Bernstein (eds.), *Neurosurgical Ethics in Practice: Value-based Medicine*,   265
DOI 10.1007/978-3-642-54980-9_24, © Springer-Verlag Berlin Heidelberg 2014

Ethical challenges in international surgery initiatives have been discussed sporadically in the context of specific missions such as Operation Smile (Ott and Olson 2011), otolaryngologists in Ethiopia (Isaacson et al. 2010), and neurosurgery in Indonesia (Bernstein 2004). Systematic categorization of ethical issues confronted while teaching and operating in a developing country has been attempted on a limited scale (Bodnar 2011; Howe et al. 2013a). While surgical education in developing countries is a wonderful practice, it is imperative that it is done as ethically as possible. We must aim to achieve the maximum "bang for the buck" in terms of ensuring the human and fiscal resources expended are used in the best and most ethically appropriate way to produce the greatest result.

> **Pearl**
>
> In spite of excellent and generous work being done by many to help improve the care in less fortunate neurosurgical environments, there are many ethical dilemmas which both visitors and hosts need to think about and attend to.

24.2   Illustrative Case (Ethical Breaches for Neurosurgeon Teaching in the Developing World)

A 48-year-old neurosurgeon in academic practice is making his first visit to a developing country to help. He was recently feeling like he needed to "reinvent" himself and international work seemed interesting. He was deciding between two or three countries and ultimately chose country A, probably because it had the most pleasant climate. He brought equipment passed their expiry dates – they were all confiscated at the airport. He is not too upset though as he wonders if the local surgeons would be have been able to use them anyway. The first day the local surgeons present him with a young man with a five-segment cervical intramedullary tumor. He is concerned about doing the case with the locals as there is no ultrasonic aspirator, microscope, or neurophysiological monitoring available at the hospital and the patient cannot afford to go to another country with a sophisticated neurosurgery unit. He is not sure what to do. A few days later they all decide to perform the first transsphenoidal operation. The locals ask, and expect, the visitor to just scrub in and do the entire case as opposed to his using his regular teaching model of helping the locals do it. The visitor agrees to do this. While the case is on, there is a film crew from a local television news show not dressed properly in scrubs, wielding large cameras and hovering over the case. During the case the visitor grows impatient with one of the local surgeons who is slow to pick up on a technique being taught. After the case, the visitor tells himself the locals will not likely do this procedure when he is gone. The next day the anesthetist that the visitor brought as part of his team gets a little ill – he had not realized she was a fussy traveler and has been unwilling to eat any of the local foods. On the last day a young boy presents to the clinic blind with severe headaches, with a huge posterior fossa tumor and hydrocephalus. He asks his local colleagues for follow-up about this child (Fig. 24.1). After the surgeon returns

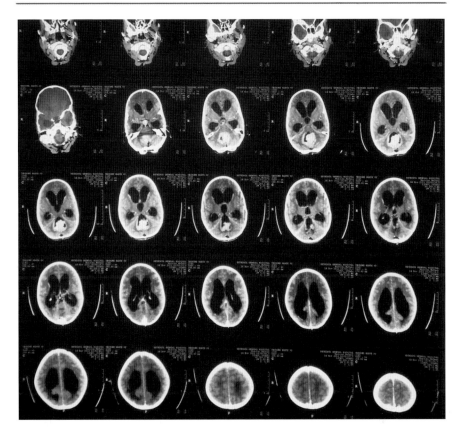

Fig. 24.1 Enhanced CT of an 8-year-old boy with subacute blindness and severe headaches who presented to a neurosurgery clinic in a sub-Saharan African city. The figure shows (*1*) advanced stage neurosurgical diseases present in resource-poor settings and (*2*) *hard copy* of images indicating the lack of electronic imaging systems. The boy was admitted urgently to the teaching hospital, but various problems caused delays getting him into the OR and he died on the seventh hospital day

home to his hospital in the United States, he tells his colleagues whenever he gets a chance about how wonderful the experience was, he lets the hospital public relations team do a story on him, and he shows many interesting photos from his experience embedded within every talk he gives.

24.3   Approach to the Case

The case above illustrates a few of the many ethical dilemmas encountered when neurosurgeons from resource-rich countries try to help neurosurgeons in resource-poor countries. In order of appearance they are (1) questionable motives, (2) which countries to support, (3) inappropriate equipment donations, (4) doing "second best",

(5) mismatched expectations, (6) the "operating room circus", (7) "white knight syndrome", (8) insensitivity, (9) sustainability, (10) inappropriate team selection, (11) anxiety about and difficulty obtaining follow-up on patients, and (12) personal gain.

Many of these issues are easily avoidable using common sense and previous experience, but many others are not, especially because it is difficult to predict equipment availability, local "politics," and how the locals will react and what chemistry will develop between visitor and host especially on a visitor's first visit to a new venue. The bioethics principles and the ethical theories can also be brought to bear on these issues. Ultimately, international surgical exchange and collaboration is about the principle of justice – an attempt to minimize the differences and gaps in care between resource-rich and recourse-poor settings. A common overriding theme blocking effective knowledge transfer is paternalism on the art of the visitors and unrealistic expectations by both visitors and hosts.

24.4   Discussion

Some of the leading ethical challenges in international neurosurgical collaboration are described below; there is overlap among many of them. This is by no means an exhaustive list – more comprehensive analyses have been done and they are not complete yet (Howe et al. 2013a).

24.4.1   Choice of Location

The issue of which sites visitors/organizations choose to help with human and fiscal resources is a matter of resource allocation and fairness. What is the decision-making process going into the selection of a host country that will receive benefit from a given surgical educational mission? Beyond a valuable medical exchange, these missions also typically provide donated resources, educational materials, and exposure to new skills that together can lead to regional inequity when distributed unfairly. How then do we determine where to allocate these human and fiscal resources? Why does site A in sub-Saharan Africa have a lot of outside help whereas no one goes to sites B and C? While no specific data exist on selection method, anecdotal evidence suggests location of surgical missions has been facilitated by ease of access such as safe travel, available infrastructure, a common language, and networking between organizations or friends.

To approach the decision from the ethical principle of justice as fairness, it would seem desirable to perform a needs assessment and have a transparently visible list of networks or institutions that are targeted for help over a specific timeline. While sociopolitical contexts will influence decisions, a solution might be for visiting surgeons to keep a 10-year plan that enables selection to vary based on regional stability, influx of new resources, or increased need. In this way, those requesting help can feel ethically satisfied that their request will receive consideration.

Ultimately we must all be globally accountable. Human and fiscal resources are valuable and finite and merit being shared as broadly and fairly as possible, avoiding duplication of efforts. Without a centralized repository of past and ongoing surgical missions, accountability has been lacking. Responsibility for ensuring fair resource allocation must be shared, between visitors and hosts. It is promising to see online access to surgical education initiatives (Canadian Network of International Surgery 2011) and records of surgical equipment donations or subsidized costs made available by the World Federation of Neurosurgical Societies (World Federation of Neurosurgical Societies 2012). A shared process must be obtained wherein visiting teams must ensure they only go where they are wanted and/or needed and where the local surgeons have expressed a desire for engagement in international surgical education.

> **Pearl**
> Choosing where neurosurgical human and financial resources are directed is often done arbitrarily. Some rationalization, central repository of information and monitoring, and equitable distribution of such efforts would be preferable to and more ethical than the current model.

24.4.2 Sustainability of Knowledge/Equipment Transfer

Sustainability is critical in global health development and international surgery specifically. A key issue that arises is the question of whether a new technique or piece of equipment can be sustained after departure of the visiting team (Haglund et al. 2011; Howe et al. 2013a, b). Skill translation is only one aspect of sustainability; success also depends on other issues such as technology-based needs (e.g., imaging or surgical drills), surgical supplies (e.g., surgical hardware), system capability and infrastructure, and institutional commitment. Often equipment that is brought cannot be properly maintained or serviced or is brought for demonstration purposes but not left behind. An example would be a cortical stimulator to teach awake craniotomy which is transported back home because they are too costly to leave behind.

The ethical principle of maleficence arises when we ignore our initial plan and albeit unintentionally embark on surgeries that leave patients incompletely treated, hosts incompletely trained, and ultimately produce a greater societal burden. Planning for sustainability is possible and might include a feasibility assessment that determines how well a given technique can be implemented in resource-limited settings where infrastructure is inadequate or is unpredictable. The simplest procedures to teach are likely the best – those that are less invasive, need less equipment, need less operating and recovery time, and produce less complications. Similarly, sustainability in surgical education might include skill enhancement in the domains of related disciplines like nursing, anesthesia, administration, and management practices to build broad-based capacity. Operation Smile has demonstrated the effectiveness of surgical educational missions on creating local sustainability and capacity building by showing that the number of patients treated by international surgical teams has decreased from 100 % initially to the current 33 % worldwide during a 20-year term (Magee et al. 2012). We need to strive for the same in neurosurgery although the metrics will be challenging.

Another important piece in knowledge transfer includes bringing colleagues from resource-poor settings, residents, and consultants to our hospitals in resource-rich settings for observation periods or clinical fellowships. This can help complete the training of a neurosurgeon. This will require expenditure of human and financial resources on the part of surgeons committed to overseas collaborations.

> **Pearl**
> Teaching/performing surgery that is not likely to be sustainable after the visitor leaves is not an effective use of resources and is ethically dubious.

24.4.3 Mismatched Expectations

Expectations can be mismatched or even unfair on both sides. Expectations of hosts placed upon the visitor performing in conditions less optimal that what he/she is used to or performing surgeries for which he/she no longer feels qualified are problematic, but visitors should prepare as best as possible for these situations. Often, the visiting specialist is seen as an outright authority and expert, as opposed to a colleague with whom clinical problems can be discussed and solved in a shared manner. In this setting, we must balance the idea of doing "good" with the ethical principle of non-maleficence.

On the other side the visitors often place expectations on the local surgeons like being as organized as the visitor, being as timely with e-mail responses, and providing excellent preparation of the cases and other activities relating to the visitor's time. When expectations of either group are not adequately met, it can lead to frustration and tension which can impede the desired effective transfer of knowledge.

24.4.4 Selection of the Visiting Team

This relates to the ethical dilemma of appropriate team selection for an educational surgical mission in a resource-poor country and again relates to resource allocation. To date, very few groups have described the rationale or criteria for which types of health-care professionals to include, but it would seem to be obvious. Regarding the makeup of the team, would it be beneficial to take anesthetists, operating room nurses, and/or residents? Evidence is emerging indicating the benefits of surgical education for residents in a resource-limited setting (Jarman et al. 2009).

In some cases, however, a more useful team member might be a biomedical engineer. The above can play a key role in ensuring sustainability and capacity. When a medical student goes on a mission with a surgeon, the experience will likely be of benefit to them, but how much can they contribute to the local surgeons?

Regarding the quality of the team, culturally sensitive team members who can promote good cultural exchange are essential. Team members must be skilled, knowledgeable, have the capacity for good cultural rapport, and be open to experiencing different cultures. While team selection is specific to the goals of a given mission, it is critical to acknowledge the existence of ethical dilemmas faced during this process and address them. Above all, team members must want to participate for the right reasons, be capable of good teamsmanship, and be open to new cultures and interactions that may require adaptive behavior in unfamiliar settings (Welling et al. 2010; Howe et al. 2013a). Appropriate preparation of the team members by the team leader is essential.

> **Pearl**
> Visiting team members must be skillful in their field, dedicated to the cause of international teaching, open to new cultures, and flexible to adapt to new situations.

24.4.5   The "White Knight"

An egregious example of unsustainable teaching is when the visitor falls into the "white knight" syndrome. In this case, the surgeon performs a few difficult cases and then leaves, without teaching the procedure and with essentially no chance of the procedure being done after he/she leaves. The ethical principle of beneficence is being ignored when we fail to do what is best for the host medical system and staff – to facilitate sustainability. Instead, the "white knight" syndrome reinforces paternalism through the idea that visiting staff can do the tough cases. The hosts have obviously requested that more complex cases to be tackled in the presence of the "white knight" which might be altruistic as the hosts truly want the unfortunate patient(s) to be helped, and they also want to learn by watching him/her. But it might also be self-serving to the hosts as it will elevate their profile and institutional reputation, especially if the case is covered by the media, which often happens in resource-poor settings.

The "white knight" may return home from such a mission enjoying a boost to the ego, without having effected knowledge translation, or reinforcing the skills gap between the visitor's and hosts' situation. Avoiding these situations on teaching missions will help promote sustainable new techniques locally and promote the development of more self-sufficiency in the developing country. Finally, avoiding this scenario ultimately ensures more fairness and justice to all patients in the host institution.

24.4.6   Cultural Sensitivity

This relates to the ethical principle of respect for persons. Regardless of where surgical teaching takes place, or with whom, mutual respect is critical. In the operating room in particular, visiting surgeons can provide more sustainable skills through positive feedback and patiently supporting host surgeons while they learn the technique. Situational insensitivities occur, for example, when a visiting surgeon demands his/her way must be followed without modification or question or when he/she becomes visibly upset when the hosts cannot learn the technique quickly enough, or when there are communication gaps because of language or accent. Situational insensitivities can also arise when the visiting surgeon believes he/she must correct all aspects of the host system, outside the primary teaching goals he/she wishes to impart.

It also requires situational sensitivity when visitors must accept the limits of the host system. One can easily see where ethical issues arise when different cultures work together in an intimate, but typically authoritative, environment where host staff surgeons are rarely in a "trainee" role or where a visiting surgeon must sit idly knowing lives might be saved if he/she intervened. For example, if the anesthetist blocks a case because the patient's temperature is a little high or a ventilator is not immediately available, and the risk benefit ratio favors doing the surgery today, how hard should the visitor push the local surgeons to push their anesthetist? Situational sensitivity not only requires being aware of tone of voice and body language, but requires acceptance of the limitations of a system in which the visiting team finds themselves working and adaptation to cultural norms very different than those back home. It also important to remember that on many levels the visiting team has as much to learn from the hosts as the other way around.

24.4.7   Settling for Doing a "Second Best" Job

This scenario involves the ethical principles of beneficence and non-maleficence. In our example above, is it acceptable for a visiting surgeon to do a procedure which would be considered malpractice at home like removing an intramedullary spinal cord tumor with no microscope or ultrasonic aspirator? An argument can be made for being satisfied that patients who would otherwise go untreated are at least given a chance, despite an increased risk of a suboptimal operation that would never occur at home. In the developing world, equipment is often inadequate (Rose 2011) and lack of consistent electrical power without a reliable generator also creates risk that would be intolerable back home, and the visiting surgeon may find himself/herself working under these conditions. Surgical missions should at minimum work within the limits of the host country's ability, and if visiting surgeons are not technically or ethically comfortable with this compromise, they are not well suited for international teaching. Additionally, the visiting surgeon may find himself/herself involved with cases where follow-up treatment such as radiation therapy is unavailable, making the role of surgery almost futile.

The issue of doing second best can also arise when the visiting surgeon operates on pathologies for which his/her experience is significantly lacking, for example, a tumor surgeon who has not done vascular neurosurgery for 15 years, helping clip an aneurysm – a situation that would be inexcusable back home. It also obtains for the execution of clinical research in resource-poor settings (Wendler et al. 2004).

> **Pearl**
> Doing a "second best" job that the surgeon would not do at home may pose ethical challenges for him/her, but it is morally acceptable if the patient has no other chance for care.

24.4.7.1   Personal Gain

Finally, we must acknowledge the ethical dilemma of surgeons enjoying personal gain. Regardless of the motives of an educational mission, nothing is 100 % altruistic. Each mission will likely contain interesting travel, adventure, novelty, exceptional surgical cases, and cultural exchange, which greatly benefit the visitor and his/her team (Bernstein 2011). The visiting surgeon will also learn much more than he/she imagined possible if their mind is wide open.

The surgeon must recognize the primary motivators of the projects by asking whether he/she is serving the greatest need with full host engagement and likelihood of sustainability, or whether personal gains are driving selection of location and team selection. Is there a small part of every visiting surgeon that enjoys the "white knight" effect and/or the escapism and elevation of one's profile in one's home community, hospital, or university? Self-reflective honesty is required to heighten our ethical awareness. It is ethically acceptable for visiting surgeons to enjoy themselves, as long as that was not the prime driver for the mission. As current and future generations of surgical residents with interest in global health develop, training should perhaps include self-reflective practice and open discussion forums to promote self-awareness and ethical practice in these unique settings.

24.5   Recommendations

There are many ethical challenges facing visiting surgeons/institutions/organizations and also local surgeons in resource-poor settings accepting such help. A few have been touched on above. Below are some questions for visitors involved in international teaching before, during, and after a mission.

Before and During

1. Has the surgeon learned about the sites he/she intends to visit?
2. Is the resource-poor host venue genuinely interested in international collaboration and is the visiting surgeon a good fit?

3. Has the surgeon had some discussions with international surgeons with more experience than he/she has?
4. Has there been ample communication with the host surgeons to discuss goals and expectations? Is it ongoing during the visit?
5. Has a needs assessment been done and is it ongoing during the mission?
6. Has an appropriate team been selected?
7. Is there support for the mission from colleagues/institution/family?
8. Has an analysis of where the funding is coming from been done?
9. Has knowledge translation been effected?

After

1. Is there ongoing communication?
2. Is there evidence of sustainability of what was taught?
3. Is everyone satisfied that goals are being met?
4. Are there future plans for return missions by the visitor, or to bring the local surgeons to the visitor's institution as observers or fellows?

Conclusion

International neurosurgical teaching and collaborations are to be applauded and encouraged. When neurosurgeons and organizations in resource-rich settings embark upon such initiatives, it is with the best of intentions. However, good intentions are not enough just as they are not enough in clinical neurosurgery – one must have the knowledge and skills to support the good intentions to do an excellent operation. Similarly some simple education about international work and some reflection on the ethical dilemmas outlined in this chapter may better prepare the neurosurgeon to make a better and more ethically sound impact.

References

Ablin G, Fairholm DJ, Kelly DF (1999) Report of FIENS activities. Foundation for International Education in Neurological Surgery. J Neurosurg 90(5):986–987

Bagan M (2010) The Foundation for International Education in Neurological Surgery. World Neurosurg 73(4):289

Bernstein M (2004) Ethical dilemmas encountered while operating and teaching in a developing country. Can J Surg 47(3):170–172

Bernstein M (2011) Out of Africa, for now. Can J Neuro Sci 38(2):373–374

Bodnar BE (2011) So you think you want to save the world. Yale J Biol Med 84(3):227–236

Canadian Network for International Surgery (CNIS) (2011) Global Network in International Surgery: CNIS. http://www.cnis.ca/what-we-do/safer-surgical-and-obstetrics-program/gnis-global-network-international-surgery/

El Khamlichi A (2001) African neurosurgery: current situation, priorities, needs. Neurosurgery 48:1344–1347

Haglund MM, Kiryabwire J, Parker S et al (2011) Surgical capacity building in Uganda through twinning, technology, and training camps. World J Surg 35(6):1175–1182

Howe KL, Malomo AO, Bernstein M (2013a) Ethical challenges in international surgical education, for visitors and hosts. World Neurosurgery 80:751–758

Howe KL, Zhou G et al (2013b) Teaching awake craniotomy in resource-poor settings and implementing it sustainably. World Neurosurg 80:171–174

Isaacson G, Drum ET, Cohen MS (2010) Surgical missions to developing countries: ethical conflicts. Otolaryngol Head Neck Surg 143:476–479

Jarman BT, Cogbill TH, Kitowski NJ (2009) Development of an international elective in a general surgery residency. J Surg Educ 66(4):222–224

Magee WP, Raimondi HM, Beers M, Koech MC (2012) Effectiveness of international surgical program model to build local sustainability. Plast Surg Int 2012 Oct 22 (Epub ahead of print)

Mathers CD, Loncar D (2006) Projections of global mortality and burden of disease from 2002 to 2030. PLoS Med 3(11):2011–2030

Ott BB, Olson RM (2011) Ethical issues of medical missions: the clinicians' view. HEC Forum 23:105–113

Rose AD (2011) Questioning the universality of medical ethics: dilemmas raised performing surgery around the globe. Hastings Cent Rep 41(5):18–22

Tollefson TT, Larrabee WF (2012) Global surgical initiatives to reduce the surgical burden of disease. JAMA 307(7):667–668

Weiser TG, Regenbogen SE, Thompson KD et al (2008) An estimation of the global volume of surgery: a modelling strategy based on available data. Lancet 372:139–144

Welling DR, Ryan JM, Burris DG, Rich NM (2010) Seven sins of humanitarian medicine. World J Surg 34:466–470

Wendler D, Emanuel EJ, Lie RK (2004) The standard of care debate: can research in developing countries be both ethical and responsive to those countries' health needs? Am J Public Health 94(6):923–928

World Federation of Neurosurgical Societies (WFNS) (2012) Neurosurgical equipment dispatched: WFNS. http://www.wfns.org/pages/neurosurgical_equipment_dispatched/207.php

World Health Organization (2012) The World Health Report 2008 – primary health care (now more than ever): World Health Organization. http://who.int/whr/2008/whr08_en.pdf

Index

A. Ammar, M. Bernstein (eds.), *Neurosurgical Ethics in Practice: Value-based Medicine*,   277
DOI 10.1007/978-3-642-54980-9, © Springer-Verlag Berlin Heidelberg 2014

Printing: Ten Brink, Meppel, The Netherlands
Binding: Stürtz, Würzburg, Germany